Coconut-Based Nutrition and Nutraceutical Perspectives

S. V. Ramesh • Shelly Praveen
Editors

Coconut-Based Nutrition and Nutraceutical Perspectives

Springer

Editors
S. V. Ramesh
ICAR-Central Plantation Crops Research Institute, Kasaragod, Kerala, India

Shelly Praveen
ICAR-Indian Agricultural Research Institute (ICAR-IARI), New Delhi, Delhi, India

ISBN 978-981-97-3975-2 ISBN 978-981-97-3976-9 (eBook)
https://doi.org/10.1007/978-981-97-3976-9

This Springer imprint is published by the registered company Springer Nature Singapore Pte Ltd.
The registered company address is: 152 Beach Road, #21-01/04 Gateway East, Singapore 189721, Singapore

Preface

This book is a maiden attempt that dedicatedly presents authoritative information on coconut-derived biomolecules and their stellar roles in conferring human wellness. The various parts of coconut (fruits, kernel, nut water, inflorescence sap, etc.) are packed with a wide spectrum of nutrients, including health-promoting lauric acid, as well as wellness-conferring phenolics, flavonoids, and antioxidant-rich biomolecules. The chapters in the book are segregated into three major sections: (i) a comprehensive coverage on the nutritional potential of coconut, (ii) elaborations on food and nutraceutical products and their underlying biochemical basis, and (iii) deliberations on the global reach and policy issues pertaining to coconut and future perspectives.

The introductory chapter on coconut, often referred to as the "tree of life" or "*Kalpavriksha*," sets the tenor by introducing the crop, coconut and emphasizing its nutritional potential, covering multiple aspects including its global reach, traditional utilities, and emerging trends in the field of functional foods. A chapter on the bio-nutritional constituents of coconut describes various biomolecules and their nutritional potential, followed by a chapter on the metabolic fate and bioavailability of coconut nutrients and the factors affecting it. These introductory chapters provide the reader with an array of coconut-derived biomolecules and their metabolic fate within human system. Incisive perspectives on diverse primary and secondary products of coconut, namely coconut kernel, milk, coconut protein powder or coconut flour, coconut water, coconut oil and virgin coconut oil, coconut inflorescence sap (*neera*), coconut inflorescence sap-based sugar, and its manifold food products, form the crux of this anthology. This section on multiple coconut-derived products enable the reader to relish the assorted health conferring products and offers a wholesome reading experience on diverse products possibly the coconut palm could offer. Furthermore, the potential of coconut as a powerhouse or a repertoire of nutraceutical products and its implications for human nutrition are discussed in a subsequent chapter. More specifically, it highlights the way forward for coconut in the realm of functional foods. Finally, a chapter deliberates on the global trade potential of coconut and its products in the wake of its ever-increasing demand worldwide. Editors have presented their insights on the future perspective of coconut biomolecules in a final chapter to stimulate evocative discussions in the field of coconut biochemistry, coconut nutraceuticals, and value addition.

It has been a great privilege to collaborate with experts in the field of plant biochemistry, coconut food processing, nutrition scientist, policymakers, among others, while crafting this book. We are greatly indebted to the authors and peer-reviewers who have contributed to shaping up this compilation, and we are thankful for their time and expertise. We hope that this will definitely serve as a reference for researchers working in the fields of coconut and human nutrition interface, coconut-based food products, and students yearning to learn about coconut nutrition and its impact on human wellness.

Kasaragod, Kerala, India S. V. Ramesh
New Delhi, Delhi, India Shelly Praveen

Contents

Editors and Contributors

About the Editors

S. V. Ramesh Dr. S. V. Ramesh is currently serving at the ICAR-Central Plantation Crops Research Institute (ICAR-CPCRI) in Kasaragod, Kerala, India, as a Senior Scientist (Biotechnology). His area of expertise is plant biochemistry and molecular biology, and he holds Master's and Doctorate degrees in Plant Biochemistry. Dr. Ramesh conducted post-doctoral research at Washington State University, USA, focusing on plant and viral small non-coding RNAs. This research was sponsored under the DBT-CREST Fellowship (2013–2014), and he also received training at the J. Craig Venter Institute (JCVI), Maryland, USA, in legume bioinformatics. His current research is centered on nutritional biochemistry and bioactives with nutraceutical potential in plantation crops. Dr. Ramesh has made significant contributions to the development of quality standards for virgin coconut oil and coconut testa oils, as well as in the field of adulteration detection in coconut oil. Dr. Ramesh is the recipient of DBT-CREST Award (2013), DBT-CTEP Travel Award (2013), the AABSc-sponsored Young Plant Biotechnologist Award (2015), and the DST-ITS Travel Award (2022). He has authored numerous scholarly articles spanning diverse fields such as plantation biology, nutritional biochemistry, and plant–virus interactions, published in international and national journals of repute. He has five edited books to his credit. Dr. Ramesh has also presented his research findings at several international scientific fora such as the World Soybean Research Conference, Durban, South Africa; the American Phytopathological Society- Canadian Phytopathological Society (APS-CPS) Joint Meeting, Minneapolis, Minnesota, USA; the International Symposium on Cocoa Research (ISCR), Montpellier, France among others. Furthermore, he serves on the Editorial Boards of international journals, including *PLOS One*, *Measurement: Food*; *Journal of Plantation Crops*.

Shelly Praveen Dr. Shelly Praveen has an illustrious career in research, teaching, program management, and research policy development at ICAR-Indian Agricultural Research Institute, India spanning over 25 years in the field of plant biochemistry. Her original scientific contributions have led to the publication of more than 100 peer-reviewed and high-quality research articles. As a leader of Division of Biochemistry, IARI, she unlocked the industry-academia synergy and launched a portfolio of developing millet-based fortified foods under "Public-Private-Partnership" mode. Earlier, Dr. Praveen led a multi-disciplinary team in the development of virus-resistant transgenic tomato. Her research collaborations with international academia, namely Universidad Politécnica de Madrid, Spain (2017); King Saud University (KSA), Kingdom of Saudi Arabia (2014–2015); Scottish Crop Research Institute (2006); CIB, CSIC, Spain (2010–2013) and CREC, Florida, USA (2001) have ensued in the development of transgenic crops to combat phytopathogenic viruses besides building a group of trained scientific personnel. Her contributions in the academia as a Head, Division of Biochemistry, ICAR-IARI, New Delhi (2016–2021) and Director, Centre for Advanced Faculty Training (2016–2019) are immense. Dr. Praveen is a recipient of coveted Awards and Fellowships including Fellow-National Academy of Sciences India, Fellow-National Academy of Agricultural Sciences, Associate-The World Academy of Sciences, Dr. P. Sheel Memorial Lecture Award (2015), Panjabrao Deshmuk Outstanding Woman Scientist Award, ICAR (2017) among others. Currently, she channelizes her research experience in the field of nutritional science for the health management through service in nutritionally important foods across globe.

Contributors

Steve W. Adkins School of Agriculture and Food Sustainability, The University of Queensland, Gatton, QLD, Australia

The Queensland Alliance for Agriculture and Food Innovation, Centre for Horticultural Science, The University of Queensland, Indooroopilly, QLD, Australia

Amirhossein Bazrafshan School of Agriculture and Food Sustainability, The University of Queensland, Gatton, QLD, Australia

P. P. Shameena Beegum ICAR-Central Plantation Crops Research Institute, Kasaragod, Kerala, India

Muskan Beura Division of Biochemistry, ICAR-Indian Agricultural Research Institute (IARI), New Delhi, Delhi, India

Department of Plant Science, School of Biological Sciences, Central University of Kerala, Kasaragod, Kerala, India

Carolina B. Castro Murdoch University, Perth, WA, Australia

Centre of Excellence for Alzheimer's Disease Research and Care, Perth, WA, Australia

Juliana Chen Macquarie University, Sydney, NSW, Australia

University of Sydney, Sydney, NSW, Australia

Nilesh Choudhary Department of Chemical Engineering, Indian Institute of Technology Tirupati, Andhra Pradesh, India

Shaun Eslick Macquarie University, Sydney, NSW, Australia

Malika G. Fernando Macquarie University, Sydney, NSW, Australia

Manohar Garg Macquarie University, Sydney, NSW, Australia

Murali Gopal ICAR-Central Plantation Crops Research Institute, Kasaragod, Kerala, India

K. B. Hebbar ICAR-Central Plantation Crops Research Institute, Kasaragod, Kerala, India

Gunawan Indrayanto School of Medicine, Ciputra University, Surabaya, Indonesia

Anjitha Jacob Physiology, Biochemistry and Post-Harvest Technology Division, ICAR-Central Plantation Crops Research Institute, Kasaragod, Kerala, India

S. Jayasekhar ICAR-Central Plantation Crops Research Institute, Kasaragod, Kerala, India

Nimanthi Jayathilaka University of Kelaniya, Kelaniya, Sri Lanka

Sundaravelpandian Kalaipandian School of Agriculture and Food Sustainability, The University of Queensland, Gatton, QLD, Australia

The Queensland Alliance for Agriculture and Food Innovation, Centre for Horticultural Science, The University of Queensland, Indooroopilly, QLD, Australia

C. S. Keerthana Division of Biochemistry, ICAR-Indian Agricultural Research Institute (IARI), New Delhi, Delhi, India

Eveline Y. Y. Kong The Queensland Alliance for Agriculture and Food Innovation, Centre for Horticultural Science, The University of Queensland, Indooroopilly, QLD, Australia

V. Krishnakumar ICAR-Central Plantation Crops Research Institute (ICAR-CPCRI), Regional Station, Kayamkulam, Kerala, India

Veda Krishnan Division of Biochemistry, ICAR-Indian Agricultural Research Institute, New Delhi, Delhi, India

M. R. Manikantan Physiology, Biochemistry and Post-Harvest Technology Division, ICAR-Central Plantation Crops Research Institute, Kasaragod, Kerala, India

Tashmi Manilgama University of Kelaniya, Kelaniya, Sri Lanka

Ralph N. Martins Macquarie University, Sydney, NSW, Australia

Centre of Excellence for Alzheimer's Disease Research and Care, Perth, WA, Australia

Edith Cowan University, Perth, WA, Australia

Kiran Mishra Department of Microbiology, SIES College of Arts, Science and Commerce, University of Mumbai, Mumbai, Maharashtra, India

Selvakumar Murugesan Department of Chemical Engineering, Indian Institute of Technology Tirupati, Andhra Pradesh, India

Yumnan Nandan Department of Chemical Engineering, Indian Institute of Technology Tirupati, Andhra Pradesh, India

Van Anh Nguyen The Queensland Alliance for Agriculture and Food Innovation, Centre for Horticultural Science, The University of Queensland, Indooroopilly, QLD, Australia

Naga Prafulla Chandrika Nulu School of Agriculture and Food Sustainability, The University of Queensland, Gatton, QLD, Australia

R. Pandiselvam Physiology, Biochemistry and Post-Harvest Technology Division, ICAR-Central Plantation Crops Research Institute, Kasaragod, Kerala, India

N. Sai Prasanna Department of Chemical Engineering, Indian Institute of Technology Tirupati, Andhra Pradesh, India

Shelly Praveen ICAR-Indian Agricultural Research Institute (ICAR-IARI), New Delhi, Delhi, India

K. S. M. S. Raghavarao Department of Chemical Engineering, Indian Institute of Technology Tirupati, Andhra Pradesh, India

S. V. Ramesh ICAR-Central Plantation Crops Research Institute, Kasaragod, Kerala, India

Abdul Rohman Center of Excellence, Institute for Halal Industry & Systems, Universitas Gadjah Mada, Yogyakarta, Indonesia

Department of Pharmaceutical Chemistry, Faculty of Pharmacy, University of Gadjah Mada, Yogyakarta, Indonesia

Kapila N. Seneviratne University of Kelaniya, Kelaniya, Sri Lanka

S. Sudharshana ICAR-Central Plantation Crops Research Institute, Kasaragod, Kerala, India

Vimala Thomas ICAR-Central Plantation Crops Research Institute, Kasaragod, Kerala, India

W. N. M. T. D. N. Weerakoon University of Kelaniya, Kelaniya, Sri Lanka

Chongxi Yang School of Agriculture and Food Sustainability, The University of Queensland, Gatton, QLD, Australia

Abbreviations

AA	Amino acids
AAB	Acetic acid bacteria
ABTS	2,2-azinobis(3-ethyl-benzothiazoline-6-sulfonic acid) diammonium salt
ACE	Angiotensin-I Converting Enzyme
acetyl-CoA	acetyl-coenzyme A
AChE	Acetylcholinesterase
acyl-CoA	acyl-coenzyme A
AD	Alzheimer's Disease
AI	Artificial Intelligence
AgNPs	Silver nanoparticles
ALP	Alkaline phosphatase
ALT	Alanine aminotransferase
AMPs	Antimicrobial peptides
APCC	Asian and Pacific Coconut Community
ASEAN	Association of Southeast Asian Nations
AST	Aspartate aminotransferase
ATR	Attenuated total reflectance
a_W	Water activity
BAT	Brown adipose tissue
BC	Bacterial cellulose
BP	Blood pressure
CAGR	Compound annual growth rate
CAT	Catalase
CCAH	Coconut Cake Albumin Hydrolysate
CCGH	Coconut Cake Globulin Hydrolysate
CCO	Copra coconut oil
CCW	Concentrated coconut water
CD or Cdots	Carbon dots
CE-MS/MS	Capillary electrophoresis-mass spectrometry
CnAMADH2	*Cocos nucifera* Amino aldehyde dehydrogenase 2

CO	Coconut oil
COD	Chowghat orange dwarf
CO-DAG	Coconut oil-derived diacyl glycerol
COX-2	Cyclooxygenase-2
COVID-19	Corona Virus Disease of 2019
CP	Coconut proteins
CPC	Coconut protein concentrate
CVD	Cardiovascular diseases
CW	Coconut water
CWK	Coconut water kefir
DCP	Desiccated coconut powder
DCR	Defatted coconut residue
DPPH	1,1-Diphenyl-2-picrylhydrazyl
DxT	Dwarf x Tall hybrids
ECF	Extracellular fluids
EDG	Expelled from dried gratings
EFSA	The European Food Safety Authority
EGD	Equatorial Guinea Green Dwarf
EPSs	Exopolysaccharides
ET – 1	Endothelin-1
FA	Fatty acids
FAAs	Free amino acids
FAOSTAT	Food and Agriculture Organization's Statistics
FDA	Food and Drug Administration
FTIR	Fourier-transform infrared
GA3	Gibberellic acid3
GABA	Gama-aminobutyric acid
GCW	Green coconut water
GI	Glycemic index
GIT	Gastrointestinal tract
GMO	Genetically modified organism
GMP	Good manufacturing practices
GOAT	Ghrelin O-acyltransferase
GPE	Grape pomace extract
GPx	Glutathione peroxidase
GR	Glutathione reductase
GSH	Glutathione
Hb	Hemoglobin
HDL-C	High-density lipoprotein cholesterol
HMF	Hydroxymethyl furfural
HMG – CoA	3-Hydroxy-3-methylglutaryl coenzyme A
IAA	Indole-3-acetic acid
IBS	Irritable bowel syndrome
ICC	International Coconut Community
IL-6	Interleukin-6

IMC	Immature coconuts
iNOS	Inducible nitric oxide synthase
IOT	Internet of Things
iP	Isopentenyladenine
kDa	Kilo Dolton
LAB	Lactic acid bacteria
LCFAs	Long-chain fatty acids
LC–MS	Liquid chromatography mass spectrometry
LCT	Laccadive Ordinary Tall
LCTs	Long chain triglycerides
LDA	Linear discriminant analysis
LDL-C	Low-density lipoprotein cholesterol
MC	Mature coconuts
MCFAs	Medium chain fatty acids
MCTs	Medium-chain triglycerides
MCW	Mature coconut water
MCWK	Mature coconut water kefir
MELs	Mannosylerythritol lipids
MGD	Malayan yellow dwarf
MGs	Monoglycerides
MR	Maillard reactions
MRSA	Methicillin-resistant *Staphylococcus Aureus*
MSG	Monosodium glutamate
MUFA	Monounsaturated fatty acid
NaCl	Sodium chloride
NaOH	Sodium hydroxide
NDF	Neutral detergent fiber
NMR	Nuclear magnetic resonance
NOS	Nitric acid synthase
O/W	Oil-in-water emulsion
OMC	Over mature coconuts
PCA	Principal component analysis
PCR	Principal component regression
PLS-R	Partial least squares regression
PO	Palm oil
POD	Peroxidase
PPO	Polyphenol oxidase
PUFA	Polyunsaturated fatty acid
R2	Coefficient of determination
RBC	Red blood cells
RBD	Refined-bleached-deodorized
RH	Relative humidity
RMSEC	Root mean square error of calibration
RMSEP	Root mean square error of prediction
RTD	Ready-to-drink

SARS-CoV-2	Severe Acute Respiratory Syndrome Coronavirus 2
SBTN	Snow ball tender nut
SCTNP	Sequential Coconut Toddy and Nut Production
SDS-PAGE	Sodium dodecyl-sulfate polyacrylamide gel electrophoresis
SFE	Super critical fluid extraction
SOD	Superoxide dismutase
T2DM	Type II diabetes mellitus
TBARS	Thiobarbituric acid reactive substance
TCP	Tricalcium phosphate
TCW	Tender coconut water
TE	Trolox equivalent
TG	Triglyceride
TLR	Toll-like receptor
TMP	Transmembrane pressure
TPC	Total phenolics content
TSS	Total soluble solids
TxD	Tall x Dwarf hybrids
UCP1	Uncoupling protein 1
UF	Ultra-filtration
UHT	Ultra-high temperature
UN	United Nations
VCO	Virgin coconut oil
VCO-Cen	VCO from centrifugal process
VCO-Fer	VCO from fermentation process
VCO-Hot	VCO from hot process
VLDL	Very low-density lipoprotein
WAT	West African tall
WBC	White blood cells
WCT	West Coast tall
WHO	World Health Organization
WTA	World Trade Agreement
^{13}C-NMR	Carbon-nuclear magnetic resonance
2-AP	2-Acetyl-1-pyrroline

Chapter 1
Coconut ('Kalpavriksha'-'Tree of Life'): A Prologue

Naga Prafulla Chandrika Nulu, Chongxi Yang, Eveline Y. Y. Kong, S. V. Ramesh, Amirhossein Bazrafshan, Van Anh Nguyen, Sundaravelpandian Kalaipandian, and Steve W. Adkins

Abstract Palms, belonging to the family Arecaceae, are a renowned and diverse plant family encompassing about 2600 recognized species worldwide. Historically, palms have offered a wide array of benefits to humanity and have played a vital role in promoting biodiversity, particularly in tropical regions. Their significance extends to being ecological keystone species, as they provide crucial support to various organisms reliant on their fruits, roots, and flowers for sustenance. Among the economically significant palms of nutritional importance are coconut (*Cocos nucifera* L.), date palm (*Phoenix dactylifera* L.), oil palm (*Elaeis guineensis* Jacq.), and other palms of neotropics. This chapter delves into the remarkable nutritional characteristics of palms in general, with a special focus on coconut. It also discusses the traditional product range of coconut and explores emerging trends in the valorization and development of novel food products with enhanced nutritional value for human consumption. Also, recent research priorities or human nutritional approaches adopted in other related economically important palms are discussed to provide a holistic view of palm-based human nutrition.

N. P. C. Nulu · C. Yang · A. Bazrafshan
School of Agriculture and Food Sustainability, The University of Queensland, Gatton, QLD, Australia

E. Y. Y. Kong · V. A. Nguyen
The Queensland Alliance for Agriculture and Food Innovation, Centre for Horticultural Science, The University of Queensland, Indooroopilly, QLD, Australia

S. V. Ramesh
ICAR-Central Plantation Crops Research Institute, Kasaragod, Kerala, India

S. Kalaipandian · S. W. Adkins (✉)
School of Agriculture and Food Sustainability, The University of Queensland, Gatton, QLD, Australia

The Queensland Alliance for Agriculture and Food Innovation, Centre for Horticultural Science, The University of Queensland, Indooroopilly, QLD, Australia
e-mail: s.kalaipandian@uq.edu.au; s.adkins@uq.edu.au

S. V. Ramesh, S. Praveen (eds.), *Coconut-Based Nutrition and Nutraceutical Perspectives*, https://doi.org/10.1007/978-981-97-3976-9_1

Keywords Palm nutrition · Neotropical palms · Palm food industry · Palm oleochemicals · Non-dairy foods

1.1 Introduction

Palm trees encompass a diverse range of perennial plants, including lianas, shrubs, and trees. They belong to the Arecaceae family and are distributed from the 44° N latitude to the 44° S latitude. Tropical and warm temperate zones host nearly 2600 species of palm trees, making them one of the most abundant plant families in these regions. Palms are among the oldest flowering plants in the world. They have contributed to the production of various common products and foods, including seed oils, palm head, fruits, traditional fresh juices, and fermented beverages. Additionally, palms are a source of concentrated sugar such as palm sugar and syrup, which are derived by processing of sap from various palm species (Hebbar et al. 2018). Thus, palms are important sources of healthy foods as dietary preferences are undergoing a transformation due to health concerns arising from changing lifestyles and work cultures. Palm products represent a cost-effective source of nutrients, encompassing carbohydrates, proteins, amino acids, and essential dietary minerals such as selenium, potassium, calcium, magnesium, manganese, and iron. They also provide dietary fiber, vitamins, carotenoids, and fatty acids. Additionally, palm products contain various bioactive compounds such as polyphenols, anthocyanins, carotenoids, tannins, procyanidins, sterols, flavonols, flavones, anthocyanidins, isoflavones, phytoestrogens, phenolic acids, cinnamic acid derivatives, and volatile compounds, contributing to their strong antioxidant potential (Hussain et al. 2020). Individuals are increasingly inclined to adjust their diets if provided with sufficient fat-free and/or sugar-free ingredients integrated into their meals. Additionally, there is a growing preference for natural and fresh foods in these regions, reflecting an emerging trend towards healthier eating habits. Hence, enhanced health consciousness and improved nutrition education have the potential to substantially boost the demand for palm-based food products (Jamshed and Ahmad 2018).

Recent efforts have focused on valorizing the palm fruit as a rich source of carotenoids and starch. Additionally, there are promising developments in utilizing a neotropical palms. For example, peach palm (*Bactris Gasipaes* Kunth.) derived lignocellulosic by-products are used to create valuable biotechnological products such as prebiotics, enzymes, cellulose nanofibrils, and high-fiber flours (de Cássia Spacki et al. 2022; Graefe et al. 2013). In addition to peach palm (*B. gasipaes* Kunth.), *Mauritia flexuosa* L., and *Oenocarpus bataua* are key palm species in the Amazon region, valued for both culinary and medicinal applications. The primary products derived from these palms are fruits and oil. Palm fruits are particularly utilized for oil extraction due to their abundant content of saturated fatty acids, fiber, provitamin A, carotenoids, tocopherols, macro and microelements, and polyphenols

(Jaramillo-Vivanco et al. 2022). Apart from the fruits and oils, other parts of palm trees are utilized by Amazonian communities for various purposes though they are not as widely recognized. These include roots, seeds, palm hearts, flowers and flower sap (Agostini-Costa 2018).

Investigations focusing on the fatty acid, flavonoid, and carotenoid contents of the primary fruits from Cerrado palm trees, including Licuri (*Syagrus coronata* (Mart.) Becc.), guariroba (*Syagrus oleracea* (Mart.) Becc.), buriti (*Mauritia flexuosa* L.), buritirana (*Mauritiella armata* Mart.), macaúba (*Acrocomia aculeata* (Jacq.) Lodd.), butiá (*Butia odorata* Barb. Rodr.), and coquinho-azedo (*Butia capitata* (Mart.)), revealed β-carotene as the predominant carotenoid, while the main flavonoids identified were catechin, rutin, and quercetin. In addition, several fruits contain saturated, monounsaturated, and polyunsaturated fatty acids. These findings suggest that the utilization of Cerrado palm fruit compounds for potential industrial applications (Nunes et al. 2023). In this backdrop, this chapter delves in to the nutritional potential of coconut palm and current product trends and proposes a way forward.

1.2 Coconut-*Kalpavriksha*

Coconut (*Cocos nucifera* L.) is one of the important palms in the tropical and subtropical regions of the world. Although its origin is unknown, it is believed to be in the earth over 80 million years. Currently, coconut is cultivated in more than 90 countries with a total area over 12 million hectares around the world (Kalaipandian et al. 2024). India ranks on top with over 20 million fruits followed by the Philippines and Indonesia with over 14 million fruits (ICC 2022). Top ten coconut producers are presented in Table 1.1 (Kalaipandian et al. 2024). Coconut is one of the main sources of lipids and proteins in the tropical countries. It is rich in nutrients, and believed to possess antibacterial, antifungal, antioxidant, antiparasitic, and antiviral properties (Ramesh et al. 2021a). In addition, it is also reported to have a positive effect on antihypertensive, anti-inflammatory, antimicrobial, antioxidant, cardioprotective, antiseizure, cytotoxicity, hepatoprotective, vasodilation, nephroprotective, and anti-osteoporosis (Lima et al. 2015).

Coconut tree in India, is popularly called as '*Kalpavriksha*' (a mythological tree supposed to grant all desires) that means "the tree provides all the necessities of life" or 'tree of life' as each part of the palm is useful for one or the other. It is believed that coconut has been used by human for about half a million years as a source of food, drink, oil, shelter, and wood (Foale 2003). Coconut palm gives several products such as food, activated carbon, shell powder, fibre, charcoal, handicrafts, fuel, furniture, and roofing. Kernel and water are the important food sources in coconut which are used for culinary preparations, and several products used to be processed from them. The palm offers wide diversity in terms colour of the nuts or fruits and in morphoforms such as talls and dwarfs are observed (Fig. 1.1). Coconut meat from the fruit is the main source of food products. Coconut fruit is botanically

Table 1.1 Production of coconuts in whole nuts from top ten countries and total production in the world from 2015 to 2020(Million Nuts)

Country	2015	2016	2017	2018	2019	2020
India	20,440	22,167	23,904	23,798	21,288	20,309
Philippines	14,735	13,825	14,049	14,726	14,765	14,491
Indonesia	14,603	14,521	14,272	14,201	14,140	13,994
Sri Lanka	3056	3011	2450	2623	3086	2792
Brazil	2679	2634	2210	2345	2349	2459
Vietnam	1434	1471	1499	1572	1677	1677
Papua New Guinea	1483	1483	1483	1483	1483	1483
Mexico	893	926	927	926	908	895
Thailand	723	708	666	686	645	591
Malaysia	506	505	517	495	537	561
Total production in the world						
Total	66,758	67,534	68,255	69,325	67,308	65,671

Source: Kalaipandian et al. (2024)

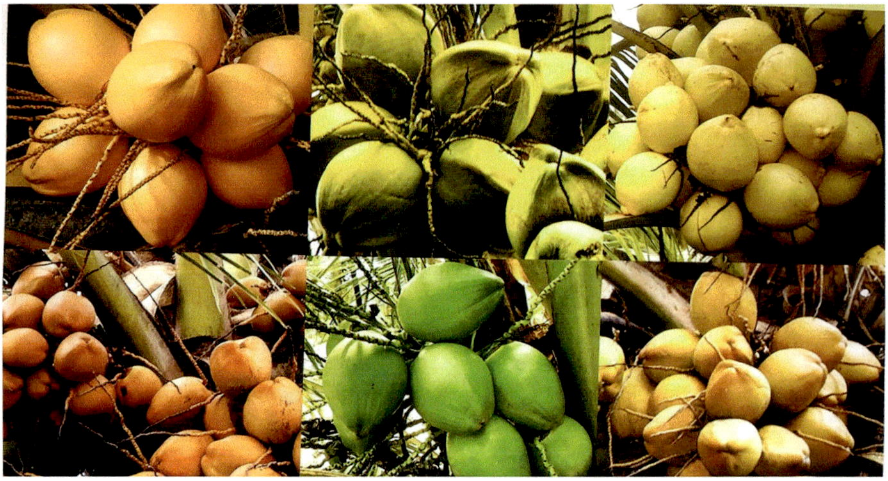

Fig. 1.1 Harnessing coconut fruit diversity for human nutrition. (Photo Credits: ICAR-CPCRI)

a drupe and Fig. 1.2 shows the different layers of the coconut fruit. Coconut fruit has three major parts including exocarp (a thin outer layer, 0.1 mm thick), mesocarp (a fibrous thick middle layer, 1 to 5 cm thick) and the endocarp (a hard lignified layer, 3 to 6 mm thick), and then inside endocarp testa (a thin seed coat layer), and endosperm (solid or kernel and liquid) are present (Beveridge et al. 2022).

Coconut food products are currently replacing several foods from animal source. For example, coconut milk and coconut yoghurt are the best alternative to people who have allergy with dairy products. In addition, coconut water is the natural hydrant to the body, and it is now used to produce sports drinks. Apart from kernel, the coconut inflorescence is tapped to collect phloem sap, which is used to produce

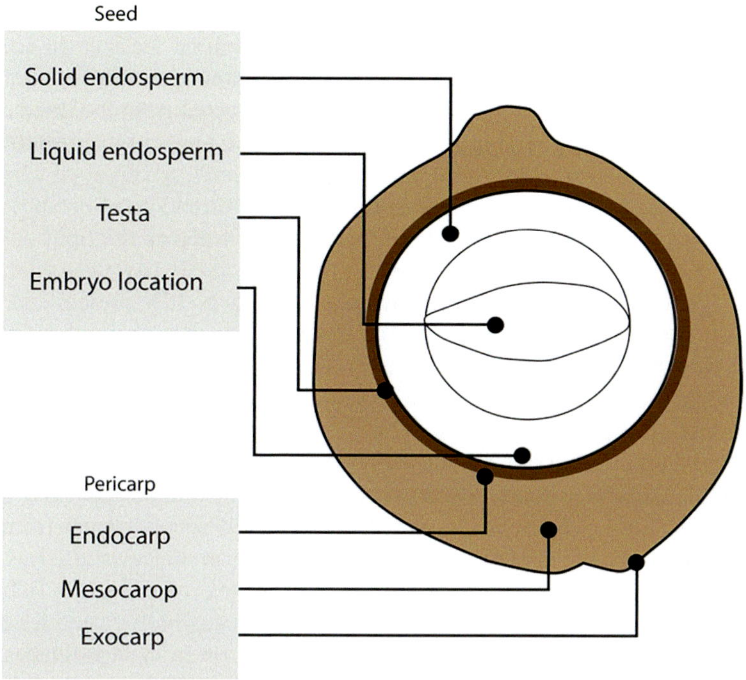

Fig. 1.2 Different layers of coconut fruit. (Source: Beveridge et al. 2022)

coconut sugar, coconut drink (*neera*), coconut syrup, coconut spirits and coconut vinegar. Recently, several coconut products are promoted as functional foods due to its numerous health benefits. Functional foods offer health benefits or disease prevention beyond their nutritional value. For example, coconut products with nutrient-rich ingredients like fruits and vegetables, or they may be fortified with vitamins, minerals, probiotics, and fiber. Among coconut-based functional foods, coconut water, virgin coconut oil (VCO) and the desiccated coconut with nutraceutical value are gaining new markets as functional foods.

1.3 Traditional Coconut Products

The edible portions of the coconut are coconut meat (solid endosperm) and water (liquid endosperm) (Abdul and Iqbal 2011). Traditionally, coconut consumed as fresh/dried coconut, coconut oil and water. Matured coconut kernel or meat processed to produce number of by-products. Coconut kernel contains great source of carbohydrate, lipids, crude fiber, proteins, vitamins, and minerals (Samarajeewa 2024). Kernel is consumed as fresh or dried or used to prepare several by-products. Coconut milk and powder are produced from fresh coconut kernel. Copra and desiccated coconut are produced from dried coconut. Oil extracted from Copra and the by-product (cake) are used for animal feed preparations. Desiccated coconut is the source of the extraction of VCO and the production of several cosmetics and confectionary products. In general, coconut oil is extracted from the dried coconut kernel, and the percentage of oil is the measure of the richness of the meat (Ng et al. 2021). Fresh or dried kernel (copra) has higher lipids and carbohydrate when compared to protein. The protein content of the fresh and dried kernel is ranging from 6.2% to 7.5% and from 8.1% to 10.2%, respectively whereas the lipid content of fresh and copra is 34.7–38.8% and 59.8–63.4%, respectively (Appaiah et al. 2014). Coconut kernel was found to have an average of about 6–10% protein and 6–11% crude fiber content (Appaiah et al. 2014). Coconut kernel has a mixture of essential and non-essential amino acids. It also has several vitamins such as ascorbic acid, niacin and pantothenic acid are present more than other vitamins. It is rich in several minerals including potassium, sodium, calcium, iron and zinc (Appaiah et al. 2014).

The liquid endosperm or coconut water is naturally rich in nutrition. It is rich in total soluble solids, carbohydrates, proteins, vitamins, minerals, and phenols (Parmer et al. 2021). Water is consumed as such, and coconut meat from tender coconut is used for jelly and ice cream preparations (Samarajeewa 2024). Coconut water is sterile until the coconut is opened, the volume of the water is found to reduce depending on the maturity. Tender coconut is usually extracted for coconut water, and the water is preserved after filter sterilization in most instances, or the water undergoes thermal or non-thermal treatments prior to packaging. It is one of the healthiest beverages across tropical countries. Coconut water is consumed in several non-coconut growing countries. Currently, it is consumed all over the world for its health benefits. The sucrose content of the coconut water can reach even up to 90% of the total sugar content (Solangi and Iqbal 2011). Coconut water has several water-soluble vitamins such as ascorbic acid (vitamin C), thiamin, riboflavin, niacin, pantothenic acid, pyridoxine, and folic acid. It is also a rich source of potassium and low in sodium, magnesium, calcium, and iron which provides a better alternative to sports drinks and hydrates the body during exercise (Saat et al. 2002).

As mentioned above, the white flesh or meat of the nut is edible, and it is used as fresh or dried for cooking. The dried meat is called copra, which is traditionally used for the extraction of crude coconut oil. In India, two types of copra are produced such as milling and edible copra (Ramakumar 2001). Coconut oil is extracted from ground milling copra, and the edible copra is consumed as dry fruit. Copra was found to have highest oil content when compared with other oilseeds. Processing and extraction of oil from copra are usually near the coconut plantations. The shell is removed from the coconut meat and dried with heat, using fire, smoke, sun, kiln, or hot air dryer (Divya et al. 2023). After the extraction of crude coconut oil from the copra, the copra cake remains called copra meal. This is widely used for animal feed. Desiccated coconut is the grated and shredded coconut obtained from dehydrated coconut meat (Jayasekara and Gunathilake 2007). It is widely used in confectionery and other food sectors worldwide to replace shredded coconut in several dishes. Coconut milk is produced by mixing two types of liquids from the flesh of the coconut (Henrietta et al. 2022). The coconut flesh is ground to paste and then this is passed through a screw press and vibrating screens to produce coconut milk on a commercial scale (Sudheer et al. 2018). Coconut water and pure water added to dilute this milk and then sugar, stabilizer, and emulsifier is added for packing and sold to consumers.

Coconut oil is the main constituent of the copra, and it possesses numerous uses and health benefits. Coconut oil is traditionally used as a hair oil in many countries including south India, Malaysia, Indonesia, Sri Lanka, coastal regions and south American countries. Although coconut oil mainly contains saturated fatty acids, they are short and medium chain fatty acids (MCFAs) which are ready to be used as an energy source rather than stored as a fat in the body (Kiyasu et al. 1952). The short and medium chain triglycerides account about 61% of the total fatty acids in coconut oil. Scientifically, such fatty acids are nutritionally positive which are arising from differences in metabolic pathways taken by fatty acids in the human body (Samarajeewa 2024). Coconut oil has C12:0 and C10:0 fatty acids which are responsible for the antiviral, antibacterial and antiprotozoal properties (Bhatnagar et al. 2009). Further, coconut oil contains less mono and poly unsaturated fatty acids which provides high stability towards oxidation thus the food products prepared in coconut oil have longer shelf-life (Senevirathne and Dissanayake 2005). It was believed that the coconut oil may be linked to cardiovascular diseases because of its lipid content. However, recent studies found that no evidence is available to link coconut oil consumption and cardiovascular diseases (Schwingshackl and Schlesinger 2023). In ancient times, coconut inflorescence was widely used for medicinal purposes (Ahuja et al. 2014). Coconut blossoms were consumed together with curd to manage diabetes (Henrietta et al. 2022). In the Pacific Island country, Kiribati, coconut blossom is used to cut to get delicious juice, and fresh juice is consumed for breakfast and supper.

1.4 Global Reach and Novel Products

In general, coconut meat and water are used for fresh consumption by the domestic consumers (Grass Ramírez et al. 2023). Coconut oil and toddy (fermented sap or coconut wine) are some other primary food products from coconut industry. However, the demand for coconut has grown substantially up to 500% over the last decade because every part of this palm offers multiple value-added products. For instance, apart from coconut fruit, coconut inflorescence sap is used to produce coconut sugar, neera (coconut nectar juice), vinegar, confectionery, beverage, and jelly. The product diversification, value addition and byproduct utilization led to an annual global export of coconut products exceeding US$ 1.2 billion. Mostly, only about ten food products are exported at a commercial scale, and these includes copra (dried meat or kernel), coconut oil, virgin coconut oil, coconut milk, coconut water, desiccated coconut, cream, milk powder, neera, and coconut sugar (Jayasekara and Gunathilake 2007; Rethinam 2018). Other food products derived from coconut can be found as snacks, chips, coconut butter, flour, and medicinal compounds

(Grass Ramírez et al. 2023). Coconut oil remains the major product being imported by European and American countries, but the growth rate is unstable over the years.

In recent time, virgin coconut oil has been the global attention due to its myriad properties in terms of health benefit (Rethinam 2018). It is now packaged not only in bottles or jars, but also in the form of soft gel capsules, and as flavoured VCO offering different tastes (Manohar et al. 2007) (Fig. 1.3.). The lauric acid contained in VCO was found to be good for immune system (Rethinam 2018), hence VCO has been gaining popularity as healthy nutritive oil that could also be used as functional food and ingredient in the pharmaceutical, nutraceutical and cosmetic industries (Angeles-Agdeppa et al. 2021; Rethinam 2006; Rethinam and Idroes 2006). As VCO is rich in MCFAs that can be rapidly absorbed without participating in cholesterol transport, these fatty acids provide a quick source of energy that is integral for infants as well as people recovering from chronic illness, making it a potential healthy addition to normal diet and reducing cardiovascular disease risk (Babu et al. 2014). Similarly, palm oil from the mesocarp of *E. guineensis* Jacq. holds a significant position in the global oils and fats market accounting for approximately 40% of all traded vegetable oil attributed to its competitive pricing and its versatility in various food applications, including frying, specialty fats, margarines, shortenings, and vegetable ghee. Palm oil is essential dietary component for over three billion people, primarily in Asia, and has diverse non-food applications such as in cleansing and sanitizing products. Globally, oil palm crops yield approximately 81 million tonnes of oil annually from around 19 million hectares of land (Murphy et al. 2021). Approximately 85% of palm oil produced globally is utilized in food products, underscoring the importance of understanding its nutritional properties through research. The fatty acid profile of palm oil, consisting of nearly 50% saturated fatty acids (SFA), has garnered attention in assessing its nutritional adequacy and its

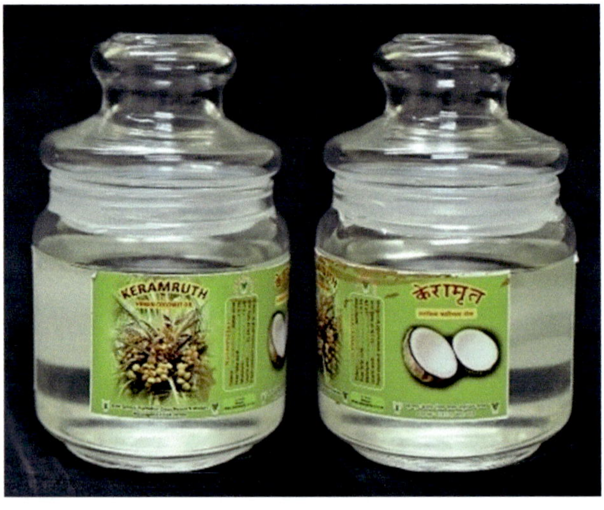

Fig. 1.3 Virgin coconut oil produced from hot process. (Photo credits: ICAR-CPCRI)

potential impact on coronary heart disease risk. Palmitic acid, comprising 44% of SFAs in palm oil, is balanced by approximately 39% monounsaturated oleic acid and 11% polyunsaturated linoleic acid. Notably, palm kernel oil, a co-product derived from the kernel, is notably higher in saturated fats, with almost 80%. Fractionation of palm oil yields palm olein (POo), a more fluid form containing up to 44% oleic acid and 13% linoleic acid. Beyond its balanced fatty acid composition, palm oil is rich in various phytonutrients, including carotenoids, tocopherols, tocotrienols, sterols, squalene, coenzyme Q10, phospholipids, and polyphenols. Despite constituting less than 1% of the oil, these minor components significantly contribute to its stability and quality. Additionally, these phytonutrients exhibit antioxidant properties and offer nutritional and health benefits beyond their antioxidant function (May and Nesaretnam 2014). Development of palm oil-based infant formula further underscores the significance of this oil in mimicking the fatty acid composition of human milk more specifically beta-palmitate (sn-2-palmitate) in infant formula (Padial-Jaudenes et al. 2020). Crude palm oil contains several valuable minor components, including carotenes, tocols (comprising 30% tocopherols and 70% tocotrienols), sterols, and squalene. In the past, many of these minor components were lost during the refining process, with all carotenes being destroyed and approximately 30% of vitamin E being condensed in palm fatty acid distillate, a by-product of palm oil refining. However, processes have been developed to recover these minor components, leading to the emergence of the nutraceutical industry. This industry produces capsules containing tocopherols and tocotrienols, carotene-rich palm oil, and palm carotene concentrate (Basiron 2001). In this context, the coconut oil or virgin coconut oil derived minor constituents such as phytosterols, phenolic acids warrant novel product formulation to harness the nutritional benefits of these minor components (Beegum et al. 2024).

The majority of readily available anti-obesity products have traditionally targeted the restriction of fat digestion and/or absorption, achieved through the use of structured lipids or nondigestible fats, or by enhancing fat catabolism, leading to fatty stools and reduced absorption of fat-soluble vitamins. However, newer products, such as those rich in diacylglycerols (DAGs), have shifted the focus away from limiting fat digestion and absorption. Instead, they concentrate on how edible oils influence fat metabolism, thereby impacting body weight. The development of coconut oil-based diacylglycerols (DAGs) as a non-dairy alternative represents a valuable addition to the range of food products available (Liu et al. 2023).

Coconut milk, milk powder and desiccated coconut are found in the market as the components in functional food, as the lauric acid provided can help in strengthening immunity against diseases. For instance, coconut water is now marketed as functional drink as it is like soft drink with added health benefits. The increasing demand for coconut drink not only attributed to the low calories and cholesterol free properties, but also the benefits of having packed with vitamins, minerals, and electrolytes. A rising trend in European Union countries and America is expected to reach US $ 4 billion in the next 5 years. Organic coconut water and other organic foods of coconut are expected to have a cutting edge in the market due to the increased consumer awareness as well as emerging evidence for the benefits of coconut water on skin and hair. Frozen coconut water with relatively longer shelf life is now offered and powdered form is also made available to allow easier global access of organic coconut water market (Rethinam 2018).

Coconut sugar made from crystallizing palm syrup into fine granules is another global product widely accepted (Rethinam 2018). Coconut blossom sugar has gained high interest among the European markets and kitchens, with its strong caramel smell and taste, in addition to the health benefits (Wrage et al. 2019). It is produced in local industry for domestic use, involving small and medium scale companies, supporting women workers. Over 7000 small scale farmers supply organic-certified coconut sugar (Benjamin-Ripple 2012), led by coconut producing countries including the Philippines, Thailand, and Indonesia. The expanding demand for coconut sugar lies in health benefits as an alternative sweetener due to the low glycemic index and highly nutritive attributes. Hence, it can be safely used by patients with diabetes as an alternative sugar and its market value is estimated to be a US $ 1.3 billion industry. The Philippines is leading this industry in the global markets by exporting coconut sap sugar to Middle East, Asia, and Europe regions, including Australia and New Zealand (Rethinam 2018). In this context, it is pertinent to know the nutritional features of another related palm that is date palm (*Phoenix dactylifera* L.) Despite their high carbohydrate content, date palm (*P. dactylifera* L.) fruits exhibit a low glycaemic response owing to the quality of these carbohydrates. When compared to commonly consumed fruits like strawberries and guava, fruits of date palm possess the highest antioxidants. Date fruits effectively scavenge free radicals due to their rich content of bioactive compounds such as phenolic acids, carotenoids, flavonoids, and polyphenols. These bioactive substances have the capacity to absorb and neutralize free radicals produced during oxidation processes in the human body. The essential role of date fruits constituents significantly contribute to reducing physiological cellular damage and shielding the body against diseases associated with oxidative stress, including cardiovascular diseases, neurodegenerative disorders, and cancer (Al-Mssallem 2020). Besides research has successfully isolated hemicelluloses type polysaccharides from the leaflets and midribs of date palm presents novel opportunities for utilizing the pruned products of date palm. Similarly, date palm midribs were converted into sizing agents for use in yarn sizing, valorisation of date palm pruning products yielded cellulose fibres, fracture sealing material from date palm seeds are some of the non-conventional products from this palm. These studies explored innovative ways to utilize date palm by-products, potentially reducing waste and creating economic and environmental benefits (EL-Mously et al. 2023)., As the huge quantum of bio-waste generated in tender coconut processing industries or vending kiosks, similar approaches of waste to wealth could be followed for coconut as like in date palm industry. In addition, novel coconut-based products are emerging that include superior protein-rich chickpea and coconut-based vegan milk (Rincon et al. 2020); fermented coconut water product as a novel functional beverage enriched with both probiotics and electrolytes (Olaide et al. 2020); spray dried coconut powder, coconut water based vinegar, coconut jam, coconut syrup, coconut based margarine, mayonnaise, coconut honey, coconut cheese among others (Hebbar et al. 2022).

These approaches could serve as an excellent platform for the development of a diverse range of innovative products.

1.5 Nutritional Potential of Coconut Products

Coconut water is rich in nutrients like sugars, minerals, vitamins, and electrolytes, and also contains enzymes and phytohormones. It is particularly abundant in potassium and antioxidants (Dayrit and Nguyen 2020; Chavalittamrong et al. 1982; Bhagya et al. 2010). Coconut oil has high content of saturated fatty acids, especially lauric acid, and also contains unsaturated fatty acids (Rajamohan and Archana 2018). It's associated with several health benefits including the reduction of heart disease risk and antimicrobial, and neuroprotective properties (Silalahi 2020; Sandupama et al. 2022; Ramesh et al., 2021b; Deen et al. 2021). Coconut Kernel offers a variety of macro and micronutrients including vitamins, minerals, dietary fiber, and proteins. It is particularly notable for its high content of L-arginine and neutral detergent fiber. Coconut milk is a nutrient-rich liquid containing carbohydrates, fat, protein, and various vitamins and minerals, including lauric acid (Tulashie et al. 2022). Coconut yogurt contains carbohydrates, fat, protein, vitamins, and minerals, with live bacterial cultures like *Lactobacillus* species and other healthy bacteria, like *Bifidobacterium bifidum* and *Streptococcus thermophilus*. Coconut Inflorescence Sap (neera) is rich in carbohydrates, amino acids, vitamins, and minerals, with a neutral pH (Aalbersberg et al. 1997; Hebbar et al. 2015) and the coconut sugar derived from the inflorescence sap through various drying methods contains carbohydrates, proteins, minerals, and antioxidants (phenolics and flavonoids), with a low glycemic index (Purnomo 1992; Hebbar et al. 2022). Each product offers unique nutritional benefits and can be incorporated into various diets for their health-promoting properties.

1.6 Emerging Trends in Coconut Products

Coconut fruit is rich in dietary fiber, vitamins, and minerals, and it is classified as a highly nutritious 'functional food'. In addition to satisfying consumer's taste, if the food products are nutritious and contribute to health then they can be called as functional foods. Recently, a symbiotic functional drink has been developed from coconut water. Coconut water has been fermented with *Lactobacillus rhamnosus* SP1 and inulin as a source of soluble fiber. After 8 h of fermentation and storage at refrigerator for 14 days, the drink had a pH of 3.48 and probiotic content was about 82×10^8 CFU/mL (Segura-Badilla et al. 2020). Coconut oil is rich in MCFAs which is considered as a functional food due to its positive effects on the lipid and glucose metabolism (Dias et al. 2018; Batista et al. 2018). In addition, coconut oil also contains vitamins, polyphenols and phytosterols which are important for antioxidant properties to scavenge the reactive oxygen species in the cells. Coconut inflorescence sap is rich in nutrients, and several health promoting vitamins, phenolics and flavonoids which can be consumed as fresh or value-added product to make them functional food (Hebbar et al. 2015). This organic sap is found to possess various health benefits including anti-diabetic, anti-ageing, anti-rheumatic, anti-electrolyte imbalance (Hebbar et al. 2015). Coconut sugar derived from the coconut inflorescence sap is one of the important food products that is gaining traction in the arena of functional foods worldwide owing to its rich mineral nutrition, and antioxidant capacity (Hebbar et al. 2022). Coconut testa contains several natural antioxidants including tocopherols, tocotrienols and phenols when compared with coconut oil, and it offers greater health benefits to be included in the diet as a functional food (Ramesh et al. 2023).

Research evidence strongly supports the cardioprotective and neuroprotective effects of coconut. Numerous clinical trials have demonstrated the anti-obesity and hypoglycemic effects of coconut oil and coconut-derived products. The high levels of myocardial antioxidants and the unique metabolism of MCFAs contribute to the cardioprotective effects of coconut. Additionally, the ketogenic effect of coconut-derived products provides neuroprotective benefits and enhances energy expenditure through the metabolism of MCFAs. Polyphenolic antioxidants found in coconut are suggested to offer anti-obesity effects. While the health advantages of coconut and its derivatives are apparent, there is a requirement for long-term clinical trials to better understand their effects (Beegum et al. 2024).

1.7 Concluding Remarks

Improving quality, adding value, and implementing targeted marketing strategies can significantly enhance the revenue and profit potential of the palm industry. Developing premium value-added products from palm resources has the potential to address numerous nutrition and health-related challenges in both developed and developing nations. Introducing such products, including food and beverages, food additives and ingredients, and industrial materials derived from palms, as premium offerings can position the industry competitively in the market. Employing niche marketing tactics will attract the appropriate audience to these products, maximizing the full potential of date palm wealth.

As stated in the beginning of this chapter, coconut can be claimed as 'Kalapavriksha' of health benefits. Because numerous food products are produced from coconut and they are highly nutritious and possess abundant health benefits. Consumption of medium chain fatty acids-rich foods reported to reduce the body fat, and also reduces the risk of heart disease, diabetes, increase mother's milk quality and active as potential antibacterial agent. Recent studies uncovered several scientific evidences on the beneficial effects of coconut. For example, coconut has been reported in number of recent studies that coconut may be beneficial in the treatment of obesity, dyslipidaemia, elevated low-density lipoprotein, insulin resistance and hypertension which are the risk factors for cardiovascular disease, type 2 diabetes, and Alzheimer's disease. Virgin coconut oil has been reported to treat or recover patients from COVID 19 which are very positive effects of the coconut. Likewise, several compounds of coconut need to be isolated and tested for their potential treatment of diseases. This will enable to consumers to include such a nutritious coconut in their diet to lead a healthy life.

References

Abdul HS, Iqbal M (2011) Chemical composition of meat (kernel) and nut water of major coconut (Cocos nucifera L.) cultivars at coastal area of Pakistan. Pak J Bot 43:357–363

Agostini-Costa T d S (2018) Bioactive compounds and health benefits of some palm species traditionally used in Africa and the Americas—a review. J Ethnopharmacol 224:202–229

Al-Mssallem MQ (2020) The role of date palm fruit in improving human health. J Clin Diagn Res 14:1–6

Aalbersberg B, Rohinee Singh RS, Praveen Ravi PR (1997) Nutrient analysis of coconut toddy. Trop Sci. 37(3):160–163

Ahuja SC, Ahuja S, Ahuja U (2014) History, uses and folklore. Asian Agri-History 18(3):221–248

Angeles-Agdeppa I, Nacis JS, Capanzana MV, Dayrit FM, Tanda KV (2021) Virgin coconut oil is effective in lowering C-reactive protein levels among suspect and probable cases of COVID-19. J Funct Foods 83:104557

Appaiah P, Sunil L, Prasanth Kumar PK, Gopala Krishna AG (2014) Composition of coconut testa, coconut kernel and its oil. Journal of the American Oil Chemists' Society 91(6):917–924

Babu AS, Veluswamy SK, Arena R, Guazzi M, Lavie CJ (2014) Virgin coconut oil and its potential cardioprotective effects. Postgrad Med 126(7):76–83

Basiron Y (2001) New palm-based products. J Oleo Sci 50(5):295–303

Batista KS, Alves AF, Lima MDS, Da Silva LA, Lins PP, De Sousa Gomes JA, Silva AS, Toscano LT, De Albuquerque Meireles BRL, De Magalhães Cordeiro AMT, Da Conceição ML, De Souza EL, Aquino JDS (2018) Beneficial effects of consumption of acerola, cashew or guava processing by-products on intestinal health and lipid metabolism in dyslipidaemic female Wistar rats. Br J Nutr 119(1):30–41

Beegum PS, Ramesh SV, Pandiselvam R, Neema M, Manikantan MR, Hebbar KB (2024) Perspectives on the cardioprotective, neuroprotective and anti-obesity functions of coconut (Cocos nucifera L.). Food. Bioscience:103756. https://doi.org/10.1016/j.fbio.2024.103756

Benjamin-Ripple (2012) Coconut palm sweetners—tripple bottom line sustainability. Paper presented at 45th Cocotech meeting of the Asian & Pacific Coconut Community (APCC) countries held in Kochi, 2–6 July 2012

Beveridge FC, Kalaipandian S, Yang C, Adkins SW (2022) Fruit Biology of Coconut (Cocos nucifera L.). Plants 11(23):3293

Bhagya D, Prema L, Rajamohan T (2010) Beneficial effects of tender coconut water on blood glucose and lipid levels in experimental hypertension. J Cell Tissue Res 10(1):2139–2144

Bhatnagar AS, Prasanth Kumar PK, Hemavathy J, Gopala Krishna AG (2009) Fatty acid composition, oxidative stability, and radical scavenging activity of vegetable oil blends with coconut oil. J Am Oil Chem Soc 86(10):991–999

Chavalittamrong B, Pidatcha P, Thavisri U (1982) Electrolytes, sugar, calories, osmolarity and pH of beverages and coconut water. Southeast Asian J Trop Med Public Health 13(3):427–431

Dayrit FM, Nguyen Q (2020) Improving the value of the coconut with biotechnology. In: Adkins S, Foale M, Bourdeix R, Nguyen Q, Biddle J (eds) Coconut biotechnology: towards the sustainability of the 'tree of life'. Springer International Publishing, Cham, pp 29–50

de Cássia Spacki K, Corrêa RCG, Uber TM, Barros L, Ferreira ICFR, Peralta RA, de Fátima Peralta Muniz Moreira R, Helm CV, de Lima EA, Bracht A et al (2022) Full exploitation of peach palm (*Bactris gasipaes* Kunth): state of the art and perspectives. Plan Theory 11:3175
Deen A, Visvanathan R, Wickramarachchi D, Marikkar N, Nammi S, Jayawardana BC, Liyanage R (2021) Chemical composition and health benefits of coconut oil: an overview. J Sci Food Agric 101(6):2182–2193
Dias MDM, Siqueira NP, da Conceição LL, dos Reis SA, Valente FX, dos Santos Dias MM, Rosa CDOB, de Paula SO, da Matta SLP, de Oliveira LL, Bressan J (2018) Consumption of virgin coconut oil in Wistar rats increases saturated fatty acids in the liver and adipose tissue, as well as adipose tissue inflammation. Journal of functional foods 48:472–480
Divya PM, Roopa BS, Manusha C, Balannara P (2023) A concise review on oil extraction methods, nutritional and therapeutic role of coconut products. J Food Sci Technol 60(2):441–452
EL-Mously H, Midani M, Darwish EA (2023) Date palm byproducts in other fields of applications. In: Date palm byproducts: a springboard for circular bio economy, Materials horizons: from nature to nanomaterials. Springer, Singapore
Foale MA (2003) The coconut odyssey: The bounteous possibilities of the Tree of Life. ACIAR Monograph. No. 101, 132 p
Graefe S, Dufour D, van Zonneveld M et al (2013) Peach palm (*Bactris gasipaes*) in tropical Latin America: implications for biodiversity conservation, natural resource management and human nutrition. Biodivers Conserv 22:269–300
Grass Ramírez JF, Muñoz RC, Zartha Sossa JW (2023) Innovations and trends in the coconut agroindustry supply chain: a technological surveillance and foresight analysis. Front Sustain Food Syst 7:1048450
ICC (International Coconut Community) (2022) Global Scenario of Coconut. In: Presented at the 58th ICC Session and Ministerial Meeting. ICC. and Government of Kingdom of Tonga, Jakarta, India
Jayasekara C, Gunathilake KDPP (2007) Processing technologies for virgin coconut oil and coconut based Confectionaries and beverages. Proceedings of international cococnut summit:7–11
Hebbar KB, Arivalagan M, Manikantan MR, Mathew AC, Thamban C, Thomas GV, Chowdappa P (2015) Coconut inflorescence sap and its value addition as sugar—collection techniques, yield, properties and market perspective. Curr Sci 109(8):1411–1417
Hebbar KB, Pandiselvam R, Manikantan MR, Arivalagan M, Beegum S, Chowdappa P (2018) Palm sap—quality profiles, fermentation chemistry, and preservation methods. Sugar Tech 20(6):621–634
Hebbar KB, Pandiselvam R, Beegum PP, Ramesh SV, Manikantan MR, Mathew AC (2022) Seventy five years of research in processing and product development in plantation crops-Coconut, arecanut and cocoa. Int J Innov Hortic 11(1):103–119
Henrietta HM, Kalaiyarasi K, Raj AS (2022) Coconut tree (Cocos nucifera) products: a review of global cultivation and its benefits. J Stabil Environ Mgt 1(2):257–264
Hussain MI, Farooq M, Syed QA (2020) Nutritional and biological characteristics of the date palm fruit (Phoenix dactylifera L.)—a review. Food Biosci 34:100509
Jamshed M, Ahmad S (2018) Niche marketing of date palm based food and beverages as health products. J Econ Cooperat Dev 39(2):49–67
Jaramillo-Vivanco T, Balslev H, Montúfar R, Cámara RM, Giampieri F, Battino M, Cámara M, Alvarez-Suarez JM (2022) Three Amazonian palms as underestimated and little-known sources of nutrients, bioactive compounds and edible insects. Food Chem 372:131273
Kalaipandian S, Biddle J, Adkins SW (2024) Global coconut trade, economy and the value chain. In: The coconut: botany, production and uses. CABI Publishers, Boston
Kiyasu JY, Bloom B, Chaikoff IL (1952) The portal transport of absorbed fatty acids. J Biol Chem 199(1):415–419
Lima EBC, Sousa CNS, Meneses LN, Ximenes NC, Santos Júnior MA, Vasconcelos GS, Lima NBC, Patrocínio MCA, Macedo D, Vasconcelos SMM (2015) Cocos nucifera (L.) (Arecaceae): a phytochemical and pharmacological review. Braz J Med Biol Res 48(11):953–964

Liu X, Xu W, Wang W, Luo R, Yang B, Lan D, Wang Y (2023) Physicochemical properties and feasibility of coconut oil-based diacylglycerol as an alternative fat for healthy non-dairy creamer. Food Chem X 19:100749

Manohar EC, Masa D, Carpio CB (2007) State of the art: virgin coconut oil production in the Philippines. Virgin coconut oil: state of the art. In: Proceedings of the NAST Symposium, Manila

May CY, Nesaretnam K (2014) Research advancements in palm oil nutrition. Eur J Lipid Sci Technol 116(10):1301–1315

Murphy DJ, Goggin K, Paterson RRM (2021) Oil palm in the 2020s and beyond: challenges and solutions. CABI Agric Biosci 2:39. https://doi.org/10.1186/s43170-021-00058-3

Ng YJ, Tham PE, Khoo KS, Cheng CK, Chew KW, Show PL (2021) A comprehensive review on the techniques for coconut oil extraction and its application. Bioprocess Biosyst Eng 44(9):1807–1818

Nunes BV, Ramos ALCC, Mendonça HOP, Reis MC, Ribeiro LV, Silva VDM, Coelho VS, de Melo AC, Reina LDCB, Melo JOF, de Araújo RLB (2023) Integrative review on the content of fatty acids, carotenoids and flavonoids of the Arecaceae of the Cerrado. Contribuciones a Las Ciencias Sociales 16(11):27477–27497

Olaide A, Lihan S, Husain AA, Saat R, Mohammad F, Adewale I, Abideen W (2020) Use of the lactococcus lactis IO-1 for developing a novel functional beverage from coconut water. Ann Univ Dunarea De Jos Galati Fascicle VI Food Technol 44(1):118–131

Padial-Jaudenes M, Castanys-Munoz E, Ramirez M, Lasekan J (2020) Physiological impact of palm olein or palm oil in infant formulas: a review of clinical evidence. Nutrients 12(12):3676

Purnomo H (1992) Sugar components of coconut sugar in Indonesia. ASEAN Food Journal 7(4):200–201

Rajamohan T, Archana U (2018) Nutrition and health aspects of coconut. In: Krishnakumar V, Thampan PK, Nair MA (eds) The coconut palm (Cocos nucifera L.)—research and development perspectives. Springer, Singapore, pp 757–777

Ramakumar R (2001) Costs and margins in coconut marketing: some evidence from Kerala. Indian Journal of Agricultural Economics 56(4):668–682

Ramesh SV, Pandiselvam R, Hebbar KB, Manikantan MR, Beegum PPS, Praveen S, Sruthi NU (2021a) Antiviral potential of coconut (Cocos nucifera L.) oil and COVID-19. COVID 2(4):405–410

Ramesh SV, Krishnan V, Praveen S, Hebbar KB (2021b) Dietary prospects of coconut oil for the prevention and treatment of Alzheimer's disease (AD): A review of recent evidences. Trends in Food Science & Technology 112:201–211

Ramesh SV, Pandiselvam R, Shameena Beegum PP, Saravana Kumar RM, Manikantan MR, Hebbar KB (2023) Review of Cocos nucifera L. testa-derived phytonutrients with special reference to phenolics and its potential for encapsulation. J Food Sci Technol 60(1):1–10

Rethinam P (2006) Strategic solutions to improve coconut production, processing and value addition. Paper presented in 42nd Cocotech meeting of the Asian & Pacific Coconut Community (APCC) countries in Manila, Philippines, 21–25 Aug 2006

Rethinam P (2018) International scenario of coconut sector. In: Krishnakumar V, Thampan PK, Nair MA (eds) The coconut palm (Cocos nucifera L.)—research and development perspectives. Springer, Singapore, pp 21–56

Rethinam P, Idroes A (2006) Generation of creative income and development opportunities through coconut industry in Pacific countries. Paper circulated at the special body on Pacific islands developing countries, 62nd ESCAP session and Asia—Pacific Business Forum 2006, Jakarta, Indonesia, 4–5 Apr 2006

Rincon L, Botelho RBA, de Alencar ER (2020) Development of novel plant-based milk based on chickpea and coconut. LWT 128:109479

Saat M, Singh R, Sirisinghe RG, Nawawi M (2002) Rehydration after exercise with fresh young coconut water, carbohydrate-electrolyte beverage and plain water. J Physiol Anthropol 21(2):93–104

Samarajeewa U (2024) Coconut: nutritional and industrial significance. In: Marc RA, Mureşan CC, Postolache AN (eds) Nut consumption and usefulness in the modern world. IntechOpen, Rijeka

Sandupama P, Munasinghe D, Jayasinghe M (2022) Coconut oil as a therapeutic treatment for Alzheimer's disease: a review. J Fut Foods 2(1):41–52

Schwingshackl L, Schlesinger S (2023) Coconut oil and cardiovascular disease risk. Curr Atheroscler Rep 25(5):231–236

Segura-Badilla O, Lazcano-Hernández M, Kammar-García A, Vera-López O, Aguilar-Alonso P, Ramírez-Calixto J, Navarro-Cruz AR (2020) Use of coconut water (Cocus nucifera L) for the development of a symbiotic functional drink. Heliyon 6(3):e03653

Senevirathne KN, Dissanayake DMS (2005) Effect of method of extraction on the quality of coconut oil. J Sci Univ Kelaniya 2:63–71

Silalahi J (2020) Nutritional values and health protective properties of coconut oil. IDJPCR 3(2):1–12

Solangi AH, Iqbal MZ (2011) Chemical composition of meat (kernel) and nut water of major coconut (Cocos nucifera L.) cultivars at coastal area of Pakistan. Pakistan Journal of Botany 43(1):357–363

Sudheer KP, Claudia KL, Sankalpa KB et al (2018) Prospects in value addition of coconut. Technical Bulletin No. CE-PHT/2018/22

Tulashie SK, Amenakpor J, Atisey S, Odai R, Akpari EEA (2022) Production of coconut milk: A sustainable alternative plant-based milk. Case Studies in Chemical and Environmental Engineering 6:100206. https://doi.org/10.1016/j.cscee.2022.100206

Wrage J, Burmester S, Kuballa J, Rohn S (2019) Coconut sugar (*Cocos nucifera* L.): production process, chemical characterization, and sensory properties. LWT 112:108227

Chapter 2
Bio-nutritional Constituents of Coconut

S. V. Ramesh and Shelly Praveen

Abstract The coconut (*Cocos nucifera* L.) palm, belonging to the *Arecaceae* family, is known for its multi-fold utilities among other fruits. Coconut products are highly recognized in various culinary and nutritional applications due to their rich nutritive metabolites, and distinct flavors. For instance, the tender coconut water is a nutritive-rich, and refreshing beverage packed with minerals and other beneficial compounds. The mature coconut kernel, abundant in fat and protein, offers coconut milk, serving as a key ingredient in virgin coconut oil (VCO) extraction. The brown coloured mesocarp of coconut fruit, commonly called testa, is rich in polyphenols and flavonoids of nutritional significance offering yet another possibility of utilizing it in the extraction of testa oils and production of nutraceuticals. Elite variants of coconut kernel such as Makapuno' (or macapuno)- or 'kopyor' and aromatic counterparts offer significant advantages for value addition processes. In addition, the expansion of coconut milk as a vegan alternative for dairy milk in the utilization in the food and beverage sectors holds a considerable market potential. Additionally, coconut's by-product, coconut flour, packed with high protein and dietary fiber content, presents opportunities for the development of functional foods. The phloem sap or coconut inflorescence sap or *neera* is another major offering of coconut palm with a potential for nutrition rich products such as *neera*-based beverage, mineral rich sugar and second line of value added products. This chapter discusses bionutritional constituents of coconut and its derivates in light of our improved understanding of human nutrition.

Keywords Nutritive metabolites · Coconut biomolecules · Tender nut water · Virgin coconut oil · Testa oil · Coconut flour · Elite kernels

---

S. V. Ramesh (✉)
ICAR-Central Plantation Crops Research Institute (ICAR-CPCRI), Kasaragod, Kerala, India
e-mail: ramesh.sv@icar.gov.in

S. Praveen (✉)
ICAR-Indian Agricultural Research Institute (ICAR-IARI), New Delhi, Delhi, India

S. V. Ramesh, S. Praveen (eds.), *Coconut-Based Nutrition and Nutraceutical Perspectives*, https://doi.org/10.1007/978-981-97-3976-9_2

2.1 Introduction

Coconut palm (*Cocos nucifera* L.) is a monotypic genus that belongs to the Palmae or Arecaceae family. Thriving in sandy soils with a pH range of 5.0 to 8.0 and exhibiting high salt tolerance, coconut palms prefer regions with copious sunlight and well distributed precipitation (1500 to 2500 mm/annum). Optimal growth also requires high humidity levels (70–80%). As one of the foremost palm crops, the coconut plays a crucial role in providing both sustenance and necessary income for millions of farm families in the tropics and sub-tropics. Spanning 12.2 million hectares across 90 countries, the worldwide cultivation of coconuts yields an estimated output of 66.67 million metric tons The major contributors of coconut production in the world scenario are the Philippines, Indonesia, India, Brazil, and Sri Lanka (Source: International Coconut Community (ICC) Statistical Year Book 2022). Renowned for its diverse array of products, the coconut palm contributes significantly to food, beverages, structural materials, and energy resources. The oil yields a broad spectrum of industrial and edible goods, complemented by derivatives from the desiccated kernel, coconut water, inflorescence sap, sugar, haustorium, testa, and dietary fiber with processing technology investments influencing production in various locations. Throughout history, the coconut has served as a valuable source of health and nourishment as every part of the palm has multiple uses and serves human kind. The kernel, also known as the endosperm, holds economic significance in the coconut fruit. Besides, various other parts, such as inflorescence sap, tender coconuts, and mature coconuts, coir, fibre and pollen find applications in food, industrial uses, nutraceutical and traditional medicinal preparations. Coconut serves various medicinal purposes across diverse countries, showcasing its versatility in traditional healing practices (Lima et al. 2015). This chapter delves into various nutritional composition of coconut and its products and highlights the nutritional benefits of food products of coconut (Table 2.1).

Table 2.1 Biochemical composition of coconut parts and derivatives

Sl.No.	Coconut component	Biochemical features	Contents	Bioactives	References
1	Liquid endosperm or tender nut water	Water	94.18–94.99%	Sugars, minerals, phytohormones, Vitamin C and Riboflavin, anti-microbial peptides	Yong et al. (2009), Santoso et al. (1996), Prades et al. (2012), Kumar et al. (2021), Chen et al. (2018)
		pH	5.16 (4.7 to 5.97)		
		Titrable acidity	0.08 (0.04 to 0.19) mEq·100 mL^{-1}		
		Protein	0.12–0.72%		
		Fat	0.07–0.2%		
		Ash	396.6 (282–864) mg/100 mL		
		Amino acids	1.67 (0.8 to 2.2) mg/100 mL		
		Total sugars	5.22 (2.69 to 7.00) g/100 mL		
		Reducing sugars (glucose, fructose)	3.8 (1.2 to 5.1) g/100 mL		
		Minerals			
		(a) Calcium	27.35 mg/100 g		
		(b) Iron	0.02 mg/100 g		
		(c) Magnesium	6.4 mg/100 g		
		(d) Phosphorus	4.66 mg/100 g		
		(e) Potassium	2029 (338 to 3080) mg/kg		
		(f) Sodium	25.6 (10 to 38) mg/kg		
		Vitamin C	7.41 mg/100 dm^3		
		Vitamin B2	0.01 mg/100 dm^3		
		Polyphenols	46.03 mg GAE/L		
		Free amino acids	30 mg %		

(continued)

Table 2.1 (continued)

Sl.No.	Coconut component	Biochemical features	Contents	Bioactives	References
2	Mature coconut water	pH	5.5 ± 0.3	Minerals, sugars, vitamins and proteins	Sandhya and Rajamohan (2008)
		Total solids	4.5 ± 0.7		
		Total sugars	2.7 ± 0.8 g/100 mL		
		Reducing sugars	1.3 ± 0.4 g/100 mL		
		Total protein	0.25 to 0.45 g/100 mL		
		Total fat	0.51 ± 0.3 g/100 mL		
		Ash	0.43 ± 0.04 g/100 mL		
		L-arginine	150 mg/100 mL		
		Vitamin C	20–40 mg/100 mL		
		Nicotinic acid	0.64 μg/mL		
		Pantothenic acid	0.52 μg/mL		
		Magnesium	7.8 to 15.0 mg/100 mL		
		Potassium	164–356 mg/100 mL		
		Sodium	4.1 to 48 mg/100 mL		
		Calcium	18.2 to 47.7 mg/100 mL		
3	Coconut Milk	Protein	1.99 g/100 mL	Lauric acid, medium chain triglycerides, Vitamin E	Ramesh et al. (2023)
		Fat	4.12 g/100 mL		
		Carbohydrate	10 g/100 mL		
		Total sugars	7.92 g/100 mL		
		Minerals			
		(a) Calcium	145.83 mg/100 mL		
		(b) Iron	0.75 mg/100 mL		
		Vitamin A	10 (% daily value)/per serving of 240 mL		

4	Coconut kernel	Moisture	3.94–4.3%	Lauric acid, medium chain triglyceride, proteins, phenolics, flavonoids	Appaiah et al. (2014)
		Fat	59.8–71.62%		
		Protein	8.80–10.2%		
		Carbohydrates	7–24%		
		Crude fibre	7%		
		Ash	1.5%		
5	Copra oil			Medium chain fatty acids (C10:0 Capric acid; C12:0 Lauric acid; C14:0 Myristic acid; C16:0 Palmitic acid)	Ramesh et al. (2021)
		SFAs	89.75%		
		MUFAs	6.45%		
		PUFAs	1.72%		
		MCFAs	60.73%		
		Tocopherols	2–6 (μg/g)		
		Phytosterols	0.5–1.0		
		Total polyphenols content	150–250 (μg/g)		
6	Virgin coconut oil			Medium chain fatty acids (C10:0 Capric acid; C12:0 Lauric acid; C14:0 Myristic acid; C16:0 Palmitic acid), polyphenols, phytosterols	Ramesh et al. (2021)
		SFAs	84.8%		
		MUFAs	6.5%		
		PUFAs	1.5%		
		MCFAs	56.3%		
		Tocopherols	15–30 (μg/g)		
		Phytosterols	2.5–3.0		
		Total polyphenols content	500–700 (μg/g)		

(continued)

Table 2.1 (continued)

Sl.No.	Coconut component	Biochemical features	Contents	Bioactives	References
7	Coconut Testa			Phenolic acids, flavonoids, anti-oxidants	Marasinghe et al. (2019), Arivalagan et al. (2018b), Ramesh et al. (2021)
		Fat	7.93–59%		
		Protein	9.3–32.22%		
		Carbohydrates	26.3–9.24%		
		Crude Fibre	11.6%		
		Phenolic acids			
		salicylic acid	54.0–2642 μg/g		
		4-hydroxy benzoic acid	19.9–3094 μg/g		
		protocatechuic acid	65.5–34,015 μg/g		
		vanillic acid	11.5–591 μg/g		
		gallic acid	18.5–5654 μg/g		
		Flavonoids			
		Catechin	6.4–3451 μg/g		
		Kaempferol	1187–9271 μg/g		
		Apigenin	33.0–3881 μg/g		
		Hesperetin	37.2–1022 μg/g		
8	Coconut inflorescence sap	Total sugars	16.20 ± 0.33 g/100 mL	Sucrose, vitamins including ascorbic acid and niacin, polyphenols	Hebbar et al. (2020)
		Reducing sugars	0.68 ± 0.01 g/100 mL		
		Free amino acids	1.03 ± 0.10 g/100 mL		
		Total phenolic content	21.7 ± 0.48 mg GAE/100 mL		
		Total flavonoid content	0.817 ± 0.19 mg CE/100 mL		
		Vitamin C	19.6 ± 0.95 mg/100 mL		
		Niacin	14.9 ± 2.80 μg/100 mL		
		Pantothenic acid	3.99 ± 0.08 μg/100 mL		
		Tocopherol	7.20 ± 0.93 μg/100 mL		
		Vitamin K1	1.73 ± 0.19 μg/100 mL		

9	Coconut sugar	Total sugars	91.8 ± 1.01 g/100 mL	Sucrose, vitamins, fibres, polyphenols, minerals	Hebbar et al. (2020)
		Reducing sugars	4.69 ± 4.60 g/100 g		
		Proteins	2.6 g/100 g		
		Dietary Fiber	3.1 g/100 g		
		Free amino acids	3.05 ± 0.07 g/100 g		
		Total phenolic content	47.2 ± 20.7 mg GAE/100 g		
		Total flavonoid content	4.76 ± 1.21 mg CE/100 g		
		Vitamin C	3.98 ± 1.12 mg/100 g		
		Thiamine	14.3 ± 1.16 µg/100 g		
		Niacin	34.7 ± 2.1 µg/100 g		
		Pantothenic acid	3.99 ± 0.08 µg/100 g		
		Tocopherol	19.6 ± 3.5 µg/100 g		
		Vitamin K1	7.35 ± 0.95 µg/100 g		
		Vitamin K2	5.57 ± 0.61 µg/100 g		
		Minerals			
		Sodium	568 mg/100 g		
		Potassium	1002 mg/100 g		
		Iron/Zinc	2.2 mg/100 g		
		Essential amino acids			
		Lysine	136.5 mg/100 g		
		Phenylalanine	57.6 mg/100 g		
		Methionine	54.55 mg/100 g		
		Valine	40.68 mg/100 g		
		Threonine	45.81 mg/100 g		

2.2 Coconut Water

Coconut water, also known as coconut juice or the liquid endosperm primarily comprises mineral elements, sugars, which constitutes the 2–5% of solid matter content. It is a clear, colourless liquid found inside tender coconuts and possesses a mildly sweet and acidic flavour with a pH of 5–6. In its natural state, the liquid endosperm is enclosed within a hermetic cavity and is sterile (Prithviraj et al. 2021). Coconut water is a natural and refreshing beverage finding numerous applications. This revitalizing beverage is consumed globally due to its nutritional richness and health benefits. Traditionally the water has been successfully used as a growth media supplement in plant *in vitro* culture and regeneration approaches owing to its phytohormone contents. Despite its composition, the unique qualities and flavors of coconut water are not solely determined by sugars and minerals. The nutritional composition of coconut water is subject to variations influenced by factors such as nut maturity, coconut genotype or variety, location of growth, edaphic conditions, fertilizer application, stage of harvesting and other environmental factors (Prades et al. 2012; Naik et al. 2022). Furthermore, after the extraction of water from the inner fruit cavity, it undergoes rapid deterioration. Spoilage is primarily attributed to the vigorous activity of microorganisms, contaminants, keeping conditions, and the kinds of materials used for packaging the water. In addition, the activities of anti-oxidant enzymes such as peroxidase (POX) and polyphenol oxidase (PPO) are found to be high in the process of handling although aseptic environment is maintained during processing of coconut water. These enzymes can significantly impact the water quality, leading to reduced shelf life, generation of off-flavor, loss of nutrients, and physical changes such as turbidity and discoloration. Coconut water's broad range of applications is substantiated by its distinctive chemical composition. It includes a blend of sugars, vitamins, minerals, amino acids, and phytohormones, collectively contributing to the beverage's unique properties (Yong et al. 2009; Prades et al. 2012). Coconut water, often considered an excellent alternative to traditional athletic drinks, provides low-calorie content (17.4 kcal/100 g). Nutritional composition of coconut water reveals it is rich in vitamins, electrolytes, free amino acids, phytohormones and other organic acids. The minerals present in coconut water mimics human blood and create a similar osmotic pressure. Thereby the coconut water serves as a suitable alternative for intravenous rehydration or fluid replacement in human under acute conditions. Coconut water is rich in water-soluble vitamins such as B1, B2, B3, B5, B6, B7, B9, and Vitamin C. These vitamins are vital coenzymes for multiple cellular enzymatic activities and ensure appropriate functioning of cellular metabolic pathways. Abundant inorganic ions, including calcium, copper, iron, magnesium, manganese, phosphorous, potassium, sodium, zinc, and other trace minerals, play crucial roles in supporting the antioxidant system of human body. In addition, coconut water is a rich source of organic acids such as acetic, citric, malic, tartaric acids and other biocatalysts such as POX, catalase (CAT), RNA polymerase, acid phosphatase, and diastase. Coconut water contains organic acids, enzymes, and phytohormones like auxin, cytokinin, kinetin, trans-zeatin, and gibberellic acid. These components play specific roles in human nutrition and physiological functions. For instance, the antioxidants in coconut water help prevent oxidative damage to cell membranes. Indole-3-acetic acid (IAA), found in coconut water, exists both in free form and conjugated with amino acids and peptides (Bhagya et al. 2012). While conjugated IAA is biologically inactive and stored in seeds for hormonal homeostasis, free IAA contributes to various physiological processes. Additionally, coconut water contains cytokinins like Trans-Zeatin and Trans-Zeatin riboside, which are used in plant tissue culture for plantlet regeneration and have potential applications in treating neuronal dysfunctions (Srinivasan et al. 2021). Coconut water also exhibits anti-aging effects on human fibroblast cells. Gibberellins GA1 and GA3, enumerated in coconut water, stimulate the elongation of shoots and stems in plants. In recent times, there has been a notable increase in scientific support for recognizing the significance of therapeutic applications of coconut water and promoting human wellness (Tuyekar et al. 2021).

Sugars in coconut water demonstrate significant variability across different stages of coconut maturity. As the fruit matures, sucrose content tends to increase at the expense of glucose and fructose, providing a potential marker for the coconut's stage of maturity. Thus the ratio of reducing sugars to total sugars can be informative in this regard. Turbidity is another factor that tends to increase with coconut maturity. Therefore, visual screening based on turbidity could serve as an indicator, with young or tender coconut water expected to be visually clear. Sorbitol concentrations and formol values have also been explored as useful parameters for characterizing young versus mature coconut water (Burns et al. 2020). These factors collectively offer potential means for distinguishing between water from tender or young and mature coconuts. The metabolomics approach has pinpointed eight differential biomarkers common to both the 'COD' and 'MYD' coconut varieties, which include chlorogenic acid, ferulic acid, lauric acid, oleic acid, palmitic acid, shikimic acid, succinic acid, and sucrose. Additionally, the 'COD' variety showed two extra biomarkers, caffeic acid, and myristic acid, whereas the 'MYD' variety exclusively exhibited fumaric acid and stearic acid (Kumar et al. 2021). Earlier LC–MS analysis identified 14 metabolites from mature coconut water, including L-isoleucine, L-leucine, L-valine, L-threonine, 5-oxo-D-proline, l-proline, gamma-aminobutyric acid, taurine, dibutyl phthalate, and 4-hydroxyphenylacetic acid. These identified metabolites have the potential to serve as biomarkers for distinguishing between different stages of mature coconut water (Chen et al. 2018). While tender nut water and mature coconut water possess similar nutritional profiles, consumers typically opt for tender coconut water as a healthful beverage, whether consumed freshly harvested or processed into various packaged drinks. One serving (240 mL) of coconut water contains approximately 46 calories, 12 g of carbohydrates including simple sugars, 1 g of protein, and a little fat. It also offers a considerable amount of dietary fiber, providing around 2.6 g/cup (Naik et al. 2022). To maximize nutritional and sugar content in the coconut liquid endosperm, coconuts are ideally harvested during the 7th and 8th month of development. In the initial stage of ripening when the endosperm is forming, invert sugar and amino acids accumulate in the coconut water. Tender nut water exhibits higher levels of total phenolics and sugar compared to mature nut water. As a healthy sports beverage, coconut water boasts significant rehydration capabilities (Cappelletti et al. 2015).

The nut water is effective in relieving urinary tract infections, gastric discomfort, preventing heat induced skin irritations, and maintaining the body's pH balance (Rajashri et al. 2020). Moreover, it shares similarities with blood plasma, making it suitable as a substitute (Rajashri et al. 2020). Additionally, consumption of coconut water help protects the heart against myocardial infarction, lowers high blood pressure, and mitigates hypertension. It also proves beneficial in alleviating severe conditions such as sickle cell anemia (Ekpenyong and Okafor 2018; Rethinam and Krishnakumar 2022).

2.3 Coconut Kernel

As the coconut matures, the coconut water is gradually replaced by the coconut kernel. Coconut milk, a sweet, milky aqueous extract from the mature coconut meat or kernel derives its colour and rich flavour the oil and sugar components of the kernel. This milk is nutritionally different from coconut water, containing a complex mixture of sugars, coenzymes, and minerals (Patil and Benjakul 2018). Remarkably, the coconut kernel or pulp, due to its high-fat content, has been a source of economic value for over a century, extending beyond its role as an oil seed. The dried kernel, commonly referred to as copra, holds a significant global value. Lauric acid (45–53%), extracted from copra, serves a variety of purposes, with the chemical and food industries processing it into detergent or margarine, respectively. In the past 20 years, the fresh coconut market has seen an impressive 300% growth, highlighting coconut's dual role as both a globally traded oil commodity and a profitable fresh fruit. Coconut oil, extracted from mature coconut meat, has served as a primary nutrient source in the diets of millions worldwide for generations. Renowned for its heat stability, coconut oil is an excellent choice for cooking and frying, boasting a smoke point of around 180 °C (360 °F). Its slow oxidation and resistance to rancidity contribute to a longer shelf life of up to 2 years owing to its highly stable saturated fatty acid components (Fife 2013). Coconut copra stands out for its high potassium content, surpassing many other foods. Various phytochemicals, such as saponins, alkaloids, tannins, glycosides, flavonoids, and phenols, have been identified in copra. These phytochemicals play a significant role in imparting health promotional attributes namely anti-inflammatory, antioxidant, and reducing properties to the copra. The protective layer surrounding the coconut, known as testa, is an outer, thin, brown-coloured layer surrounding the endosperm. Coconut serves as both a co-product and by-product in the manufacturing processes of haustorium and the coconut processing industry. Coconut proteins, oil, and water are essential components, along with various derived products such as coconut palm sugar, inflorescence sap, haustorium, coconut testa, and various nutraceuticals. These derived products, including dietary supplements, help prevent nutrient deficiencies and provide health benefits. Beyond its use as a cooking oil, coconut oil holds significant medical value, serving both cosmetic and therapeutic purposes for skin care. In modern times, coconut is acknowledged as a valuable source of comprehensive nutrients, assisting in addressing malnutrition and enhancing overall health. Coconut oil contains fatty acids like lauric acid and medium-chain, both renowned for their medicinal and nutritional attributes (Twishsri et al. 2011; Beegum et al. 2024).

2.3.1 Elite Kernel Variants

The coconut endosperm is typically consumed as a dessert when it's around 6–7 months old exhibiting a soft, mucous-like consistency. As the coconut matures beyond 7 months, the endosperm becomes more solid, developing a tougher texture. Besides the correlation of biochemical features of coconut endosperms across the various maturity stages there are instances of edible coconut endosperms, which are mutation-induced variations, and are often called as "elite" kernel variants.

2.3.1.1 'Makapuno' (or Macapuno)- or 'Kopyor'

Macapuno/makapuno and Kopyor represent mutant varieties of coconuts. In the case of the Kopyor coconut, it features a brittle endosperm that is believed to undergo deformation in the early stages of solid endosperm formation. On the contrary, the Makapuno coconut exhibits a gelatinous endosperm, characterized by galactomannan-rich solid part and a phytohormone IAA-rich liquid portion, both resulting from the absence of enzymatic production (Wicaksono et al. 2021). In a normal endosperm, the reserve glucomannans undergo enzymatic degradation into simple sugars namely fructose, galactose and mannose which ultimately nourishes the embryo. In the case of the makapuno coconut endosperm, an increase in the β-mannase activity, results in the accumulation of disaccharides or oligosaccharides such as galactomannobiose, mannobiose, mannotriose. However, the lack of downstream acting enzymes, specifically α-D-galactosidase and β-mannosidase in macapuno coconut causes the lack of simple sugars (galactose and mannose) as a source of nutrition for the developing embryo, thereby impeding the growth of embryo. Also, the lack of enzymes peroxidase and IAA-oxidase leads to the upregulation of IAA biosynthesis in makapuno coconut (Nguyen et al. 2016). Thus the abundant accumulation of IAA coupled with the presence of high quantities of galactomannan derived sugar compounds imparts a characteristic jelly-like consistency to the makapuno endosperm. Additionally, Makapuno coconut experiences disrupted cytokinesis in endosperm cells, leading to the formation of polyploid cells. Both the mutant coconut variants Makapuno and Kopyor are highly regarded as delicacies. In addition, the fatty acid profile of Makapuno nuts was quite different from normal kernel since the percentages of medium chain fatty acids [caproic acid (<1%), capric acid (7%), lauric acid (50%), and myristic acid (18%)] are relatively high (Castillo 1986). Besides other mutant variants such as wax coconut (Indonesian: "kelapalilin"), and canary coconut (Indonesian: "kelapakenari") are also recognized. The endosperm of wax coconut is edible but poses a melting wax like features. On the other hand canary coconut is characterized with crispy brittle endosperm (Wicaksono et al. 2021).

2.3.1.2 Aromatic Coconut

Aromatic coconut is a distinct variant of the green dwarf coconut, distinguished by the pleasing "pandan-like" aroma in its liquid endosperm, attributed to the presence of 2-acetyl-1-pyrroline (2AP) (Luckanatinvong et al. 2018). Biochemical characterization of aromatic coconut revealed a change in single nucleotide position within the coding region of gene, *CnAMADH2*, resulting in biosynthesis of 2AP. Intriguingly, this specific nucleotide variation was undetected in another aromatic yellow dwarf coconut disclosing an alternative allele of the gene *CnAMADH2*. Besides the pleasing fragrance of water and kernel, the aromatic coconut variants also possess other traits of economic importance such as early maturity and high yield potential. The kernel of aromatic coconut is recognized as a superior naturally sourced green food, attributed to its high sugar content and fine aroma. The interplay of sugars and fatty acids plays a crucial role in shaping the intense flavor profile of aromatic coconut. A comprehensive analysis of aromatic coconut and a wild type coconut kernel indicated a significant three to fourfolds increase of sugars (fructose and glucose) in the former compared to the latter at 11 months of age. This marked difference underscores the distinctive composition of sugars in the aromatic coconut meat. Furthermore, a multitude of genes responsible for the accumulation and metabolism of sugars and fatty acids in both aromatic coconut and non-aromatic coconut meat was identified shedding light on the underlying genetic mechanisms contributing to the unique flavor characteristics of aromatic coconut (Zhou et al. 2024).

2.4 Coconut Milk

Coconut milk is derived from the grated kernel of mature coconuts typically aged between 12 to 14 months. It has a creamy white appearance and is characterized as an oil-in-water emulsion, separating naturally into a dense aqueous phase and a lighter cream phase (Seow and Gwee 1997; Tansakul and Chaisawang 2006). It is a mixture characterized primarily by lipid carbohydrates and proteins, forming an emulsion. Alongside these major components, it includes various minor compounds such as phenolic substances. Assessment of anti-oxidant potential of coconut milk through the ferric reducing power (FRAP) and the 1,1-diphenyl-2-picrylhydrazyl (DPPH) assays suggests that the coconut milk exhibits superior antioxidant qualities. Coconut milk shows anti-ulcerogenic effects in rodent models (Nneli and Woyike 2008). Coconut milk is significantly low in fiber and contains protein (3.3%) and fat (27%) (USDA 2018). The freshly extracted coconut milk also comprises little quantities of vitamin B and vitamin C. The primary carbohydrate of coconut milk is sucrose, which is also accompanied by traces of starch. In the wake of rise in the demand for vegan milk alternatives, the worldwide market potential of coconut milk powder has crossed a staggering 59 million USD in the year 2020.

2.5 Coconut Testa

Coconut testa or mesocarp is generated as a by-product in the production of dehydrated coconut powder, coconut milk, and virgin coconut oil. Unfortunately, it is often overlooked, yet it holds value and is utilized as feed for animals. Appaiah et al. (2014) showcased the abundant antioxidants in coconut testa oils, attributed to their high levels of phenolics, tocotrienols, and tocopherols. The health promotional properties of coconut testa oils, as demonstrated through its antioxidant potential and protection against hydrogen peroxide-induced oxidative damage on human serum albumin, divulge it as a promising source for functional foods (Zhang et al. 2016). The phytochemical profile and antioxidant activity of testa extracts uncovered various bioconstituents such as amino acids, carbohydrates, flavonoids, glycosides, phenolics, saponins triterpenes and tannins (Appaiah et al. 2016). Additionally, the biochemical analysis of coconut testa identified 16 phenolic acids and 12 flavonoids as primary components, further confirming its innate potential as a natural antioxidant. Among the major phenolic acids were protocatechuic acid, p-coumaric acid, and ferulic acid, while significant flavonoids included catechin, apigenin, and kaempferol (Arivalagan et al. 2018b). This underscores the potential significance of utilizing testa as a valuable resource in various applications. Concentrated phenolics derived from coconut testa play a significant role in conferring cardioprotective effects in laboratory animal models that underwent high-fat diet by reducing the accumulation of fatty acids (Geetha and Kumar 2022). Consequently, the phenolics derived from coconut testa contribute significantly to alleviating risk factors associated with obesity. Also, coconut testa-based concentrates were shown to confer DNA protection properties further highlighting their potential in mitigating or diminishing stress-induced ailments (Geetha et al. 2016). The testa bioflavonoid based nano-encapsulated nutraceutical product development emerges as a crucial research priority, aiming to substitute synthetic antioxidants in food formulations with these natural compounds (Ramesh et al. 2021) (Fig. 2.1).

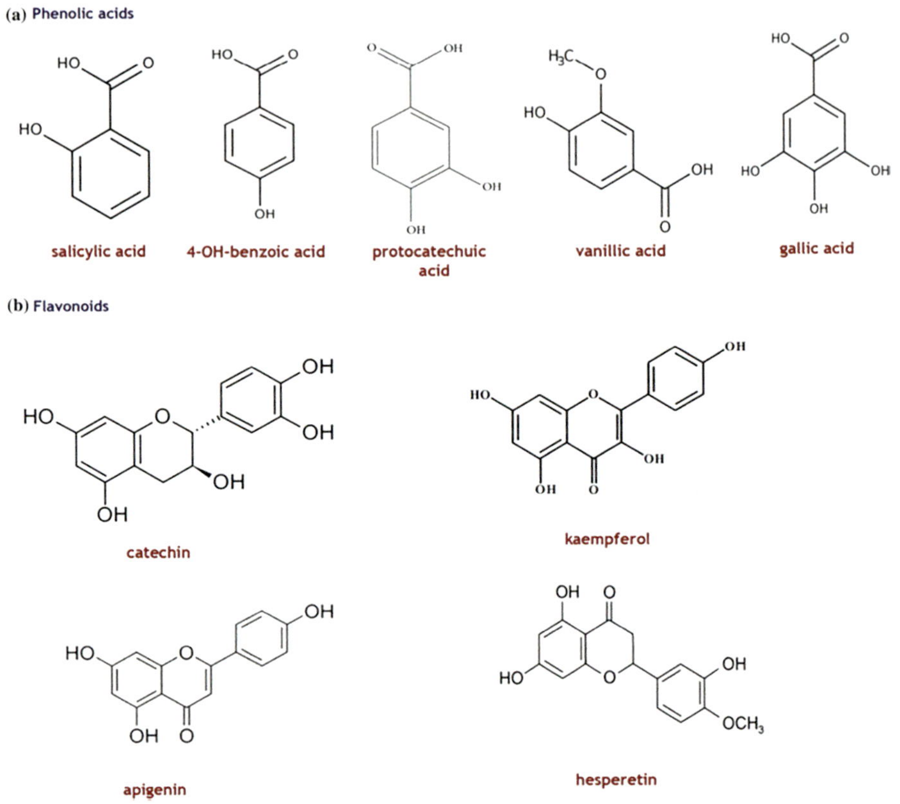

Fig. 2.1 The phenolics and flavonoids profile of coconut testa. (Source: Ramesh et al. 2021, https://doi.org/10.1007/s13197-021-05310-2. Reprinted with permission from Springer Nature)

2.6 Coconut Haustorium

In the coconut germination process, the embryo undergoes growth in two directions. The basal portion of the embryo transforms into an absorbent tissue referred to as a haustorium or coconut apple. Haustorium facilitates the mobilization of nutrients initially from the liquid endosperm and subsequently from the solid endosperm, providing nourishment to the emerging embryo. The outer yellow region is oil rich whereas the inner white portion is rich in carbohydrates. Therefore, it is presumed that haustorium tissue is a reservoir of readily available nutrients. The white portion of coconut haustorium shows a low total fat (1.01–3.18%), protein (4.95–6.25%), and significant carbohydrate (59.2–75.6%). Soluble and insoluble fiber ranged from 4.96–6.20% and 17.1–23.2%, respectively. In contrast to the matured coconut endosperm, the haustorium displayed lower total fat (2% vs. 63%), high carbohydrates (67% vs. 29%), soluble sugars (44% vs. 12%), and dietary fibers (26% vs. 17%). The fatty acid profile of the haustorium showed lauric acid (43.2 ± 2.5%), followed by myristic (18.8 ± 0.7%) and palmitic acid (12.6 ± 1.0%). Oleic acid is highest among long-chain fatty acids (9.42 ± 2.0%), followed by stearic (5.54 ± 0.4%) and linoleic acid (1.68 ± 0.5%).The amino acid composition of haustorium revealed high levels of aspartic acid (9.32%), proline, and glutamic acid (6.35%). Essential amino acid scores of the haustorium revealed that amino acids histidine, valine, and lysine are present in abundance with reference to the recommended FAO/WHO values, whereas the contents of threonine corresponded with the recommended reference values. However, haustorium showed significantly low quantities of aromatic amino acids (amino acid score of 33%), leucine (46%), sulphur-containing amino acids (58%), and isoleucine (68%) (Arivalagan et al. 2018a). This highlights the need for formulating a nutritionally balanced food by combining the goodness of coconut haustorium with pseudo-cereals and millets. The high aspartate and glutamate content (36%) suggests potential flavor-enhancing properties, indicating its use in food formulations. Similarly identification of characteristic flavor compounds in coconut haustorium revealed five acids, eleven aldehydes, three alcohols, three ketones, two esters, and a pyrazine (Zhang et al. 2022). The flavor compounds identified in coconut haustorium include isomeric forms of ethanol, acetone, 2-butanone, acetoin, acetic acid, hexanal, butyrolactone, 2-propanol, 2-methyl-propanal, 2-methylbutanal, 3-methylbutanal, propionic acid, pentanal, methyl pyrazine, hexanoic acid, n-nonanal, and isobutyric acid. The coconut haustorium derived compounds could serve as enhancers of mineral elements. Also it can be used a raw material in the production of weaning food or medicine owing to its sugar, amino acids profile and antioxidant potential, respectively.

2.7 Coconut Inflorescence Sap and Derivatives

The phloem sap of coconut or inflorescence sap, also called as *neera* is tapped from unopened spadix. The sap, being a type of phloem sap, contains a rich combination of sugars, amino acids, minerals, vitamins, proteins, and phenolics, showcasing significant antioxidant potential. Depending on the palm's health and existing climatic conditions, the coconut palm characteristically produces 10 to 14 spadices in a year. On average, a single spadix can yield 2 liters of sap per day, and a coconut tree has the potential to produce 400 liters per year. The unfermented sap can be marketed as a nutritious beverage, or it can be easily converted into syrup or neera concentrate or coconut sugar or coconut jaggery. In contrast to the traditional method of tapping sap into open earthen pots, the use of a specially designed double-jacketed box known as the Cocosap chiller guarantees the collection of sap in a hygienic and non-fermented manner (Hebbar et al. 2022). The sap obtained through the Cocosap chiller exhibits a golden-brown hue, possesses a delightful taste, and is devoid of impurities such as insects, ants, pollen, and dust particles. This sap is abundant in health-promoting biochemicals, as the unfermented sap not only has elevated sugar levels but also boasts higher concentrations of amino acids, polyphenols, flavonoids, and antioxidants. Specifically, these components are 1.5 to 2.5-folds greater compared to the traditionally collected neera. Besides being an excellent health beverage, it serves as an ideal substrate for producing premium natural value-added products (Hebbar et al. 2013). The nutritional composition of coconut sugar encompasses vital nutrients including Vitamin E and Vitamin C and elemental nutrition such as like potassium, iron, zinc, and phosphorus. Moreover, the sap comprises multiple health promoting components such as flavonoids, phenolics, and anthocyanidins (Hebbar et al. 2020). Coconut sugar derived from the sap contains a significant quantity of inulin (4.7%), a crucial component involved in the synthesis of short-chain fatty acids (SCFAs) (Trinidad et al. 2016). This conversion of fermentable inulin into SCFAs enhances the functional properties of coconut sugar and syrup, with the latter containing both dietary fiber and inulin. Moreover, coconut inflorescence sap serves as a substrate for the synthesis of silver nanoparticles (Rajesh et al. 2020). Also a metagenomic approach has unveiled that the sap is characterized with microorganisms that offer probiotic properties (Gopal et al. 2021).

2.8 Coconut Biomolecules

Coconut and its derivatives offer multitude of health promoting biomolecules ranging from virgin coconut oil, testa oil, coconut protein, coconut fibre, coconut sugar among others. Coconut is inherently packed with a wide array of nutrients and known for its adaptability, with each component of the fruit offering valuable nutritional advantages.

2.8.1 Virgin Coconut Oil

Virgin coconut oil (VCO) is an exemplary value added product among the economically impactful output of a coconut industry. VCO is extracted mechanically from fresh, mature coconut kernels or coconut milk and it precludes the processes of refining, bleaching, or deodorization (RBD) to safeguard its innate biochemical qualities. The oil yield of coconut milk exhibits a direct correlation with the age of the mesocarp. Besides the stage and genotype of coconut, the coconut milk's composition is determined by the physical or chemical or biological methodologies employed to extract the milk from the coconut. In general the extraction of coconut oil from the mature kernel entails various chemical approaches, including alkaline treatment and bleaching. VCO, on the other hand, is extracted through multiple methods such as hot process, cold processes either through application of centrifugal force or microbial fermentation, physical treatments involving chilling, freezing and thawing, low-pressure extraction, supercritical fluid carbon dioxide and use of enzymes. Analysis of physical and biochemical characteristics of various types of VCOs derived from different processes such as hot extraction, fermentation, extraction from dried gratings, centrifugation, and comparing them with copra coconut oil

Table 2.2 Phenolics and antioxidant potential of variants of virgin coconut oil (VCOs)

Biochemical parameters	VCO-Hot	VCO-Fer	VCO-EDG	VCO-Cen	CCO
Total phenol (mg GAE/100 g)	2.867 ± 0.152	0.566 ± 0.020	0.63 ± 0.121	0.446 ± 0.041	1.946 ± 0.041
CUPRAC (mM TE/kg)	11.31 ± 0.495	4.67 ± 0.064	4.69 ± 0.468	3.87 ± 0.085	9.01 ± 0.446
ABTS IC50 (mg/mL)	17.42	57.36	44.37	64.78	28.64

Reprinted with permission from John Wiley and Sons. Source: Ramesh et al. (2020). Total phenolics and antioxidant potential of various vCO's including VCO-hot (VCO produced from hot process), VCO-Fer (VCO fermentation process), VCO-EDG (VCO from expelled from dried gratings), VCO-Cen (VCO from centrifugal method), and coconut copra oil are being compared

revealed that total phenolic content (mg GAE/100 g) varied from 0.446 ± 0.041 in VCO samples from centrifugation process to 2.867 ± 0.152 VCOs produced in hot process. The corresponding antioxidant potential of all the VCO types ranged from 3.87 mM Trolox equivalent (TE) in the VCO samples of centrifugation process to 11.31 mM TE in samples derived from hot extraction methodology (Ramesh et al. 2020) (Table 2.2). These diverse extraction methods contribute to the unique characteristics and qualities of the resulting coconut oil. This process results in a protein rich solid known as 'VCO cake or VCO meal'. Lauric acid (12:0) stands out as the predominant fatty acid, comprising roughly 45–50% of the total fatty acids irrespective of the preparation method. Its significance lies in its notable antimicrobial, antiviral, and anti-inflammatory properties. Conspicuously, Dayrit's research has elucidated that numerous beneficial properties associated with coconut oil can be traced back to the presence of lauric acid. They demonstrate potential antibiotic components against infections and antidiabetic properties (Dayrit 2015; Beegum et al. 2022; Srivastava et al. 2016; Siddalingaswamy et al. 2011). Investigations regarding the phenolic compounds present in coconut oil have observed variations in phenolic acids such as caffeic acid, ferulic acid, gallic acid, and p-coumaric acid depending on the extraction method used (Seneviratne and Dissanayake 2008). Currently there has been considerable interest in sterols due to their potential benefits in reducing the risk of cardiovascular disease. According to Schwartz et al. (2008), coconut oil contains the lowest sterol content at 1.14 mg/g compared to other oils. Despite its lower sterol content, β-sitosterol, which is known for its potential anticancer properties, constitutes the major sterol, accounting for 70.4% of the sterols found in coconut oil. The metabolic significance of medium-chain fatty acids (MCFAs) obtained from coconut oil or VCO is widely acknowledged. MCFAs are rapidly converted into ketone bodies thereby providing an alternative source of energy to the brain tissues. Emerging evidence supports the understanding of how coconut oil plays a role in mitigating the symptoms of Alzheimer's Disease. The biochemical mechanisms underlying coconut oil's ability to alleviate AD symptoms include its dietary impact on reducing neuro-inflammation, reversing neurodegeneration, promoting cell survival pathways, and inhibiting the secretion of Aβ peptides are delineated (Ramesh et al. 2021) (Fig. 2.2.)

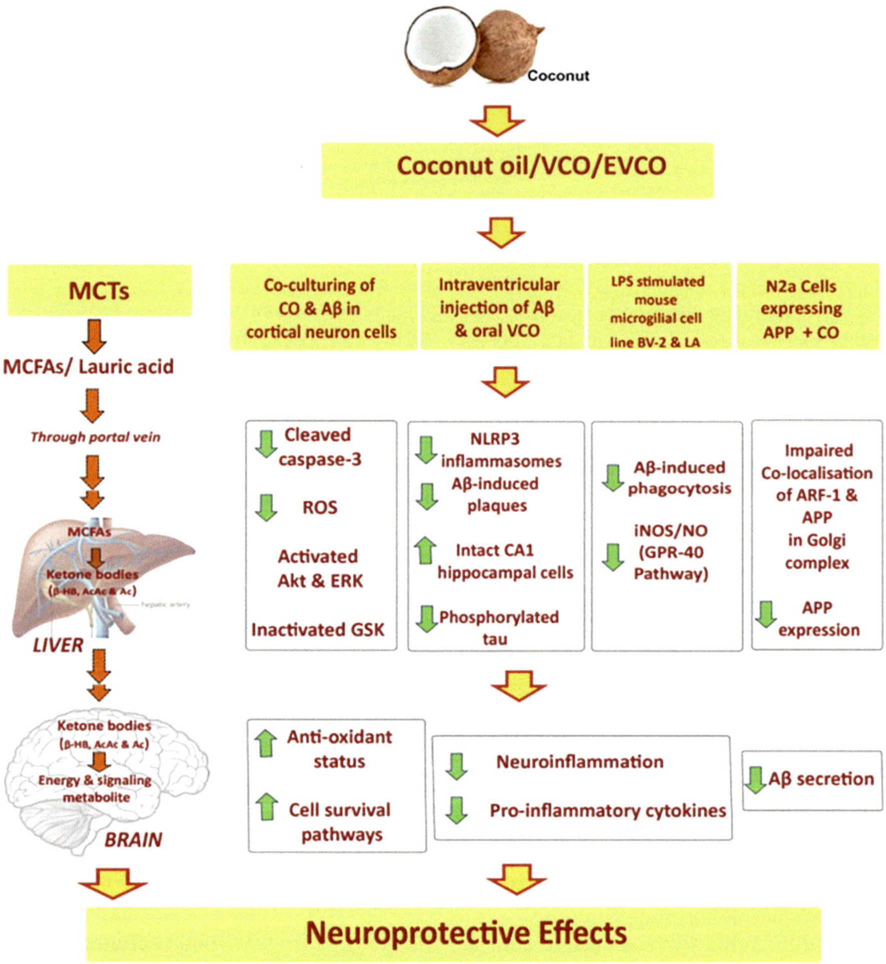

Fig. 2.2 Multiple modes of action of coconut oil derived medium chain fatty acids (MCFAs) in conferring neuroprotective effects. (Source: Ramesh et al. 2021, https://doi.org/10.1016/j.tifs.2021.03.046. Reprinted with permission from Elsevier)

2.8.2 *Coconut Testa Oils*

Appaiah et al. (2014) conducted a comparative analysis of the phytochemical composition of testa oils derived from wet coconuts and copra, contrasting them with oils extracted from whole coconuts, as well as the white kernels of both wet coconuts and copra. The findings indicated that testa oils of coconut show appreciable richness in antioxidants, particularly tocopherols, tocotrienols (ranging from 22.3 to 100.1 mg/100 g), and phenolics (ranging from 313.9 to 389.0 μg/100 g). This composition suggests their potential to offer health benefits. The biochemical components of testa oils exhibit considerable variation depending on coconut genotypes (Ramesh et al. 2023). Proxidant elements, that accelerate lipid oxidation, specifically iron (Fe) ranging from 34.17 to 62.48 ppm and copper (Cu) from 1.63 to 2.77 ppm, showed variability. The total phenolic content ranged from 6.84 to 8.67 mg gallic acid equivalent (GAE)/100 g, while phytosterol content varied between 54.66 and 137.73 mg CE/100 g. Coconut testa oils have relatively high polyunsaturated fatty acid (PUFA) content, ranging from 7.55 to 12.78%, and monounsaturated fatty acid (MUFA) content, ranging from 11.94% to 17.63%, when compared to coconut kernel oils. Nevertheless, the relatively high phenolic content of coconut testa oils (6.84–8.67 mg GAE/100 g) reveals their antioxidant potential. The presence of health promoting phenolic acids in coconut testa oils underscores the unexploited realm of coconut testa which generally goes underutilized as animal feed (Ramesh et al. 2023).

2.8.3 Coconut Protein

The coconut palm comprises various parts, including leaves, bud, flower, fruit, and germinating nut, each offering distinct attributes. Coconut water can serve as a substrate for the production of protein rich foods in the process of fermentation utilizing yeast *Saccharomyces fragilis.* On the other hand, the crude protein content in coconut inflorescence sap has been reported to be 0.26% (Asghar et al. 2020) suggesting that the sap is not a principal protein source. These properties accentuate the variability in protein content across different parts of the coconut palm. For instance, certain parts like the coconut kernel and meal are rich in proteins, while others such as coconut milk, leaves, main trunk are poor sources of protein. The white kernel or endosperm of the coconut, which is edible, comprises approximately 4.3% protein, primarily of globulin. The proteins derived from coconut kernel have demonstrated a reduction in lipid content in experimental animal models owing to coconut proteins' low lysine-to-arginine ratio (2.13: 24.5%) (Lal et al. 2003). Moreover, the coconut endosperm contains an effective natural coagulant protein, which is water-soluble. Copra meal, derived as a protein source, has been successfully used as feed for ruminants, pigs, and poultry, yielding positive results in terms of nutrition and animal health. This highlights the versatile nutritional contributions of different components of the coconut palm. Coconut meal stands out as a rich protein source, containing approximately 21.2–21.4% protein on a dry matter basis, making it ideal for livestock feed. Coconut meal contains 22.8% crude protein, but the vital amino acids lysine (0.59%) and methionine (0.34%) are low compared to other livestock feeds such as soybean, sunflower and groundnut meals as in the latter lysine content varies from 1–2.39% and methionine content ranges from 0.5% to 0.62% indicating a potential need for supplemental balancing (Moorthy and Viswanathan 2009). Despite lower crude protein and deficiencies in some of the essential amino acids compared to other common oil seed meals, barley grain meals, and meals from cocoa by-products, coconut meal exhibits a higher biological value. Additionally, the ratio of rumen degradable protein content of coconut meal to that of the rumen by-pass protein is low compared to common ruminant feed materials. Currently, coconut meal having 18–25% crude protein is used as a protein source for ruminants owing to its cost-effectiveness. However, the limitations of coconut meal including low content of amino acids lysine and sulfur containing amino acids coupled with relatively high fiber nature restrict its use in non-ruminant diets. Therefore, there is a need for amino acid fortification for its inclusion in non-ruminant diets. The by-products of VCO production process, coconut skim milk and insoluble protein, are blended and homogenized, followed by spray drying to produce a dehydrated protein powder with high protein content (33%) and a low fat content (3%) (Naik et al. 2012). The coconut protein powder exhibits commendable emulsifying properties and sensory features, suggesting its potential application in emulsified foods and underscoring the viability of coconut protein powder as a valuable food ingredient. Similarly, coconut whey generated from VCO production unit was processed into a concentrated coconut whey protein (protein content of 46%) suggest it as a novel source of high quality functional ingredient for food processing industries (Vijayasanthi et al. 2020). The water and oil absorption capacities of protein powders derived from coconut milk residue are high, whereas protein powders obtained from oil cake showed a remarkable foaming and emulsifying properties. Additionally, protein powders extracted from both the coconut cakes display solubility in extremely acidic and alkaline solutions (Thaiphanit and Anprung 2016). Sequential extraction of protein fractions from coconut cake reveals the presence of various protein fractions such as albumin, globulin, glutelin-1, glutelin-2 and prolamine. With the exception of albumin, all these fractions displayed elevated antioxidant potential through radical-scavenging ability and also showed ability of ion chelation. Moreover, except for glutelin-2, these fractions demonstrated DNA protection capability against oxidative damage. Thus coconut protein fractions have demonstrated their ability to function as natural antioxidants or food ingredients to extend shelf life and serve as functional foods (Li et al. 2018).

2.8.4 *Coconut Flour*

The nutritional analysis of residues, coconut milk residue and coconut cell wall polysaccharides, derived from VCO production indicates that the latter exhibit higher levels of crude, neutral and acid detergent fibers (NDF and ADF), hemicelluloses contents, and metal binding capabilities. In contrast, coconut milk residue is characterized by a high fat content. Furthermore, the coconut cell wall polysaccharides demonstrate improved dietary fiber attributes compared to several commercially available fibers, presenting opportunities for the utilization of coconut-derived dietary fiber components (Yalegama et al. 2013). Proximate analysis, reveal that coconut flour contains 12.1% protein, 10.9% fat and 70.3% carbohydrates (Trinidad et al. 2006). Biochemical composition of coconut meal derived from VCO production process reveal that the meal comprises protein (14.3%), fat (54.0%), fiber (20.50%), and carbohydrates (23.4%) (Khan et al. 2015). Coconut flour, despite being high in dietary fiber (61%), [the insoluble fibre content is high (57%) compared to soluble fibres (4%)] produces short-chain fatty acids when fermented (Trinidad et al. 2006). The chemical composition of NDF derived from coconut kernel is rich in hemicellulose (45.10%), cellulose (43.28%) and a considerable quantity of lignin (8.15%) among others such as silica. Coconut flour, being a versatile ingredient, is utilized in the development of functional foods with various health benefits. Its dietary fiber content may contribute to anti-diabetic and hypocholesterolemic effects as well as in gut health. Due to its cost-effectiveness and high in vitro hypoglycemic activity, coconut flour can be a major ingredient in feed and food formulations. It exhibits effective antioxidant activity against cellular radicals, along with significant swelling, oil, and water holding capacities (Du et al. 2019). Adeloye et al. (2020) suggest that incorporating defatted coconut flour in maize flour can potentially address protein-energy malnutrition, and also promotes the use of coconut flour in various food applications. Additionally, Raczyk et al. (2021) highlight that coconut flour is an excellent ingredient for nutritionally enriched functional foods. Coconut flour has found wider applications due to its multiple beneficial effects such as in the prevention of cardiovascular disease, colon cancer and diabetes (Mat et al. 2022).

2.8.5 *Desiccated Coconut Powder (DCP)*

Desiccated coconut is the finely shredded, dehydrated flesh derived from the fresh coconut kernel. Possessing a gentle, sweet flavor and a chewy texture characteristic of coconut, it retains its inherent qualities even after dehydration. Being essentially dehydrated coconut meat, its fundamental composition closely resembles that of raw coconut flesh, particularly in the composition of Vitamin B (pantothenic acid and niacin) (Divya et al. 2023).

2.8.6 *Coconut Sugar*

Processing coconut sap into coarse-grained sugar presents a valuable opportunity for value addition, with significant potential in the neera industry. Coconut sugar offers distinct nutritional advantages over brown sugar, boasting half the copper content, fourfold higher magnesium, and over tenfold increased zinc content. Its lower glycemic index makes it a favorable alternative to conventional sugar sources, as it has a lesser impact on blood sugar levels (Hebbar et al. 2020, 2022). Furthermore, coconut sap sugar has demonstrated α-amylase inhibitory activity, aiding in the regulation of carbohydrate digestion and absorption, thus proving beneficial in managing type II diabetes mellitus (Devi et al. 2022). In a study by Srikaeo (2015) assessing wheat flour combined with various sweeteners, including coconut sugar, palm sugar, sugarcane, and sorbitol, it was found that coconut sugar exhibited lower estimated glycemic index and higher rate of starch digestion compared to cane sugar. Given its low glycemic index and rich nutrient profile, the food applications of coconut sugar are extensive.

2.9 Concluding Remarks and Perspectives

Coconut offers a diverse range of products for human consumption, including coconut oil, coconut kernel, nut water, neera or phloem sap, haustorium, testa oil, coconut sugar, desiccated coconut powder etc. Despite concerns regarding coconut oil's relatively high content of saturated fatty acids and the increased risk of cardiac diseases, numerous research findings highlight its health benefits attributable to its unique fatty acid composition especially MCFAs. VCO obtained from fresh coconut kernel in wet processing is particularly nutritious and possesses important health-promoting properties. Owing to its MCFA content, notably lauric, capric, caproic acids coconut oil exhibits multiple medicinal properties. Beyond coconut oil, the coconut kernel contains various other beneficial components. The bionutritional composition of coconut kernel, especially its protein and fibre, demonstrates cardioprotective and anti-diabetic properties. Also, the hemicelluloses component of the dietary fiber derived from coconut endosperm has a significant hypocholesterolemic effect. Additionally, coconut haustorium is highlighted for its potential health benefits and is considered a suitable ingredient for development of weaning food formulations because of its sugar and amino acids profile. Coconut water, both from mature and tender nuts, have essential micro-minerals and other vital nutrients for human health. Moreover, mature coconut water has shown a hypoglycemic effect in diabetic rats. The inflorescence sap, extracted from coconut spadix, aids digestion and boasts a low glycemic index. Research indicates that immature coconut inflorescence can decrease blood glucose levels in diabetic rats. Given its extensive utility in culinary, medicinal, cosmetic, and industrial domains, it is imperative to actively promote value-added coconut products. Moreover, there should be a focused effort on research and development to uncover novel biomolecules aimed at advancing the coconut industry.

References

Adeloye JB, Osho H, Idris LO (2020) Defatted coconut flour improved the bioactive components, dietary fibre, antioxidant and sensory properties of nixtamalized maize flour. J Agric Food Res 2:100042

Appaiah P, Sunil L, Prasanth Kumar PK, Gopala Krishna AG (2014) Composition of coconut testa, coconut kernel and its oil. J Am Oil Chem Soc 91(6):917–924

Appaiah P, Sunil L, Krishna AGK, Gurusiddaiah SK (2016) Phytochemicals and antioxidant activity of testa extracts of commercial wet and dry coconuts and cakes. Int Res J Pharm 9:9–13

Arivalagan M, Bhardwaj R, Padmanabhan S, Suneja P, Hebbar KB, Kanade SR (2018a) Biochemical and nutritional characterization of coconut (*Cocosnucifera* L.) haustorium. Food Chem 238:153–159

Arivalagan M, Roy TK, Yasmeen AM, Pavithra KC, Jwala PN, Shivasankara KS, Manikantan MR, Hebbar KB, Kanade SR (2018b) Extraction of phenolic compounds with antioxidant potential from coconut (*Cocos nucifera* L.) testa and identification of phenolic acids and flavonoids using UPLC coupled with TQD-MS/MS. LWT 92:116–126

Asghar MT, Yusof YA, Mokhtar MN, Ya'acob ME, Mohd Ghazali H, Chang LS, Manaf YN (2020) Coconut (*Cocos nucifera* L.) sap as a potential source of sugar: antioxidant and nutritional properties. Food Sci Nutr 8:1777–1787

Beegum PPS, Pandiselvam R, Ramesh SV, Thube SH, Pandian TP, Khanashyam AC, Manikantan MR, Hebbar KB (2022) A critical appraisal on the antimicrobial, oral protective, and anti-diabetic functions of coconut and its derivatives. Qual Assur Saf Crops Foods 14(2):86–100

Beegum PPS, Ramesh SV, Pandiselvam R, Neema M, Manikantan MR, Hebbar KB (2024) Perspectives on the cardioprotective, neuroprotective and anti-obesity functions of coconut (*Cocos nucifera* L.). Food Biosci 58:103756

Bhagya D, Prema L, Rajamohan T (2012) Therapeutic effects of tender coconut water on oxidative stress in fructose fed insulin resistant hypertensive rats. Asian Pac J Trop Med 5(4):270–276. https://doi.org/10.1016/S1995-7645(12)60038-8

Burns DT, Johnston EL, Walker MJ (2020) Authenticity and the potability of coconut water-a critical review. J AOAC Int 103(3):800–806

Cappelletti M, Ferrentino G, Endrizzi I, Aprea E, Betta E, Corollaro ML, Charles M, Gasperi F, Spilimbergo S (2015) High pressure carbon dioxide pasteurization of coconut water: A sport drink with high nutritional and sensory quality. Journal of Food Engineering 145:73–81

Castillo EM (1986) Chemical characterization of makapuno and normal coconut endosperms [Philippines]. Thesis, Philippines Univ., Los Banos College, Laguna, 105 p

Chen W, Zhang G, Chen W, Zhong Q, Chen H (2018) Metabolomic profiling of matured coconut water during post-harvest storage revealed discrimination and distinct changes in metabolites. RSC Adv 8(55):31396–31405

Dayrit FM (2015) The properties of lauric acid and their significance in coconut oil. J Am Oil Chem Soc 92:1–15. https://doi.org/10.1007/s11746-014-2562-7

Devi M, Ghatani K (2022) The use of coconut in rituals and food preparations in India: a review. Journal of Ethnic Foods 9(1):37. https://doi.org/10.1186/s42779-022-00150-7

Divya PM, Roopa BS, Manusha C, Balannara P (2023) A concise review on oil extraction methods, nutritional and therapeutic role of coconut products. J Food Sci Technol 60(2):441–452

Du X, Bai X, Gao W, Jiang Z (2019) Properties of soluble dietary fibre from defatted coconut flour obtained through subcritical water extraction. Int J Food Sci Technol 54:1390–1404

Ekpenyong EE, Okafor IMA (2018) Cocos nucifera water: therapeutic benefits and sickle cell anaemiaa review. Int J Innov Sci Res Technol 3(8):513–520

Fife B (2013) Health properties of coconut oil. Agro Food Ind Hi Tec 24(3):7–10

Geetha V, Kumar GS (2022) Concentrates from tender coconut water and coconut testa beneficially modulates tissue lipid profiles in high-fat fed rats. J Food Sci Technol 59:1649–1657. https://doi.org/10.1007/s13197-021-05178-2

Geetha V, Bhavana KP, Chetana R, Krishna AG, Kumar GS (2016) Studies on the composition and in-vitro antioxidant activities of concentrates from coconut testa and tender coconut water. J Food Process Technol 7:588

Gopal M, Shil S, Gupta A, Hebbar KB, Arivalagan M (2021) Metagenomic investigation uncovers presence of probiotic-type microbiome in *Kalparasa®* (fresh unfermented coconut inflorescence sap). Front Microbiol 12:662783. https://doi.org/10.3389/fmicb.2021.662783

Hebbar KB, Mathew AC, Arivalagan M, Samsudeen K, Thomas GV (2013) Value added products from neera. Indian Coconut J 56(4):28–33

Hebbar KB, Arivalagan M, Pavithra KC, Roy TK, Gopal M, Shivashankara KS, Chowdappa P (2020) Nutritional profiling of coconut (*Cocos nucifera* L.) inflorescence sap collected using novel coco-sap chiller method and its value added products. J Food Meas Charact 14(5):2703–2712

Hebbar KB, Ramesh SV, Ghosh DK, Beegum PS, Pandiselvam R, Manikantan MR, Mathew AC (2022) Coconut sugar-a potential storehouse of nutritive metabolites, novel bio-products and prospects. Sugar Tech 24(3):841–856

ICC (International Coconut Community) (2022) Coconut Statistical Yearbook 2020. International Coconut Community, Compiled by Alit Pirmansah, Market and Statistics Officer ICC, Jakarta, Indonesia

Khan M, Mahesh C, Semwal A, Sharma G (2015) Effect of virgin coconut meal (VCM) on the development of rice-based extruded snacks. Int J Adv Res 3:717–725

Kumar M, Saini SS, Agrawal PK, Roy P, Sircar D (2021) Nutritional and metabolomics characterization of the coconut water at different nut developmental stages. J Food Compos Anal 96:103738

Lal J, Kumar CS, Indira M (2003) Coconut palm. Encylopedia Food Sci Nutr 2003:1464–1475

Li Y, Zheng Y, Zhang Y, Xu J, Gao G (2018) Antioxidant activity of coconut (*Cocos nucifera* L.) protein fractions. Molecules 23(3):707. https://doi.org/10.3390/molecules23030707

Lima EB, Sousa CN, Meneses LN, Ximenes NC, Júnior S, Vasconcelos GS, Lima NB, Patrocínio MC, Macedo D, Vasconcelos SM (2015) Cocos nucifera (L.) (Arecaceae): a phytochemical and pharmacological review. Braz J Med Biol Res 48:953–964

Luckanatinvong V, Mahatheeranont S, Siriphanich J (2018) Variation in the aromatic nature of Nam-Hom coconut depends on the presence and contents of 2-acetyl-1-pyrroline. Sci Hortic 233:277–282

Marasinghe SS, Marikkar JN, Yalegama C, Wimalasiri S, Seneviratne G, Weerasooriya R, Liyanage R (2019) Comparison of inter varietal differences in chemical composition and nutritional properties of coconut testa flour. J Natl Sci Found Sri Lanka 47:349–356

Mat K, Abdul Kari Z, Rusli ND, Che Harun H, Wei LS, Rahman MM, Mohd Khalid HN, Mohd Ali Hanafiah MH, Mohamad Sukri SA, Raja Khalif RI, Mohd Zin Z (2022) Coconut palm: food, feed, and nutraceutical properties. Animals 12(16):2107

Moorthy M, Viswanathan K (2009) Nutritive value of extracted coconut (*Cocos nucifera*) meal. Res J Agric Biol Sci 5:515–517

Naik A, Raghavendra SN, Raghavarao KSMS (2012) Production of coconut protein powder from coconut wet processing waste and its characterization. Appl Biochem Biotechnol 167:1290–1302. https://doi.org/10.1007/s12010-012-9632-9

Naik M, Sunil CK, Rawson A, Venkatachalapathy N (2022) Tender coconut water: a review on recent advances in processing and preservation. Food Rev Intl 38(6):1215–1236

Nguyen QT, Bandupriya HDD, Foale M, Adkins SW (2016) Biology, propagation and utilization of elite coconut varieties (makapuno and aromatics). Plant Physiol Biochem 109:579–589. https://doi.org/10.1016/j.plaphy.2016.11.003

Nneli RO, Woyike OA (2008) Antiulcerogenic effects of coconut (Cocos nucifera) extract in rats. Phytother Res 22(7):970–972

Patil U, Benjakul S (2018) Coconut milk and coconut oil: their manufacture associated with protein functionality. J Food Sci 83(8):2019–2027

Prades A, Dornier M, Diop N, Pain JP (2012) Coconut water uses, composition and properties: a review. Fruits 67:87–107

Prithviraj V, Pandiselvam R, Babu AC, Kothakota A, Manikantan MR, Ramesh SV, Beegum PS, Mathew AC, Hebbar KB (2021) Emerging non-thermal processing techniques for preservation of tender coconut water. LWT 149:111850

Raczyk M, Kruszewski B, Michałowska D (2021) Effect of coconut and chestnut flour supplementations on texture, nutritional and sensory properties of baked wheat based bread. Molecules 26:4641

Rajashri K, Roopa BS, Negi PS, Rastogi NK (2020) Effect of ozone and ultrasound treatments on polyphenol content, browning enzyme activities, and shelf life of tender coconut water. J Food Process Preserv 44(3):e14363

Rajesh MK, Muralikrishna KS, Nair SS, Krishna KB, Subrahmanya TM, Sonu KP, Subaharan K, Sweta H, Keshava PT, Neeli C, Karunasagar I (2020) Facile coconut inflorescence sap mediated synthesis of silver nanoparticles and its diverse antimicrobial and cytotoxic properties. Mater Sci Eng C 111:110834

Ramesh SV, Pandiselvam R, Thushara R, Manikantan MR, Hebbar KB, Beegum S, Mathew AC, Neenu S, Shil S (2020) Engineering intervention for production of virgin coconut oil by hot process and multivariate analysis of quality attributes of virgin coconut oil extracted by various methods. J Food Process Eng 43(6):e13395

Ramesh SV, Pandiselvam R, Shameena Beegum PP, Saravana Kumar RM, Manikantan MR, Hebbar KB (2021) Review of *Cocos nucifera* L. testa-derived phytonutrients with special reference to phenolics and its potential for encapsulation. J Food Sci Technol 60:1–10. https://doi.org/10.1007/s13197-021-05310-2

Ramesh SV, Mary R, Beegum Puthiya PS, Pandiselvam R, Padmanabhan S, Sathyan N, Shil S, Niral V, Manikantan MR, Lokesha AN, Shivashankara KS, Hebbar KB (2023) Physicochemical characterization and fatty acid profiles of testa oils from various coconut (*Cocos nucifera* L.) genotypes. J Sci Food Agric 103(1):370–379

Rethinam P, Krishnakumar V (2022) Health benefits of coconut water. In: Coconut water: a promising natural health drink-distribution, processing and nutritional benefits. Springer International Publishing, Cham, pp 385–455

Sandhya VG, Rajamohan T (2008) Comparative evaluation of the hypolipidemic effects of coconut water and lovastatin in rats fed with fat-cholesterol enriched diet. Food Chem Toxicol 46:3586–3592

Santoso U, Kubo K, Ota T, Tadokoro T, Maekawa A (1996) Nutrient composition of kopyor coconuts (*Cocos nucifera* L.). Food Chem 57:299–304

Schwartz H, Ilainen V, Pfironen V, Lampi AM (2008) Tocopherol, tocotrienol and plant sterol contents of vegetable oils and industrial fats. J Food Compos Anal 21(2):152–161

Seneviratne KN, Dissanayake DMS (2008) Variation of phenolic content in coconut oil extracted by two conventional methods. Int J Food Sci Tech 43(4):597–602

Seow CC, Gwee CN (1997) Review-coconut milk: chemistry and technology. Int J Food Sci Technol 32:189–201. https://doi.org/10.1046/j.1365-2621.1997.00400.x

Siddalingaswamy M, Rayaorth A, Khanum F (2011) Anti-diabetic effects of cold and hot extracted virgin coconut oil. J Diabetes Mellitus 1(4):118–123. https://doi.org/10.4236/jdm.2011.14016

Srikaeo K, Thongta R (2015) Effects of sugarcane, palm sugar, coconut sugar and sorbitol on starch digestibility and physicochemical properties of wheat based foods. International Food Research Journal 22(3):923–929

Srinivasan P, Raja HD, Tamilvanan R (2021) Effect of coconut water and cytokinins on rapid micropropagation of *Ranunculus wallichianus* Wight & Arnn—a rare and endemic medicinal plant of the Western Ghats, India. In Vitro Cell Dev Biol Plant 57:365–371

Srivastava Y, Semwal AD, Majumdar A (2016) Quantitative and qualitative analysis of bioactive components present in virgin coconut oil. Cogent Food Agric 2:1–13. https://doi.org/10.1080/23311932.2016.1164929

Tansakul A, Chaisawang P (2006) Thermophysical properties of coconut milk. J Food Eng 73(3):276–280

Thaiphanit S, Anprung P (2016) Physicochemical and emulsion properties of edible protein concentrate from coconut (*Cocos nucifera* L.) processing by-products and the influence of heat treatment. Food Hydrocoll 52:756–765

Trinidad TP, Mallillin AC, Valdez DH, Loyola AS, Askali-Mercado FC, Castillo JC, Encabo RR, Masa DB, Maglaya AS, Chua MT (2006) Dietary fiber from coconut flour: A functional food. Innovative food science & emerging technologies 7(4):309–317

Trinidad TP, Mallillin AC, Valdez DH, Loyola AS, Askali-Mercado FC, Castillo JC, Encabo RR, Masa DB, Maglaya AS, Chua MT (2016) Dietary fiber from coconut flour: a functional food. Innov Food Sci Emerg Technol 7:309–317

Tuyekar SN, Tawade BS, Singh KS, Wagh VS, Vidhate PK, Yevale RP, Gaikwad S, Kale M (2021) An overview on coconut water: as a multipurpose nutrition. Int J Pharm Sci Rev Res 68(2):63–70

Twishsri W, Runheem P, Usathit S, Watanayothin S, Naka P (2011) Study on fatty acid composition and amino acid content of coconut endosperm of selected coconut cultivars in Thailand. Int Symp Trop Subtrop Fruits 1024:427–432

USDA Data (2018) Coconut products—food composition database: United States Department of Agriculture, Agriculture Research Service

Vijayasanthi J, Adsare SR, Lamdande AG et al (2020) Recovery of proteins from coconut milk whey employing ultrafiltration and spray drying. J Food Sci Technol 57:22–31. https://doi.org/10.1007/s13197-019-04025-9

Wicaksono A, Raihandhany R, Teixeira da Silva JA (2021) Kopyor versus macapuno coconuts: are these two edible mutants of Southeast Asia the same? Planta 254:86. https://doi.org/10.1007/s00425-021-03740-y

Yalegama LL, Karunaratne DN, Sivakanesan R, Jayasekara C (2013) Chemical and functional properties of fibre concentrates obtained from by-products of coconut kernel. Food Chem 141(1):124–130

Yong JW, Ge L, Ng YF, Tan SN (2009) The chemical composition and biological properties of coconut (Cocos nucifera L.) water. Molecules 14(12):5144–5164

Zhang Y, Zheng Y, Duan K, Gui Q (2016) Preparation, antioxidant activity and protective effect of coconut testa oil extraction on oxidative damage to human serum albumin. International journal of food science & technology 51(4):946–953

Zhang Y, Kan J, Tang M, Song F, Li N, Zhang Y (2022) Chemical composition, nutritive value, volatile profiles and antioxidant activity of coconut (Cocos nucifera L.) haustorium with different transverse diameter. Foods 11(7):916

Zhou L, Sun X, Yarra R, Iqbal A, Wu Q, Li J, Yang Y (2024) Combined transcriptome and metabolome analysis of sugar and fatty acid of aromatic coconut and non-aromatic coconut in China. Food Chem Mol Sci 8:100190

Chapter 3
Metabolic Fate and Bioavailability of Coconut Nutrients

Malika G. Fernando, Juliana Chen, Shaun Eslick, Carolina B. Castro, Manohar Garg, and Ralph N. Martins

Abstract Coconut (*Cocos nucifera* L.) is a tropical palm of both food and industrial importance, offering multiple products and vital resources for the sustenance of tropical ecosystems. Every part of the coconut is enriched with various phytochemicals, including medium-chain fatty acids (MCFAs), polyphenolics, phytosterols, mineral nutrients, and dietary fibers, among others. The nutrient composition of coconuts varies with the parts of the palm, maturity stage, harvest time, and other climatic and edaphic factors. Coconut-derived nutrients, especially MCFAs, are metabolized differently in the human body compared to LCFAs found in other vegetable oils. This chapter delves into the nutritional characteristics of various parts or products of coconut (including the coconut kernel, testa, and oil), and discusses their metabolic fate and bioavailability.

Keywords Bioavailability · Biochemical conversion · MCFAs · Virgin coconut oil · Saturated fatty acids

M. G. Fernando · S. Eslick · M. Garg
Macquarie University, Sydney, NSW, Australia

J. Chen
Macquarie University, Sydney, NSW, Australia

University of Sydney, Sydney, NSW, Australia

C. B. Castro
Murdoch University, Perth, WA, Australia

Centre of Excellence for Alzheimer's Disease Research and Care, Perth, WA, Australia

R. N. Martins (✉)
Macquarie University, Sydney, NSW, Australia

Centre of Excellence for Alzheimer's Disease Research and Care, Perth, WA, Australia

Edith Cowan University, Perth, WA, Australia
e-mail: r.martins@ecu.edu.au

S. V. Ramesh, S. Praveen (eds.), *Coconut-Based Nutrition and Nutraceutical Perspectives*, https://doi.org/10.1007/978-981-97-3976-9_3

3.1 Introduction

Coconut is considered a functional food due to its remarkable composition of nutrients, including medium-chain fatty acids (MCFAs) and polyphenols (Gopala et al. 2010). Coconut products including coconut oil, coconut milk, coconut water and coconut meat differ greatly in nutrient content and composition. Since the food structure (matrix) is different for various coconut products, bioavailability, and metabolic consequences of consuming these products may also differ to a large extent. The unique fatty acid profile of coconut fat, which is rich in medium-chain triglycerides (MCTs), specifically lauric acid, capric acid, and caprylic acid, have garnered considerable attention due to their distinctive bio-accessibility and metabolic behavior.

Unlike long-chain fatty acids (LCFAs), which necessitate complex processing for absorption, MCTs are absorbed directly into the portal circulation, bypassing the lymphatic system, and providing a rapid source of energy (Aoyama et al. 2007). This rapid absorption mechanism lays the foundation of the ketogenic potential of coconut, with MCTs serving as precursors to ketone bodies, including acetoacetate, β-hydroxybutyrate, and acetone. These ketone bodies play their role in providing an alternative energy source, particularly for the brain, when glucose availability is limited (Fernando et al. 2015; Chatterjee et al. 2020).

While MCFAs in the coconut products are undoubtedly the most important in their nutritional functionality, coconut is also rich in polyphenolic compounds, some vitamins, and minerals as well as fiber (Marina et al. 2009). These bioactive components of coconut contributing to antioxidant and anti-inflammatory properties have garnered attention for their potential to combat oxidative stress, inflammation, and chronic diseases. These unique fatty acids, micronutrients and phytochemicals set coconut apart from other dietary fat sources and have sparked attention for its potential health effects and applications in various contexts, including nutrition and wellness. Coconut products have gained considerable attention due to their potential health benefits and diverse culinary applications. In this chapter, we will delve into the nutritional compositions of various coconut products, including the coconut kernel/meat, testa, and oil, as well as the bioavailability and properties of coconut constituents, such as fatty acids. Additionally, the composition and uses of coconut water will be explored, shedding light on its role as a refreshing and nutritious beverage.

3.2 Nutritional Characteristics

3.2.1 Coconut Nutrients: Nutritional Composition

The nutrient composition of coconuts can vary depending on several factors, including harvesting time, growth conditions such as temperature, humidity, and the coconut's origin (Mahayothee et al. 2016). While coconuts generally have a consistent nutrient profile, there can be some variations.

Harvesting Time
The stage at which coconuts are harvested can impact their nutrient composition. Young green coconuts tend to have more coconut water and less mature coconut meat, which can affect the nutritional content. As they mature, the composition changes, with the coconut meat becoming thicker and more nutrient-dense. Green and mature coconuts differ in several aspects, including their fat content, percentage of MCFA, potassium levels, and phytochemical composition. The comparative nutrient contents of both are present below:

(a) Fat Content:

- Green Coconut: Green coconuts generally have less fat than mature coconuts and the fat content in green coconuts make up just a smaller percentage of the total weight. The fat in green coconuts is primarily in the form of oil.
- Mature Coconut: Mature coconuts have a higher fat content. The white flesh of the mature coconut, also known as the coconut meat or kernel, contains a significant amount of oil, which is commonly used for cooking and in various food products. This oil is rich in saturated fats.

(b) Percentage of MCFAs:

- Green Coconut: Green coconuts typically have a lower percentage of MCFA, such as lauric acid, caprylic acid, and capric acid compared to mature coconuts.
- Mature Coconut: Mature coconuts are known for their higher MCFA content, particularly lauric acid. Lauric acid is a medium-chain fatty acid that has various health benefits, including being antimicrobial and easily digestible.

(c) Potassium

- Green Coconut: Green coconuts are often praised for their high potassium content which is an essential mineral for maintaining proper electrolyte balance and supporting muscle and nerve function.
- Mature Coconut: While mature coconuts also contain potassium, the concentration may be slightly lower than in green coconuts.

(d) Phytochemicals:

- Green Coconut: Green coconuts contain a variety of phytochemicals, including antioxidants as flavonoids and tannins and certain vitamins.
- Mature Coconut: Mature coconuts also contain phytochemicals, but the composition may differ. The antioxidant content can vary depending on factors like the coconut's ripeness and processing methods.

Overall, green and mature coconuts have distinct differences in terms of fat content, MCFA levels, potassium, and phytochemicals. Green coconuts are typically lower in fat and MCFA, higher in potassium, and may have a different phytochemical profile compared to mature coconuts.

Growth Conditions

Environmental factors such as temperature, humidity, soil quality, including nutrients in the soil, can influence the nutrient content of coconuts. For example, coconuts grown in nutrient-rich soils may have slightly different nutrient profiles compared to those grown in less fertile soil. The nutrient content of coconuts can change based on a variety of growth conditions and factors. Factors such as coconut variety, maturity stage, environmental conditions, agricultural practices, post-harvest handling, ripeness, processing methods, and seasonal variations all play a role in determining the nutrient composition of coconuts. For instance, green coconuts contain more water and fewer solids, while mature coconuts are prized for their coconut meat and oil. Additionally, the geographic location of coconut growth and the use of different agricultural practices can influence the mineral content of coconuts. These variables underscore the need to consider the specific growth and handling conditions when assessing the nutritional value of coconuts.

The nutrient content of various parts of the coconut offers valuable insights into their bio-nutritional characteristics (Appaiah et al. 2014). The coconut testa is rich in fibers, flavonoids, and tannins, which contribute to its antioxidant properties. On the other hand, the coconut meat is a concentrated source of carbohydrates, proteins, and fats, making it a versatile ingredient for multiple value added products (Appaiah et al. 2014).

Coconut oil stands out for its unique fatty acid composition (Patil and Benjakul 2018). Research on the fatty acid composition and health effects of coconut constituents highlights the predominance of MCFAs, such as lauric acid, capric acid, and caprylic acid (Patil and Benjakul 2018). MCFA are metabolized differently than LCFA, and studies suggest that they possess antimicrobial and anti-inflammatory properties.

Furthermore, the chemical composition and biological properties of coconut water have been extensively studied and it has gained popularity for its refreshing taste and potential health benefits (DebMandal and Mandal 2011). Coconut water is a rich source of electrolytes, vitamins, minerals, and phytohormones. It contains essential minerals such as potassium, magnesium, and calcium, which are important for maintaining proper hydration and supporting various physiological functions in the body (DebMandal and Mandal 2011). It possesses antioxidant and anti-inflammatory properties mainly due to the vitamin C (ascorbic acid), flavonoids and phenolic compounds, which may contribute to its potential role in promoting overall well-being (DebMandal and Mandal 2011). A comprehensive review on coconut water has highlighted its diverse applications, ranging from its use as a functional beverage providing rehydration to its incorporation in food formulations and cosmetic products (Panth et al. 2018).

Coconut milk is a creamy, white liquid extracted from mature coconut meat. It's notably high in calories, primarily deriving from its rich fat content, which consists mainly of medium chain saturated fats like lauric acid, which can provide quick energy. A one-cup (240 mL) serving of canned, unsweetened coconut milk contains approximately 552 kcal, with 57 g of fat, 5 g of carbohydrates, and 5 g of protein. It also provides essential vitamins, such as B vitamins, and minerals like iron, magnesium, and potassium.

Understanding the nutritional compositions of coconut products, including coconut testa, meat, oil, and water offers valuable insights into their potential health benefits and culinary applications. From the antioxidant-rich properties of the coconut testa to the unique fatty acid composition of coconut oil and the electrolyte-packed goodness of coconut water, coconuts present a versatile and nutritious addition to a balanced diet.

3.2.1.1 Coconut Oil

Coconut oil is one of the major cooking oils used in many tropical and south Asian countries. The extraction methods for coconut oil primarily include two methods, which are dry processing and wet processing. The dry processing is the most common and traditional method for extracting coconut oil, in which clean, ground and steamed dry copra is pressed by wedge press, screw press or hydraulic press to obtain the oil. The extracted oil undergoes a refining, bleaching and deodorizing (RBD) process and this step often involves exposure to high heat (≤60–80 °C) and chemicals (O'Brien 2004). In contrast, during the wet processing, the cream from fresh coconut milk is extracted and consequently, the cream emulsion is fractionated without applying chemical refining, shear or high heat treatments (≤60–80 °C). Thus, the end product of wet processing is virgin coconut oil (VCO), which does not undergo RBD process (Villariano et al. 2007).

The difference in production method incorporates superior antioxidant properties into VCO compared to RBD coconut oil, due to its preserved richer profile of phenolics compounds. However, the fatty acid composition of VCO is comparable to that of RBD coconut oil, while having a higher content of preserved phenolic compounds such as caffeic acid, p-coumaric acid, ferulic acid, methyl catechin, dihydrokaempferol, gallic acid, quercetin and myricetin glycoside as well as other biologically active compounds such as tocopherols, tocotrienols, squalene and sterols (Marina et al. 2009; Illam et al. 2017). Additionally, some studies have reported that VCO tends to have a lower level of hydrogen peroxide compared to RBD coconut oil (Dayrit et al. 2007, 2011). The nutritional composition of coconut oil per 100 g is depicted in Table 3.1, based on data from the USDA food composition database. The Table 3.2 shows the standard percentages of fatty acids in RBD coconut oil and VCO as recommended by the Codex Alimentarius International Food standards and the Asian and Pacific coconut community (APCC) standards, respectively.

Coconut fat is primarily composed of saturated fatty acids, making up approximately 92% of its total fat composition. Among these saturated fatty acids, around 63.3% are MCFAs, which are characterized by having chain lengths ranging from 6

Table 3.1 Nutritional composition of coconut oil per 100 g

Nutrient	Coconut oil (per 100 g) (U.S. Department of Agriculture—Agricultural Research Service 2023)
Water (g)	0.03
Protein (g)	0
Total lipid (g)	99.1
Carbohydrate, by difference (g)	0.84
Calcium (mg)	1
Iron (mg)	0.05
Zinc (mg)	0.02
Vitamin E (alpha-tocopherol) (mg)	0.11
Tocotrienol, alpha (mg)	2.17
Vitamin K (phylloquinone) (μg)	0.6
Total saturated fatty acids (g)	82.5
4:0	0.01
6:0	0.45
8:0	6.80
10:0	5.39
12:0	41.80
14:0	16.70
16:0	8.64
18:0	2.52
20:0	0.08
22:0	0.02
24:0	0.03
Total monounsaturated fatty acids (g)	6.31
16:1	0.02
18:1	6.25
20:1	0.04
Total polyunsaturated fatty acids (g)	1.70
18.2	1.68
18.3	0.02
Total trans fatty acids	0.028

Table 3.2 Fatty acid composition (% of total fat) of RBD coconut oil and VCO

Fatty acid	RBD coconut oil (%) (Codex Alimentarius 2001)	VCO (%) (Asian and Pacific Coconut Community (APCC) 2003)
Caproic acid (6:0)	0–0.7	0.4–0.6
Caprylic acid (8:0)	4.6–10.0	5.0–10.0
Capric acid (10:0)	5.0–8.0	4.5–8.0
Lauric acid (12:0)	45.1–53.2	43.0–53.0
Myristic acid (14:0)	16.8–21.0	16.0–21.0
Palmitic acid (16:0)	7.5–10.2	7.5–10.0
Stearic acid (18:0)	2.0–4.0	2.0–4.0
Oleic acid (18:1)	5.0–10.0	5.0–10.0
Linoleic acid (18:2)	1.0–2.5	1.0–2.5
Linolenic acid (18:3)	0–0.2	<0.5

to 12 carbons (Perera 2002; Marten et al. 2006). Notably, the most abundant fatty acid is lauric acid (C12:0), which accounts for roughly half of all the fatty acids present in coconut (Chempakan 1992; Pehowich et al. 2000; Perera 2002; Marina et al. 2009; Gopala et al. 2010). On the contrary, coconut fat is a poor source of monounsaturated fatty acids (MUFA) and polyunsaturated fatty acids (PUFA). Oleic acid (C18:1) is the only MUFA, and linoleic acid (C18:2) is the only PUFA from the omega-9 and omega-6 families, respectively that is found in substantial amounts in coconut (Raheja and Bhoraskar 1999).

3.2.1.2 Coconut Water

Coconut water, also referred to as tender coconut water, has a wide application due to its unique and distinctive nutrient composition (DebMandal and Mandal 2011; Vigliar et al. 2006). Coconut water is comprised of a variety of enzymes, antioxidants, vitamins, minerals, phytohormones and phenolic compounds. As such, coconut water is reported to have a number of health benefits including anti-microbial, anti-bacterial, anti-inflammatory, anti-hypertensive, rehydration, hypolipemic and hepatoprotective effects (Rethinam and Krishnakumar 2022). Coconut water has cardio-protective effects, particularly in myocardial infarction due to its rich mineral content, specifically high content of potassium (DebMandal and Mandal 2011). Due to its impressive micronutrient content coconut water is an excellent remedy for treating dehydration (DebMandal and Mandal 2011). Coconut water contains approximately 17.4 calories per 100 g. It is primarily composed of water (~95%), sugar (4%), fat (0.01%), iron (0.5%), calcium (0.02%), phosphorus (0.01%) as well as amino acids, vitamin C, complex B vitamins and mineral salts such as potassium (Table 3.3) (Vigliar et al. 2006). Coconut water has a short shelf life and can deteriorate rapidly when exposed to sunlight and/or air, therefore it is mainly consumed in tropical coastal areas. To extend shelf-life, coconut water is typically treated using ultra-high temperature (UHT) sterilisation, however a number of nutrients are lost and taste can be diminished, potentially limiting marketability of coconut waters and hence non-thermal treatments are suggested (Prithviraj et al. 2021).

3.2.1.3 Coconut Milk

Coconut milk is the aqueous emulsion extracted from grated coconut meat after pressing or squeezing with or without the addition of water (DebMandal and Mandal 2011). Commercially, coconut milk is prepared by the addition of water to the scraped coconut kernel and blended to form an emulsion. Typically, it takes coconut fruit 12 months to be at the stage where the coconut meat can be used to make coconut milk. Fundamentally, coconut milk is an oil-in-water emulsion, where the oil droplets are surrounded by a film of interfacial active protein and emulsion stability is dependent on the quantity and quality of these proteins (Yong et al. 2009).

Table 3.3 Nutrient composition of coconut water per 100 g

	Coconut water (mg/100 g) (Vigliar et al. 2006)	
Nutrient	Young (6 months)	Mature (12 months)
Micronutrients		
Calcium	27.35	31.64
Iron	0.02	0.02
Magnesium	6.40	9.44
Potassium	203.70	257.52
Sodium	1.75	16.10
Zinc	0.07	0.02
Manganese	0.12	0.08
Vitamins		
Thiamin (B1)	2.4	
Riboflavin (B2)	0.3	
Niacin (B3)	0.057	
Pantothenic acid (B5)	0.08	
Pyridoxine (B6)	0.043	
Folate, total	0.032	
Folic acid	–	
Biotin	–	

Coconut milk is widely used in cooking to prepare a vast variety of dishes. Due to different preparation methods of coconut milk, the chemical and nutritional qualities can alter between different products (Karunasiri et al. 2020) (Table 3.4).

3.2.1.4 Coconut Meat: Fresh or Dried

Coconut meat or flesh or kernel is a staple food in many tropical regions, such as in the Pacific Islands, South-East Asia and India (Food and Agriculture Organization 2002), it has gained popularity globally due to its unique taste and diverse culinary applications (South Pacific Commission 1983). Variations in the nutritional values can be attributed to differences in coconut variety, ripeness, processing methods as well as the chemical analysis methods used by different countries (Guo et al. 2022) (Tables 3.5 and 3.6).

Coconut meat can be obtained from both the immature and mature fruit of the coconut palm (Paull and Ketsa 2015). The meat of fresh mature coconuts has a higher energy value ranging from 314 to 398 kcal, compared to 81 to 86 kcal for immature coconut meat. This is primarily due to the increased fat content ranging from 5.6% to 5.9% in immature coconut meat and increases to a range of 30.1–40% in mature coconut meat. Saturated fat is the predominant fat type in coconut meat, similar to coconut oil, and namely in the form of MCTs, particularly lauric acid (Eyres et al. 2016). As the coconut matures, the content of all MCFAs, such as caprylic acid, capric acid, lauric acid and myristic acid, have been found to significantly increase (Lima et al. 2015). Carbohydrate levels for fresh mature coconut meat range from 3.4% to 15.2% of weight and protein ranges from 3.3% to 4%. Concentration of macronutrients increases for dried coconut meat due to the dehydration process, with 6.7–23.6% increment in carbohydrate, 6.3–7.3% for protein, 64.5–67.8% for total fat. Fresh mature coconut meat and dried coconut are both considered to be excellent sources of dietary fiber with levels ranging from 7.3–9 g and 14.7–16.3 g/100 g, respectively. Coconut meat is also considered to be a source of micronutrients that contribute to overall health. Additionally, coconut meat contains water soluble vitamins, including thiamine, riboflavin, niacin and folate, which contribute to energy metabolism and neurological health. In summary, the nutrient compositions of different coconut products vary and the Table 3.7 shows the comparison of fatty acid compositions of coconut milk, oil, and meat per their 100 g edible portions.

Table 3.4 Chemical composition of coconut milk per 100 g

Nutrient	Coconut milk (/100 g) (Karunasiri et al. 2020)
Water (g)	67.6
Energy (kcal)	230
Carbohydrates (g)	5.5
Sugars (g)	3.3
Fiber (g)	2.2
Protein (g)	2.3
Total fat (g)	23.8
Total saturated fatty acids (g)	21.1
6:0	0.1
8:0	1.7
10:0	1.3
12:0	10.6
14:0	4.2
16:0	2.0
18:0	1.2
Total monounsaturated fatty acids (g)	1.0
18:1	1.0
Total polyunsaturated fatty acids (g)	0.3
18:2	0.3
Sodium (mg)	15.0
Magnesium (mg)	37.0
Potassium (mg)	263.0
Calcium (mg)	16.0
Iron (mg)	1.6
Zinc (mg)	0.7
Phosphorus (mg)	100.0
Thiamine (mg)	0.1
Niacin (mg)	0.8
Vitamin B-6 (mg)	0.1
Folate (μg)	16
Vitamin C (mg)	2.8
Vitamin E (alpha-tocopherol) (mg)	0.2

3.3 Metabolism and Bioavailability of Coconut Nutrients

3.3.1 Fatty Acids

Absorption and metabolism of fatty acids differ according to their chain length and

Table 3.5 Nutritional characteristics for fresh coconut meat per 100 g edible portion

Nutrient	Coconut, fresh, young or immature, meat[a]	Coconut, meat, immature[b]	Coconut, fresh, mature fruit, meat[a]	Coconut, meat, fresh, mature[b]	Coconut meat, raw (from mature coconut)[c]	Coconut, mature fruit, white meat, grated, fresh[d]
Water (g)	83	86	51	45	47	47
Energy (kcal)	86	81	314	398	354	371
Carbohydrates (g)	7	3.8	3.4	3.5	15.2	3.4
Sugars (g)	4	–	3.1	–	6.2	3.4
Fiber (g)	0.5	3.2	7.8	7.3	9	7.6
Protein (g)	1.6	1.8	3.4	4	3.3	4.5
Total Fat (g)	5.6	5.9	30.1	40	33.5	36.6
Saturated Fat (g)	4.9	–	26.6	–	29.7	34.7
Monounsaturated Fat (g)	0.3	–	1.5	–	1.4	1.6
Polyunsaturated Fat (g)	0.05	–	0.3	–	0.4	0.3
Sodium (mg)	6	33	10	17	20	14
Magnesium (mg)	18	30	32	57	32	52
Potassium (mg)	138	377	305	370	356	290
Calcium (mg)	18	2	8	14	14	6
Iron (mg)	0.6	1.3	0.8	2.2	2.4	1.5
Zinc (mg)	0.2	0.4	0.6	0.5	1.1	0.6
Phosphorus (mg)	29	–	62	–	113	95
Thiamine (mg)	0.005	0.11	0.005	0.04	0.07	0.02
Riboflavin (mg)	0.005	0.02	0.005	0.01	0.02	0.02
Niacin (mg)	0.6	3.6	0.6	0.6	0.5	1
Vitamin B-6 (mg)	0.02	–	0.02	–	0.1	0.06
Folate (µg)	26	–	26	–	26	21
Vitamin C (mg)	3	3.8	2	7	3.3	0
Vitamin E (alpha-tocopherol) (mg)	0	0.2	0	0.7	0.2	trace

"–" has been marked for nutrients where data is missing from certain databases

[a]AUStralian Food and NUTrient Database 2011–2013 (Australia) (Food Standards Australia New Zealand 2018)

[b]The Pacific Islands Food Composition Tables 2nd Ed. (Dignan et al. 2004)

[c]USDA FoodData Central (US) (U.S. Department of Agriculture—Agricultural Research Service 2023)

[d]The Concise New Zealand Food Composition Tables 14th Ed. (New Zealand) (New Zealand Institute for Plant and Food Research Limited and Ministry of Health (New Zealand) 2022)

the saturation level. Short chain fatty acids (SCFAs) and MCFAs are more water soluble than long chain fatty acids (LCFAs) and are easily hydrolyzed and absorbed in the gastrointestinal tract (Iber 1974). MCFA, which is the main component in

Table 3.6 Nutritional characteristics for dried coconut meat per 100 g edible portion

Nutrient	Coconut, grated & desiccated[a]	Coconut, desiccated[b]	Coconut meat, dried (desiccated), not sweetened[c]	Coconut, desiccated[d]
Water (g)	2	2	3	2
Energy (kcal)	675	656	660	691
Carbohydrates (g)	7.3	6.7	23.6	8.3
Sugars (g)	6.6	–	7.35	8.3
Fiber (g)	15.4	14.7	16.3	15.3
Protein (g)	6.6	6.3	6.9	7.3
Total Fat (g)	65.4	65.1	64.5	67.8
Saturated Fat (g)	57.7	–	57.2	63.8
Monounsaturated Fat (g)	3.3	–	2.7	2.9
Polyunsaturated Fat (g)	0.6	–	0.7	0.5
Sodium (mg)	15	18	37	29
Magnesium (mg)	72	95	90	90
Potassium (mg)	574	650	543	740
Calcium (mg)	12	12	26	15
Iron (mg)	1.7	2.6	3.3	2.7
Zinc (mg)	1.2	1.3	2	1.3
Phosphorus (mg)	125	–	206	180
Thiamine (mg)	0.002	0.02	0.06	0.03
Riboflavin (mg)	0	0.02	0.1	0
Niacin (mg)	1.3	1.3	0.6	2.1
Vitamin B-6 (mg)	0.05	–	0.3	0.1
Folate (μg)	9	–	9	20
Vitamin C (mg)	0	0	1.5	0
Vitamin E (alpha-tocopherol) (mg)	1.1	1.3	0.4	trace

"–" has been marked for nutrients where data is missing from certain databases

[a]AUStralian Food and NUTrient Database 2011–2013 (Australia) (Food Standards Australia New Zealand 2018)

[b]The Pacific Islands Food Composition Tables 2nd Ed. (Dignan et al. 2004)

[c]USDA FoodData Central (US) (U.S. Department of Agriculture—Agricultural Research Service 2023)

[d]The Concise New Zealand Food Composition Tables 14th Ed. (New Zealand) (New Zealand Institute for Plant and Food Research Limited and Ministry of Health (New Zealand) 2022)

coconut fat, is almost immediately hydrolyzed by the enzymes in saliva (lingual lipase) and gastric juices (gastric lipase) in the stomach. Thus, the absorption can take place even without catalysis by pancreatic lipase and bile salts. MCFAs are absorbed directly into the portal venous system mainly as free fatty acids and transported to liver (Vicente Valdivieso 1972; Ruppin and Middleton 1980). Then they quickly enter into the mitochondria of hepatocytes crossing the double

Table 3.7 Fatty acid compositions of coconut milk, oil, and meat per 100 g edible portion

Fatty acid	Coconut milk (g/100 g) (Karunasiri et al. 2020)	Coconut oil (g/100 g) (U.S. Department of Agriculture—Agricultural Research Service 2023)	Coconut meat (tender) (g/100 g) (Appaiah et al. 2014)	Coconut meat (mature) (g/100 g) (Appaiah et al. 2014)
Saturated				
6:0	0.1	0.45	0	0
8:0	1.7	6.80	5.6	10.6
10:0	1.3	5.39	3.5	6.0
12:0	10.6	41.80	38.2	47.5
14:0	4.2	16.70	21.9	18.8
16:0	2	8.64	13.5	8.2
18:0	1.2	2.52	0.6	0.9
Monounsaturated				
18:1	1	6.25	13.2	8.2
Polyunsaturated				
18:2	0.3	1.68	3.5	1.5

mitochondrial membrane without the assistance of carnitine shuttle that is required for transport of LCFA into mitochondria. In mitochondria, they undergo rapid beta-oxidation to produce ketones and thus, energy (Hashim 1967; Bach and Babayan 1982; Babayan 1987; Metges and Wolfram 1991; Aoyama et al. 2007). As MCFAs do not directly enter into the systemic circulation and are less prone to deposit in the arterial walls as well as in adipose tissue, unlike LCFAs, MCFAs are non-atherogenic and anti-obesogenic. They also increase the energy expenditure and causes faster satiety (St-Onge and Jones 2002; Dayrit 2003). However, the metabolic kinetics of MCFA differ depending on the MCFA type (carbon chain-length). The fatty acids 8:0 and 10:0 have demonstrated a higher ketone body production in hepatocytes than 12:0 (Fushimi et al. 2020). Furthermore, fatty acid 8:0 has demonstrated rapid conversion to acetyl-coenzyme A (acetyl-CoA) via beta-oxidation which are utilized to produce ketone bodies, citrate cycle intermediates and glycogenic amino acids, rather than utilized as a substrate for triglycerides synthesis (Fushimi et al. 2020) (Figs. 3.1 and 3.2).

On the contrary, LCFAs are hydrolyzed and absorbed in the intestines with the assistance of pancreatic lipase, which are then esterified and bound with fatty acid binding proteins forming chylomicrons (Ockner et al. 1972; Ockner and Manning 1974; Bach and Babayan 1982). In the presence of acyl-coenzyme A (acyl-CoA) synthetase enzyme, LCFAs are converted into acyl-CoA and then incorporated into triacylglycerols, which are the major components of chylomicrons. Chylomicrons are then transported into the systemic circulation via lymphatic system, mostly bypassing the liver. Lipoprotein lipase enzyme located on the interior walls of capillary blood vessels partially hydrolyses the triacylglycerol in chylomicrons, which allow extensive uptake of fatty acids into adipose tissue as well as to deposit in arterialintima leading to atherosclerosis (Tsuji et al. 2001). Eventually the

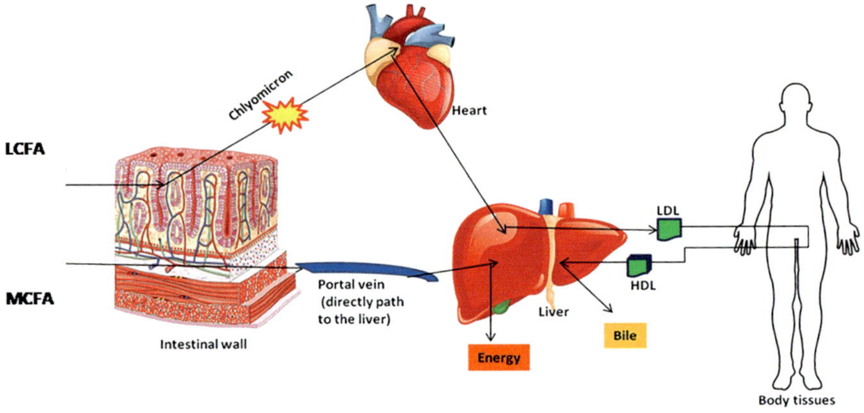

Different fatty acid metabolism: Long chain fatty acids (LCFAs) are absorbed in the intestinal wall and after combining with cholesterol and protein (to form chlyomicron), they are circulated throughout the body as a component of lipoprotein (LDL) and are eventually deposited in various organs including heart vessels. In contrast, medium chain fatty acids (MCFAs) are transported across the intestinal wall and transported directly to the liver via portal vein. In liver, the MCFAs are used for producing energy.

Fig. 3.1 Metabolic fate of coconut oil derived fats. (Source: Beegum et al. 2024, https://doi.org/10.1016/j.fbio.2024.103756)

chylomicron remnants reach the liver and most of LCFAs are packaged into triglycerides in hepatocytes (Calabrese et al. 1999; Black and DiRusso 2003) (Fig. 3.1).

In summary, the metabolic fate of MCFAs from coconut products is unique i.e. involve digestion in the mouth/stomach, do not require bile for emulsification or pancreatic amylase for hydrolysis, rapid absorption in the small intestine, transportation through the portal system, oxidation to form ketone bodies in the liver, and utilization by various tissues. The unique property of MCFAs is their rapid absorption and utilization, making them a readily available energy source and a potential substrate for ketone body production. This distinct metabolic pathway contributes to the versatility and potential health benefits associated with coconut-derived fatty acids (Fig. 3.1).

Although coconut oil is implicated in cardiovascular disease risk due to being a source of saturated fatty acids, VCO is highly studied and believed to offer promising health benefits on cardiovascular health (Murugaiha Jeyakumar et al. 2023; Beegum et al. 2024). Insulin resistance in the brain is a feature of Alzheimer's disease. MCFAs (specifically from VCO) have attracted considerable interest in the preventation and treatment of Alzheimer's disease due to their ability to rescue brain energy in the form of ketone bodies without adversely affecting body cholesterol levels (Chatterjee et al. 2020; Fernando et al. 2023). Furthermore, glycerol monolaurate (GML), which is a fatty acid monoglyceride abundantly present in coconut oil, has demonstrated antibacterial ability, potential for reducing lipid accumulation, modulating immune activity, and rebuilding intestinal barrier, that will also exert a positive impact on the nervous system (Luo et al. 2022). In addition, the gut

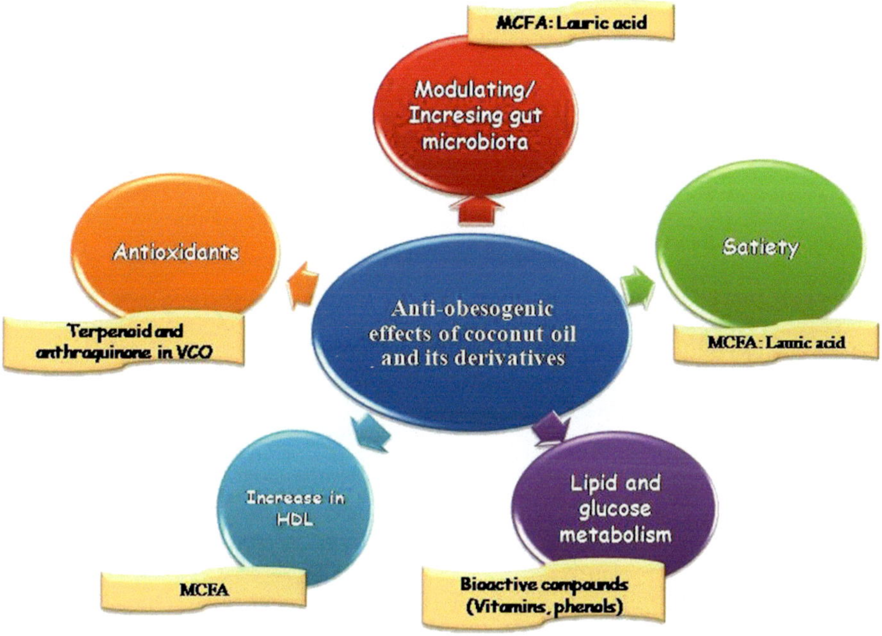

Fig. 3.2 Anti-obesogenic effects of coconut oil. (Source: Beegum et al. 2024, https://doi.org/10.1016/j.fbio.2024.103756)

hormone and neuropeptide ghrelin has been identified to exert a neuroprotective role via acylated-ghrelin-induced synaptic changes which are paralleled by enhanced spatial learning and memory (Diano et al. 2006; Shi et al. 2016). Caprylic acid (fatty acid C8:0) rich in coconut oil was shown to octanoylate ghrelin which thus provides the ghrelin O-acyltransferase (GOAT) enzyme with octanoyl-CoA co-substrates necessary for the acyl modification of ghrelin (Lemarié et al. 2018).

3.3.2 *Phytochemicals: Antioxidants and Phytohormones*

Coconut, including the water, meat or kernel, oil, husk and cotyledon (sprout) contains various phytochemicals, such as polyphenols, flavonoids, tannins, alkaloids, antioxidants and phytohormone (Lima et al. 2015; Nyayiru Kannaian et al. 2020). Figure 3.3 from Lima et al.'s review, depicts the various phytochemicals found in coconut. The presence of these phytochemicals highlights the nutritional value of coconut and its potential role as a functional food with health-enhancing properties, however, compared to other nutrients in coconut such as the fatty acids, the functional and biological acitivites of these phytochemicals in coconut are poorly understood. However, the fatty acid profiles being similar between coconut oil and VCO, the superior health benefits of VCO including antioxidant, anti-inflammatory,

Phytochemical compounds	Coconut parts/ Extract	References
Vitamin C 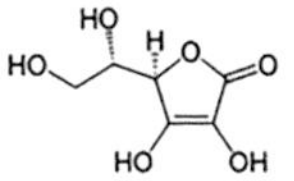	Liquid albumen	37
Lauric acid 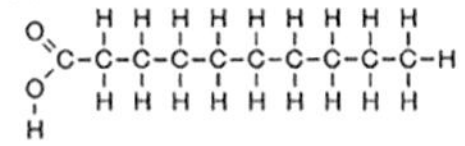	Coconut oil	39
L-arginine 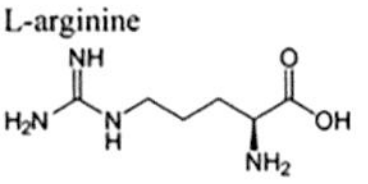	Liquid albumen Solid albumen	37, 61
a-tocopherol 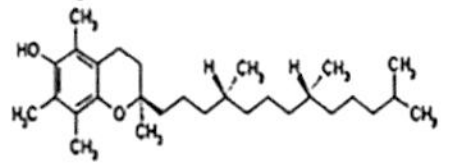	Coconut oil	40
Saponin 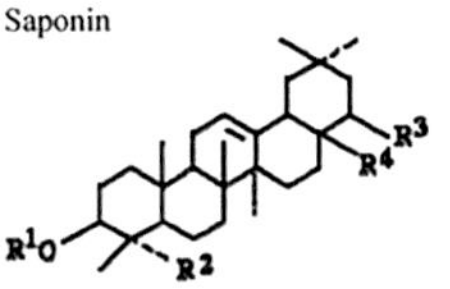	Root	41
Catechin 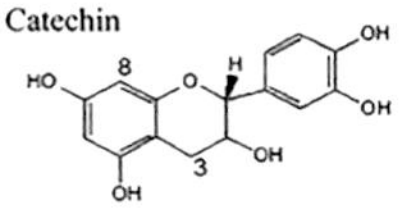	Coconut fiber	27,35
Flavonoid 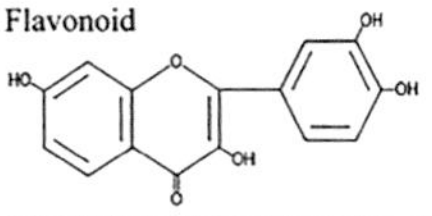	Coconut fiber Root Inflorescence	27,41,72

Phytochemical compounds	Coconut parts/ Extract	References
Tannins 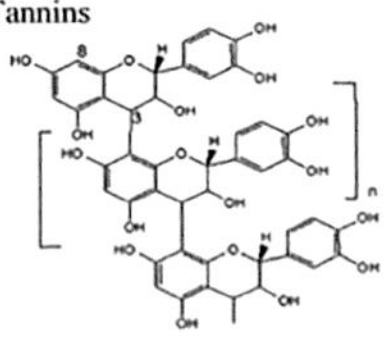	Coconut fiber Inflorescence	35,72
Lupeol-methylether 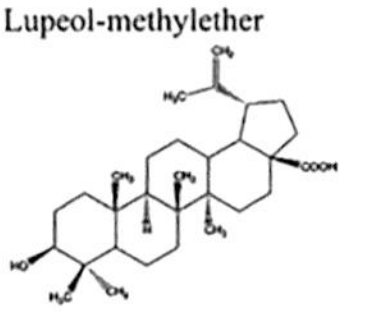	Leaves (epicuticular wax)	42
Skimmiwallin 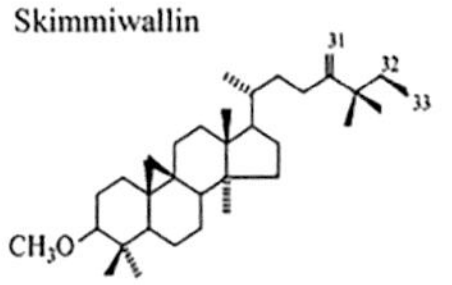	Leaves (epicuticular wax)	42
Isoskimmiwallin 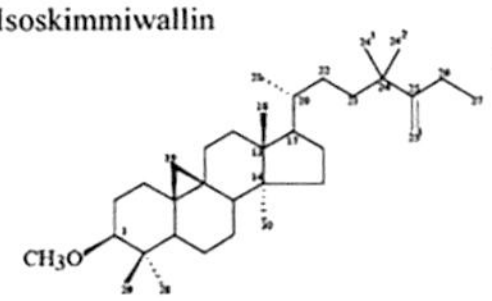	Leaves (epicuticular wax)	42

Fig. 3.3 Different phytochemical compounds from coconut (Lima et al. 2015)

lipid-lowering and cytoprotective efficacies might be possibly attributed to its higher polyphenolics contents (Narayanankutty et al. 2018), phytosterols, or vitamins (Beegum et al. 2024).

A range of antioxidant proteins and antioxidant protein-derived peptides have been identified in coconut. Ma et al. (2022) found 17 antioxidant proteins in coconut meat, which were determined to be related to the sub-networks of glutathione metabolism and peroxisome (Ma et al. 2022). It is proposed that lipid peroxidation in the human body could be inhibited by antioxidant proteins and their digested peptides through inactivating reactive oxygen species, neutralising free radicals and also reducing hydroperoxide formation (Ma et al. 2022).

Virgin coconut oil contains phenolic compounds, which are proposed to contribute to its antioxidant potential. The most abundant phenolic acids in virgin coconut oil include ferulic acid, p-coumaric acid and caffeic acid (Marina et al. 2009).

Research has indicated that coconut water contains phytohormones such as cytokinins, particularly zeatin and zeatin riboside (Ge et al. 2004, 2005, 2006a, b), as well as other acidic phytohormones, such as salicylic acid, indole-3-acetic acid, abscisic acid and jasmonic acid (Wu and Hu 2009). These phytohormones have been implicated in promoting cell division and differentiation, which may contribute to coconut water's reputed anti-aging and tissue-regenerating properties.

It is important to note that the studies of the phytochemicals in coconut have been conducted *in vitro*, and for their health functionality to be understood in humans, more research is required. Significance of consuming coconut phytochemicals as part of a regular diet providing abudndance of other polyphenols, merits further investigations.

3.3.3 Carbohydrates

Carbohydrates play a vital role in providing energy to the body and are a significant component of coconut products. The composition of carbohydrates in coconuts contain various types of carbohydrates, including glucose, fructose, and sucrose (Lima et al. 2015). The presence of these carbohydrates contributes to the sweet taste and energy content of coconut products. In a study the production processes of coconut milk and coconut oil were examined, with a specific focus on their impact on protein functionality (Patil and Benjakul 2018). This research unveiled the presence of distinct carbohydrates within coconut milk, shedding light on their potential interactions with proteins. These interactions are believed to have a significant influence on how proteins perform in a wide range of food-related applications.

3.3.4 Proteins

Coconut proteins, offer a remarkable blend of amino acids with distinctive compositions that contribute to their notable bioactivity and potential health benefits. Studies conducted by DebMandal and Mandal (2011), along with Lima et al. (2015) have provided valuable insights into the specific aspects of coconut proteins.

One notable characteristic of coconut proteins is their amino acid profile. These proteins boast a unique composition rich in essential amino acids such as leucine, isoleucine, and valine, which are pivotal for muscle development and repair (Appaiah et al. 2014). Additionally, they contain arginine, an amino acid known for its potential cardiovascular benefits and vasodilatory effects (Appaiah et al. 2014). On the other hand, coconut products are notably low in the essential amino acid methionine vital for protein synthesis, methylation reactions, antioxidant activity, and detoxification. It also plays a role in cardiovascular health and the health of hair and skin. The well-balanced essential and non-essential amino acids in coconut proteins make them an intriguing nutritional component for human consumption.

Beyond their amino acid composition, the bioactivity of coconut proteins has garnered considerable attention. They are recognized for their potential antioxidative properties, which are attributed to their ability to scavenge free radicals and reduce oxidative stress (Patil and Benjakul 2018). This antioxidant capacity may contribute to the overall health-promoting effects of coconut consumption, potentially aiding in the prevention of chronic diseases and aging-related processes (Patil and Benjakul 2018).

Furthermore, coconut proteins have been investigated for their role in modulating lipid metabolism and reducing cholesterol levels, indicating a potential benefit in cardiovascular health (Patil and Benjakul 2018). Additionally, these proteins may play a role in enhancing the immune system's defence mechanisms due to their bioactive peptides (Patil and Benjakul 2018).

In conclusion, coconut proteins stand out for their unique amino acid composition and multifaceted bioactivity aspects. Their rich essential amino acid content, coupled with potential anti-oxidative and cardiovascular benefits, underscores their significance in health promotion and disease prevention.

3.3.5 Dietary Fibre

Dietary fiber is as a crucial component within a wholesome diet, known for its vital contributions to digestive health and the prevention of various diseases. Within the realm of nutrition, coconut kernel or coconut flour emerges as notable source of dietary fiber, further enhancing their nutritional value (Lima et al. 2015).

Comprehensive investigations have illuminated the substantial presence of dietary fiber within coconuts, elucidating its potential to bolster overall fiber intake and promote digestive well-being. The dietary fiber content found in coconuts can aid in maintaining regular bowel movements, preventing constipation, and optimizing nutrient absorption within the gastrointestinal tract (Appaiah et al. 2014). This dietary fiber, predominantly composed of non-digestible plant materials such as insoluble fibers, offers a multifaceted approach to health maintenance. In summary, the inclusion of dietary fiber within coconuts enriches their nutritional profile, promoting digestive health and overall well-being.

3.3.6 Micronutrients

Delving deeper into the bioavailability and metabolism of minerals and trace elements present in coconut products broadens our understanding of their nutritional value and potential health implications. While coconut products are renowned for their versatility and wide-ranging applications, it is imperative to consider the bioavailability and metabolic fate of key minerals and trace elements they contain.

For instance, studies by Appaiah et al. (2014) have explored the composition of coconut testa, meat, and oil, shedding light on their mineral and trace element content (Appaiah et al. 2014). Understanding the bioavailability of essential minerals like magnesium, potassium, and copper within coconuts is essential, as these minerals play pivotal roles in maintaining various physiological processes, including nerve function, muscle contraction, and bone health. Furthermore, trace elements such as selenium and zinc, also present in coconut products, are known for their antioxidant properties and contribution to immune system function (Appaiah et al. 2014). While the high dietary fiber content in coconut is beneficial for various aspects of health, including digestive function, it can also interact with the bioavailability of minerals. The fiber in coconuts, particularly insoluble fiber, can bind to minerals, forming complexes that are less absorbable by the body. This can reduce the bioavailability of magnesium, potassium, and copper present in coconuts (Harland 1989).

In summary, while coconuts contain essential minerals like magnesium, potassium, and copper, their bioavailability may be low compared to other dietary sources due to factors like the chemical forms in which these minerals are present, the high fiber content in coconuts, and the influence of other dietary components. To ensure an adequate intake of these essential minerals, it's essential to maintain a balanced diet that includes a variety of foods from different sources. Additionally, a thorough exploration of the bioavailability and metabolic aspects of minerals and trace elements present in coconut products emphasizes the holistic understanding of their nutritional value and potential health benefits.

3.3.7 Coconut Nutrition and Gut Microbiome

The gut microbiome is a complex and diverse population of micro-organisms, believed to play a significant role in metabolism and modulation of immunity. Coconut has demonstrated a positive impact on gut microbiome due to its soluble and insoluble fiber content, which promotes healthy digestion and maintaining a balanced gut microbiome by exerting prebiotic effect and supporting beneficial gut bacteria growth. In addition, the easily digestible MCFA content of coconut helps to reduce inflammation in the gut and thus, improve gut microbiome balance. Antimicrobial properties of coconut also prevent growth of harmful gut bacteria leading to a healthy gut microbiome and reduce the risk of gut-related health issues. Overall, coconut helps to improve digestion in the gut and helps maintaining a healthy and balanced gut microbiome.

Polyphenols and lauric acid have been shown to have beneficial effects on gut microbiome in terms of benefiting the growth of good bacteria and discouraging harmful bacteria. VCO is a rich source of both polyphenols and lauric acid. A study that investigated the effect of VCO on changes in faecal microbiota composition in non-diabetic and alloxan-induced diabetic rats has demonstrated a significant increase in the abundance of beneficial probiotic bacteria such as *Lactobacillus, Allobaculum* and *Bifidobacterium* species (Djurasevic et al. 2018). Another study by Rolinec et al. (2020) demonstrated a positive impact of adding coconut oil to the feed of growing pigs on their intestinal microbiome diversity and bacterial abundance (Rolinec et al. 2020). A significant increase in the abundance of probiotic bacteria such as *Bifidobacterium* and *Lactobacillus* in the gastrointestinal tract was shown while decreasing some unfavorable taxa, which is desirable in pig breeding and performance (Rolinec et al. 2020). Moreover, the effect of coconut water as a gut microbiome modulator in patients with mild-moderate ulcerative colitis was evaluated (Kedia et al. 2024). Coconut water is a rich source of potassium and possesses anti-inflammatory properties which can potentially manipulate the microbiome. Findings of this study indicated that compared to a placebo, coconut water modulated gut microbiome and was more effective for induction of mild-moderate ulcerative colitis remission (Kedia et al. 2024). Currently, very few studies have investigated the impact of the effects of coconut nutrients on gut microbiome. Currently a paucity of research has examined the effect of coconut nutrients on gut microbiome in humans and thus, future studies should explore the effects of different coconut products such as coconut water, coconut milk and coconut oil.

3.4 Conclusion

The nutritional composition of coconut is primarily characterized by saturated fats, with a predominant presence of medium chain triglycerides, contributing to the ketogenic properties of coconut oil. Additionally, the rich phytochemicals composition of coconut, particularly the polyphenols found in coconut oil, meat, milk and water, highlights the potential of coconut as a functional food with antioxidative and anti-inflammatory properties. Furthermore, coconut is a rich source of vitamins, minerals, and dietary fiber, particularly reported in coconut milk, meat and water. Coconut water stands out as a popular hydrating beverage due to its abundant electrolytes, vitamins, minerals, and phytohormones. While coconut contains some carbohydrates and proteins, their quantities are relatively modest, with coconut meat being a notable source of dietary fiber. The bioavailability of these diverse nutrients in coconut makes it a functional food that offers holistic health-enhancing properties.

References

Aoyama T, Nosaka N, Kasai M (2007) Research on the nutritional characteristics of medium-chain fatty acids. J Med Investig 54:385–388. https://doi.org/10.2152/jmi.54.385

Appaiah P, Sunil L, Prasanth Kumar PK, Gopala Krishna AG (2014) Composition of coconut testa, coconut kernel and its oil. J Am Oil Chem Soc 91:917–924. https://doi.org/10.1007/S11746-014-2447-9

Asian and Pacific Coconut Community (2003) Standards for virgin coconut oil. https://old.coconutcommunity.org/viewpdf/apcc_quality_standards_for_coconut_products/3. Accessed on 25.June.2024

Babayan VK (1987) Medium-chain triglycerides and structured lipids. Lipids 22:417–420

Bach AC, Babayan VK (1982) Medium-chain triglycerides: an update. Am J Clin Nutr 36:950–962

Beegum PS, Ramesh SV, Pandiselvam R, Neema M, Manikantan MR, Hebbar KB (2024) Perspectives on the cardioprotective, neuroprotective and anti-obesity functions of coconut (Cocos nucifera L.), vol 58. Food Biosci, p 103756. https://doi.org/10.1016/j.fbio.2024.103756

Black PN, DiRusso CC (2003) Transmembrane movement of exogenous long-chain fatty acids: proteins, enzymes, and vectorial esterification. Microbiol Mol Biol Rev 67:454–472, table of contents

Calabrese C, Myer S, Munson S et al (1999) A cross-over study of the effect of a single oral feeding of medium chain triglyceride oil vs. canola oil on post-ingestion plasma triglyceride levels in healthy men. Altern Med Rev 4:23–28

Chatterjee P, Fernando M, Fernando B et al (2020) Potential of coconut oil and medium chain triglycerides in the prevention and treatment of Alzheimer's disease. Mech Ageing Dev 186:111209. https://doi.org/10.1016/J.MAD.2020.111209

Chempakan B (1992) Health hazards of coconut oil—a myth or reality? CORD J 8:18–23

Codex Alimentarius (2001) Codex standard for named vegetable oils. Codex Stan 210(8):11–25. https://doi.org/10.1017/CBO9781107415324.004

Dayrit CS (2003) Coconut oil: atherogenic or not? (What therefore causes atherosclerosis?). Philipp J Cardiol 31:97–104

Dayrit FM, Erin Buenafe OM, Chainani ET et al (2007) Standards for essential composition and quality factors of commercial virgin coconut oil and its differentiation from RBD coconut oil and copra oil. Philipp J Sci 136:119–129

Dayrit FM, Dimzon IKD, Valde MF et al (2011) Quality characteristics of virgin coconut oil: comparisons with refined coconut oil. Pure Appl Chem 83:1789–1799. https://doi.org/10.1351/PAC-CON-11-04-01

DebMandal M, Mandal S (2011) Coconut (Cocos nucifera L.: Arecaceae): in health promotion and disease prevention. Asian Pac J Trop Med 4:241–247. https://doi.org/10.1016/S1995-7645(11)60078-3

Diano S, Farr SA, Benoit SC et al (2006) Ghrelin controls hippocampal spine synapse density and memory performance. Nat Neurosci 9:381–388. https://doi.org/10.1038/nn1656

Dignan CA, Burlingame B, Kumar S, Aalbersberg W (2004) The Pacific Islands food composition tables. Food and Agriculture Organization of the United Nations, Rome

Djurasevic S, Bojic S, Nikolic B et al (2018) Beneficial effect of virgin coconut oil on alloxan-induced diabetes and microbiota composition in rats. Plant Foods Hum Nutr 73:295–301. https://doi.org/10.1007/s11130-018-0689-7

Eyres L, Eyres MF, Chisholm A, Brown RC (2016) Coconut oil consumption and cardiovascular risk factors in humans. Nutr Rev 74:267–280. https://doi.org/10.1093/NUTRIT/NUW002

Fernando WMADB, Martins IJ, Goozee KG et al (2015) The role of dietary coconut for the prevention and treatment of Alzheimer's disease: potential mechanisms of action. Br J Nutr 114:1–14. https://doi.org/10.1017/S0007114515001452

Fernando MG, Silva R, Fernando WMADB et al (2023) Effect of virgin coconut oil supplementation on cognition of individuals with mild-to-moderate Alzheimer's disease in Sri Lanka (VCO-AD study): a randomized placebo-controlled trial. J Alzheimers Dis 96:1195–1206. https://doi.org/10.3233/JAD-230670

Food and Agriculture Organization (2002) Table 51. Coconut: production. https://www.fao.org/4/ad452e/ad452e11.htm

Food Standards Australia New Zealand (2018) AUSNUT 2011–13 food nutrient database. https://www.foodstandards.gov.au/science-data/food-composition-databases/ausnut-2011-13. Accessed 22 Sept 2023
Fushimi T, Izumi Y, Takahashi M et al (2020) Dynamic metabolome analysis reveals the metabolic fate of medium-chain fatty acids in AML12 cells. J Agric Food Chem 68:11997–12010. https://doi.org/10.1021/ACS.JAFC.0C04723/SUPPL_FILE/JF0C04723_SI_002.XLSX
Ge L, Yong JWH, Tan SN et al (2004) Analysis of some cytokinins in coconut (Cocos nucifera L.) water by micellar electrokinetic capillary chromatography after solid-phase extraction. J Chromatogr A 1048:119–126. https://doi.org/10.1016/J.CHROMA.2004.07.031
Ge L, Yong JWH, Goh NK et al (2005) Identification of kinetin and kinetin riboside in coconut (Cocos nucifera L.) water using a combined approach of liquid chromatography-tandem mass spectrometry, high performance liquid chromatography and capillary electrophoresis. J Chromatogr B Analyt Technol Biomed Life Sci 829:26–34. https://doi.org/10.1016/J.JCHROMB.2005.09.026
Ge L, Yong JWH, Tan SN et al (2006a) Analysis of cytokinin nucleotides in coconut (Cocos nucifera L.) water using capillary zone electrophoresis-tandem mass spectrometry after solid-phase extraction. J Chromatogr A 1133:322–331. https://doi.org/10.1016/J.CHROMA.2006.08.027
Ge L, Yong JWH, Tan SN, Ong ES (2006b) Determination of cytokinins in coconut (Cocos nucifera L.) water using capillary zone electrophoresis-tandem mass spectrometry. Electrophoresis 27:2171–2181. https://doi.org/10.1002/ELPS.200500465
Gopala K, Gaurav R, Ajit S, Prasanth P et al (2010) Coconut oil: chemistry, production and its applications—a review. Indian Coconut J 73:15–27
Guo H, Lai J, Li C et al (2022) Comparative metabolomics reveals key determinants in the flavor and nutritional value of coconut by HS-SPME/GC-MS and UHPLC-MS/MS. Metabolites 12:691. https://doi.org/10.3390/METABO12080691
Harland BF (1989) Dietary fibre and mineral bioavailability. Nutr Res Rev 2:133–147. https://doi.org/10.1079/nrr19890011
Hashim SA (1967) Medium-chain triglycerides—clinical and metabolic aspects. J Am Diet Assoc 51:221–227
Iber FL (1974) Relative rates of metabolism MCT, LCT and ethanol in man. Z Ernahrungswiss Suppl 17:9–16
Illam SP, Narayanankutty A, Raghavamenon AC (2017) Polyphenols of virgin coconut oil prevent pro-oxidant mediated cell death. Toxicol Mech Methods 27:442–450. https://doi.org/10.1080/15376516.2017.1320458
Karunasiri AN, Gunawardane M, Senanayake CM et al (2020) Antioxidant and nutritional properties of domestic and commercial coconut milk preparations. Int J Food Sci 2020:3489605. https://doi.org/10.1155/2020/3489605
Kedia S, Virmani S, Bajaj A et al (2024) Coconut water induces clinical remission in mild to moderate ulcerative colitis: double-blind placebo-controlled trial. Clin Gastroenterol Hepatol 22(6):1295–1306.e7. https://doi.org/10.1016/J.CGH.2024.01.013
Lemarié F, Beauchamp E, Drouin G et al (2018) Dietary caprylic acid and ghrelin O-acyltransferase activity to modulate octanoylated ghrelin functions: what is new in this nutritional field? Prostaglandins Leukot Essent Fatty Acids 135:121–127. https://doi.org/10.1016/j.plefa.2018.07.009
Lima EBC, Sousa CNS, Meneses LN et al (2015) Cocos nucifera (L.) (Arecaceae): a phytochemical and pharmacological review. Braz J Med Biol Res 48:953–964. https://doi.org/10.1590/1414-431X20154773
Luo X, Liu W, Zhao M et al (2022) Glycerol monolaurate beyond an emulsifier: synthesis, in vivo fate, food quality benefits and health efficacies. Trends Food Sci Technol 127:291–302. https://doi.org/10.1016/J.TIFS.2022.05.017
Ma J, Pan C, Chen H et al (2022) Insight of the functional and biological activities of coconut (Cocos nucifera L) protein by proteomics analysis and protein-based bioinformatics. Molecules 27:2987. https://doi.org/10.3390/MOLECULES27092987

Mahayothee B, Koomyart I, Khuwijitjaru P et al (2016) Phenolic compounds, antioxidant activity, and medium chain fatty acids profiles of coconut water and meat at different maturity stages. Int J Food Prop 19:2041–2051. https://doi.org/10.1080/10942912.2015.1099042

Marina A, Che Man Y, Amin I (2009) Virgin coconut oil: emerging functional food oil. Trends Food Sci Technol 20:481–487. https://doi.org/10.1016/j.tifs.2009.06.003

Marten B, Pfeuffer M, Schrezenmeir J (2006) Medium-chain triglycerides. Int Dairy J 16:1374–1382. https://doi.org/10.1016/J.IDAIRYJ.2006.06.015

Metges C, Wolfram G (1991) Medium-and long-chain triglycerides labeled with 13C: a comparison of oxidation after oral or parenteral administration in humans. J Nutr 121:31–36

Murugaiha Jeyakumar S, Damayanti K, Ponday LR et al (2023) Assessment of virgin coconut oil in a balanced diet on indicators of cardiovascular health in non-obese volunteers: a human metabolic study. Diabetes Metab Syndr 17(9):102844. https://doi.org/10.1016/j.dsx.2023.102844

Narayanankutty A, Parathodi Illam S, Raghavamenon AC (2018) Health impacts of different edible oils prepared from coconut (Cocos nucifera): a comprehensive review. https://doi.org/10.1016/j.tifs.2018.07.025

New Zealand Institute for Plant and Food Research Limited & Ministry of Health (New Zealand) (2022) The concise New Zealand food composition tables 14th edition 2021. https://view.officeapps.live.com/op/view.aspx?src=https%3A%2F%2Fwww.foodcomposition.co.nz%2Fdownloads%2Fconcise-14-edition.xlsx&wdOrigin=BROWSELINK. Accessed 22 Sept 2023

Nyayiru Kannaian UP, Edwin JB, Rajagopal V et al (2020) Phytochemical composition and antioxidant activity of coconut cotyledon. Heliyon 6:e03411. https://doi.org/10.1016/J.HELIYON.2020.E03411

O'Brien RD (2004) Fats and oils: formulating and processing for applications, 2nd edn. CRC Press, Boca Raton. https://doi.org/10.1201/9780203483664/FATS-OILS-RICHARD-BRIEN

Ockner RK, Manning JA (1974) Fatty acid-binding protein in small intestine. Identification, isolation, and evidence for its role in cellular fatty acid transport. J Clin Invest 54:326–338. https://doi.org/10.1172/JCI107768

Ockner RK, Manning JA, Poppenhausen RB, Ho WK (1972) A binding protein for fatty acids in cytosol of intestinal mucosa, liver, myocardium, and other tissues. Science 177:56–58

Panth N, Abbott KA, Dias CB et al (2018) Differential effects of medium- and long-chain saturated fatty acids on blood lipid profile: a systematic review and meta-analysis. Am J Clin Nutr 108:675–687. https://doi.org/10.1093/AJCN/NQY167

Patil U, Benjakul S (2018) Coconut milk and coconut oil: their manufacture associated with protein functionality. J Food Sci 83:2019–2027. https://doi.org/10.1111/1750-3841.14223

Paull RE, Ketsa S (2015) Fruit, nut, and beverage crops coconut: postharvest quality-maintenance guidelines.Fruit, Nut, and Beverage Crops. College of Tropical Agriculture and Human Resources (CTAHR), University of Hawai'i at Manoa, FN-45: 1–5

Pehowich DJ, Gomes AV, Barnes JA (2000) Fatty acid composition and possible health effects of coconut constituents. West Indian Med J 49:128–133

Perera AAFLK (2002) Coconut oil—scare? Coconut Bull 10:1–7

Prithviraj V, Pandiselvam R, Babu AC, Kothakota A, Manikantan MR, Ramesh SV, Beegum PS, Mathew AC, Hebbar KB (2021) Emerging non-thermal processing techniques for preservation of tender coconut water. LWT 149:111850

Raheja BS, Bhoraskar AS (1999) Health benefits of coconut oil. Ind Coc J 11:7–11

Rethinam P, Krishnakumar V (2022) Coconut water: a promising natural health drink-distribution, processing and nutritional benefits. Springer, Cham. https://doi.org/10.1007/978-3-031-10713-9

Rolinec M, Medo J, Gábor M et al (2020) The effect of coconut oil addition to feed of pigs on rectal microbial diversity and bacterial abundance. Animals (Basel) 10(10):1764. https://doi.org/10.3390/ani10101764

Ruppin DC, Middleton WR (1980) Clinical use of medium chain triglycerides. Drugs 20:216–224

Shi L, Du X, Jiang H, Xie J (2016) Ghrelin and neurodegenerative disorders—a review. Mol Neurobiol 54:1144–1155. https://doi.org/10.1007/S12035-016-9729-1

South Pacific Commission (1983) Coconut. South Pacific Commission, Noumea
St-Onge M-P, Jones PJH (2002) Recent advances in nutritional sciences physiological effects of medium- chain triglycerides: potential of obesity. Clin Trials 132:329–332
Tsuji H, Kasai M, Takeuchi H et al (2001) Dietary medium-chain triacylglycerols suppress accumulation of body fat in a double-blind, controlled trial in healthy men and women. J Nutr 131:2853–2859
U.S. Department of Agriculture—Agricultural Research Service (2023) FoodData central. https://fdc.nal.usda.gov/. Accessed 22 Sept 2023
Vicente Valdivieso D (1972) Absorption of medium-chain triglycerides in animals with pancreatic atrophy. Am J Dig Dis 17:129–137. https://doi.org/10.1007/BF02232732
Vigliar R, Sdepanian VL, Fagundes-Neto U (2006) Biochemical profile of coconut water from coconut palms planted in an inland region. J Pediatr 82:308–312. https://doi.org/10.2223/JPED.1508
Villariano BJ, Dy LM, Lizada CC (2007) Descriptive sensory evaluation of virgin coconut oil and refined, bleached, and deodorized coconut oil. LWT Food Sci Technol 40:193–199
Wu Y, Hu B (2009) Simultaneous determination of several phytohormones in natural coconut juice by hollow fiber-based liquid-liquid-liquid microextraction-high performance liquid chromatography. J Chromatogr A 1216:7657–7663. https://doi.org/10.1016/J.CHROMA.2009.09.008
Yong JWH, Ge L, Ng YF, Tan SN (2009) The chemical composition and biological properties of coconut (Cocos nucifera L.) water. Molecules 14:5144–5164. https://doi.org/10.3390/MOLECULES14125144

Chapter 4
Coconut Kernel and Milk

W. N. M. T. D. N. Weerakoon, Tashmi Manilgama, Nimanthi Jayathilaka, and Kapila N. Seneviratne

Abstract Coconut (*Cocos nucifera* L.) is an economic crop mainly found in tropical countries. Coconut fruit consists of kernel, water and shell. There are many food products currently available in the markets which are made from coconut kernel or coconut milk. Coconut milk is the aqueous extract of coconut kernel. The focus in this chapter is to discuss biochemical properties, physicochemical properties and poorly explored health benefits of the coconut kernel and the derived products of coconut kernel. Coconut kernel products are also used in many industries such as cosmetic industry, detergent industry and culinary industry. There are many benefits of using coconut kernel products for humans due to its medium chain fatty acid composition. Due to the unique fatty acid composition with rich composition of medium chain fatty acids and phenolic antioxidants, the consumption of coconut kernel and coconut milk may lead to many health benefits. However, detailed studies on the health benefits of coconut kernel and coconut milk are limited. Further studies in this area are vital for the popularization of coconut kernel-based foods and for the processing of such foods to enhance or preserve nutritional quality. Nutrient composition, health effects and potential of developing more food items based on coconut kernel are highlighted in this chapter.

Keywords Coconut milk · Vegan alternative · Plant-based milk · Plant proteins

4.1 Introduction

Coconut, *Cocos nucifera* L., can be classified as a fruit, nut, or seed. The coconut tree belongs to the palm family and is native to Indian and Southeast Asian countries. It has become an important palm in tropical regions, with one healthy coconut tree yielding nearly a hundred coconuts a year. It takes approximately a year for the

---

W. N. M. T. D. N. Weerakoon · T. Manilgama · N. Jayathilaka (✉) · K. N. Seneviratne (✉)
University of Kelaniya, Kelaniya, Sri Lanka
e-mail: njayathi@kln.ac.lk; kapilas@kln.ac.lk

S. V. Ramesh, S. Praveen (eds.), *Coconut-Based Nutrition and Nutraceutical Perspectives*, https://doi.org/10.1007/978-981-97-3976-9_4

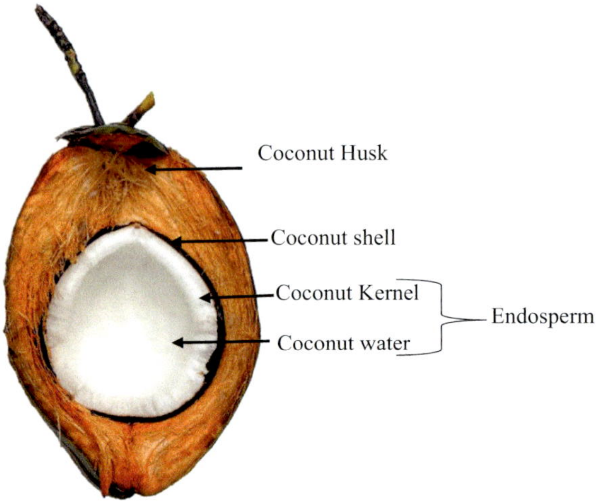

Fig. 4.1 Cross section of coconut fruit

fruit to fully ripen (Ohler 1999). The inner white portion of the coconut is called the coconut kernel or meat (see Fig. 4.1). The quality of the kernel and the size of the fruit vary with the variety or cultivar of coconut. Dwarf cultivars typically have smaller fruit sizes compared to tall tree cultivars. Coconuts from dwarf cultivars, before reaching full maturity, are mainly used as a source of coconut water. Varieties such as "King coconut" or "Thembili" in Sri Lanka, "Yellow Malayan" in Ivory Coast and Malaysia, and "Nam Hom" in Thailand are cultivated specifically for coconut water production. Tall cultivars like "Laguna" in the Philippines, "West African Tall" in Ivory Coast, and "Bali" in Indonesia are generally meant for mature coconuts (Ohler 1984; Rethinam and Krishnakumar 2002). Dwarf cultivars have the potential for self-pollination, exhibit high resistance to lethal yellowing disease, and flower early. However, they may have disadvantages such as small kernels, low productivity, and less tolerance to stress conditions. Taller cultivars typically cross-pollinate and take longer to flower (Ohler 1984). For commercial purposes, hybrid varieties are preferred for their improved quality and higher yield compared to parent plants.

Coconut has been utilized as a folk medicine for various ailments such as skin rashes, nausea, toothaches, tumors, constipation, and fever since ancient times. The water from young coconuts has been traditionally used to treat diarrhea, stomach aches, and dysentery in tropical regions. Coconut milk is prepared by extracting the white coconut kernel with water. Coconut kernels can be easily scraped and pressed with water to extract coconut milk. The pressing can be done using a blender or by hand for domestic cooking, or machine-pressed for large-scale production of coconut milk for coconut oil and canned coconut milk production (Seneviratne and Jayathilaka 2016). Coconut milk serves as the aqueous medium for cooking vegetable and meat curries and is also available as a vegan alternative to cow's milk in the market.

There are two edible parts of a coconut: the kernel and coconut water. The white coconut kernel, also known as white meat, can be considered as solid endosperm, while the coconut water can be seen as liquid endosperm. The coconut kernel, also known as the flesh of the coconut, consists of two parts: the brown layer and the fibrous white part. The brown layer covers the white fibrous part of the coconut kernel, known as the coconut testa. The fibrous white part initially starts as a thin layer and gradually develops into a thick layer over 12–14 months after flowering, reaching maturity. This mature coconut kernel is the nutritious portion known to provide various health benefits and is used in culinary, cosmetic, pharmaceutical, and other industries globally.

Coconut milk is an essential ingredient in many Asian cuisines and can be extracted manually or mechanically by grating the kernel and extracting it with or without water (De Leon and Delores 2004). Coconut milk is an oil-in-water emulsion where oil droplets are dispersed in a continuous water phase. The stability of coconut milk is determined by the proteins surrounding the oil droplets (Dendy and Timmins 1973). The nutritional content and other parameters of coconut milk depend on the properties of the extracted coconut kernel. The efficiency of coconut milk extraction depends on pressing conditions and the temperature of the water added during extraction (Grisingha 1991). The ratio of water to coconut meat typically varies from 1:1 to 20:1 during extraction (Dendy and Timmins 1973). Thungkao (1988) observed no variation in protein content of coconut milk prepared at different temperatures (30, 55, and 80 °C) when the water to coconut meat ratio was 1:1. Coconut milk contains various organic compounds, and its high moisture content and oily texture make it prone to rapid spoilage (Gonzalez 1990). Thermal processing is commonly used to increase the shelf life of coconut milk, involving heating the extracted coconut milk at 92–95 °C for 5–20 min. Homogenization of canned coconut milk is done after adding stabilizers and emulsifiers (Timmins and Kramer 1977; Gonzalez 1990; Arumughan et al. 1993).

4.2 Developmental Stages of Coconut Kernel

The endosperm tissue of the coconut fruit, along with the coconut meat and water, is edible. The development of endosperm tissues occurs in one of three main modes: nuclear, cellular, or helobial. Specifically, coconut endosperm development occurs in the nuclear mode. The primary endosperm nucleus undergoes multiple divisions without cytokinesis, producing free nuclei initially present in the liquid endosperm. Forming the cellular endosperm layer by moving from the periphery to the center, it starts as a jelly-like and translucent substance. As it ages, the cellular endosperm hardens, transforming into white flesh, known as coconut meat. In a coconut fruit, the process of cellularization leaves the embryo sac cavity partially filled with a solution, rather than completely filling it. This solution, of cytoplasmic origin, is often referred to as coconut water. Coconut water contains nutrients that are transferred symplasmically (via plasmodesmata) from the apoplasm, or surrounding cell wall, of the seed into the endosperm.

The coconut cotyledon, also known as the coconut apple, sprout, or pearl, is a spongy, white, off-white, or creamy structure that develops during the germination of a zygotic embryo. It forms the foundation of the growing plant's nutrients and consists of parenchyma cells and sparse vascular tissues (Jackson et al. 2004; Yong et al. 2009).

Coconut fruit is typically harvested by farmers around 9 months of maturity when the jelly is soft, translucent, and less than 0.5 cm thick. Beyond 9 months, the white meat (jelly) hardens, and the water content begins to decrease. The composition of the de-husked coconut fruit is approximately 47% coconut kernel, 27% shell, and 25% coconut water. Despite being predominantly saturated, coconut oil has a low concentration of the highly lipotoxic palmitic acid and a high concentration of medium-chain fatty acids, particularly lauric acid, which may have more positive effects than negative ones (Adoyo et al. 2021).

One of the main qualities of coconut water that varies with the maturity of the coconut is its volume. From stages of 7 through 9 months, the amount of water in the entire nut increases, and from the stages of 9 through 10 months, coconut water volume decreases. As the coconuts mature the crude fat content of the coconut water increases. The protein content of coconut water also increases significantly with maturity, possibly correlating with the endosperm development of the nut (Jackson et al. 2004; Purseglove 1972). The pH of the water rises with maturity from 4.7 to 5.6 (Pue et al. 1992). Total solids, a measurement of the dry matter remaining in the samples of coconut water after moisture removal, are thought to be a result of higher concentrations of ions, including phosphate, sulfate, chloride, and fluoride, found in mature coconuts. Additionally, there were no statistically significant variations in ash content with coconut maturity (Pue et al. 1992).

During maturation, the total amount of reducing and non-reducing sugars of coconut water increases significantly. Glucose and fructose content is about 75% of all the sugars in the early stages of maturity. However, in the later stages, the amount of non-reducing sugar (sucrose) increased (Jackson et al. 2004). Fructose and glucose are two types of sugars that are crucial to the delicate tender composition of coconut water. Furthermore, the sugar content in the water gradually rises from 1.5% in the early months of nut maturation to 5.0–5.5% and then gradually drops to 2% at the point of full maturity of the nut (Jayalekshmy et al. 1986; Child 1974).

Coconut water also contains various phytochemicals and hormones such as auxin, different cytokinins, Gibberellic acids (GAs), and abscisic acid (ABA) (Kobayashi et al. 1997). Indole-3-acetic acid (IAA) can be found in both free form and conjugated to other amino acids, peptides, or carbohydrates. These physiologically inert IAA conjugates appear to serve as the storage forms of IAA in seeds and likely contribute to hormonal balance. Coconut water contains cytokinins that facilitate cell division, consequently accelerating growth. Numerous cytokinins can be found in coconut water, and it also contains folate, also referred to as vitamin B9 (Goh and Koren 2008).

Phenolic compounds and antioxidant activities were evaluated in coconut water and meat of coconut fruits (the endosperm) at three distinct stages of maturity: 180, 190, and 225 days after pollination (DAP) (Mahayothee et al. 2016). Between 180 and 190 days after pollination, the coconut's total phenolic content and antioxidant activity indices increased; by 225 days after pollination, they had either decreased or remained stable. The two primary phenolic compounds detected in coconut water were catechin and salicylic acid, while the meat contained gallic acid, caffeic acid, salicylic acid, and p-coumaric acid.

As the meat reached a more mature stage, its fat content noticeably increased. The predominant amino acid was glutamic acid, followed by aspartic acid and arginine. Alanine, glycine, valine, isoleucine, leucine, histidine, and lysine were among the other amino acids found in white meat (Phonphoem et al. 2022). The predominant monounsaturated fatty acid was oleic acid (C18:1n9c), and the predominant saturated fatty acid was lauric acid (C12:0). Mature coconut meats showed no discernible omega-3 fatty acid; only omega-6 and omega-9 fatty acids were present (Phonphoem et al. 2022).

According to Kannaian et al. (2020), the cotyledon has a carbohydrate content of 12.72 ± 0.15 mg/g, a protein content of 1.93 ± 0.04 mg/g, a lipid content of 16 ± 0.03 mg/g, ash content of 1.05 ± 0.2%, soluble sugar content of 24.5 ± 3.2%, starch content of 5.50 ± 0.3%, soluble dietary fiber content of 5.72 ± 0.4%, and insoluble dietary fiber content of 20.3 ± 1.9%. The amount of potassium, magnesium, calcium, phosphorus, manganese, copper, iron, and zinc were quantified to be 145 ± 8.6, 104 ± 9.6, 33.9 ± 8.2, 30.9 ± 1.9, 9.45 ± 2.1, 0.292 ± 0.1, 2.53 ± 0.2, and 1.20 ± 0.1 mg, respectively, in 100 g coconut haustorium (dry weight basis) (Manivannan et al. 2018). Methionine + cysteine (57.6%), phenylalanine + tyrosine (32.6%), leucine (45.7%), and isoleucine (68%) are less common in the cotyledon, according to the amino acid score. Reports indicate that the protein and fat contents of coconut water and endosperm from coconuts aged 7 to 10 months apart range from 0.02% to 0.13% and 0.5% to 1.8%, respectively. It is observed that the nutritional value of the coconut's liquid endosperm and cotyledon do not differ significantly (Kannaian et al. 2020; Jackson et al. 2004). The identification of cardiac glycosides through secondary metabolite analysis supports the use of cotyledon as a dietary supplement for patients suffering from heart disease. The cotyledon's total phenolics, tannins, and alkaloids demonstrate their nutritional parity with those of coconut endosperm. Additionally, assays for free radical scavenging show their medium-to-weak antioxidant activity. The EC50 and percent inhibition values indicate that the antioxidant activity of cotyledon is comparable to that of the endosperm or coconut water. Antioxidant activities have also been reported using β-carotene bleaching and ferric thiocyanate radical scavenging assays. Quantified lipids and alkaloids only showed a positive correlation with the DPPH, NO radical scavenging, and β-carotene bleaching assays. On the other hand, the FTC and TBA assays exhibited a positive correlation with carbohydrates, proteins, and tannins extracted from cotyledon (Kannaian et al. 2020).

4.3 Biochemical Features of Coconut Kernel and Coconut Milk

Several studies have reported the nutritional value of coconut kernel. The physicochemical properties, moisture content, ash content, total dissolved matter, volatile matter and pH are listed in Table 4.1 during the maturity periods of 6 months and 12 months. Protein content of fresh coconut kernel is reported in the range of 2.6–8% on wet basis (Appaiah et al. 2014; Kwon et al. 1996a; Hagenmaier et al. 1973). According to Appaiah et al. 2014, fresh coconut kernel contains proteins (7.5%), carbohydrates (12.3%), crude fiber (14.3%), and fat (37%). Coconut kernel also contains proteins with relatively a balanced amino acid profiles (Gonzales and Tanchuco 1977; Gunetileke and Laurentius 1974). About 75% of the proteins in the skim coconut milk extracted from the coconut kernel contain globulin and the rest is albumin (Garcia et al. 2005). Arginine, aspartic acid, glutamic acid and lysine are charged amino acids present in globulin fraction of coconut kernel (Kwon et al. 1996b; Patil and Benjakul 2017). Albumin fraction in coconut kernel contains polar amino acids and the proportion of these amino acids is important for the overall nutritional value. Among the total proteins present in coconut, approximately 71–77% are essential amino acids and it has high digestibility of 86% (Hagenmaier et al. 1974; Molina and Lachance 1973). Skim milk of coconut contains amino acids tryptophan, threonine, isoleucine and methionine in limited amounts (Hagenmaier et al. 1975). Except for the amino acids, arginine, lysine and glutamic acid, most of the other amino acids are found in lower concentrations in albumin fractions (Kwon et al. 1996b). The functionality of proteins in coconut milk is important for the stability of coconut milk emulsion.

While the fat content of fresh coconut kernel is about 35% by weight, the fat content of coconut milk is about 3–5% by weight, and it varies with the water content of coconut milk (Appaiah et al. 2014; Karunasiri et al. 2020a). The water

Table 4.1 Physicochemical features of coconut kernel of 6 and 12 months maturity (Abdul and Iqbal 2011; Dendy and Timmins 1973; Grimwood and Ashman 1975; Chakraborty 1985; Kwon et al. 1996a)

	Variety	Moisture (%)	Volatile matter (%)	Ash (%)	TDS g/L	pH
6-month maturity	Sri Lankan tall variety	35–40	28–32	1–2	4.04 ± 0.028	5.5 ± 0.034
	Malayan yellow dwarf	31–35	30–38	0.5–1.1	4.21 ± 0.156	4.6 ± 0.173
	Hybrid	14–18	13–16	0.2–0.8	7.35 ± 0.242	5.06 ± 0.040
12-month maturity	Sri Lankan tall variety	61–70	40–59	0.8–1.0	4.99 ± 0.023	4.46 ± 0.086
	Malayan yellow dwarf	37–39	35–42	1.2–1.7	3.00 ± 0.115	4.43 ± 0.184
	Hybrid	55–60	52–56	0.8–1.0	5.23 ± 0.086	4.16 ± 0.086

content of coconut kernel is reduced to about 6% when dry coconut kernel is prepared. The main fatty acid of coconut milk is lauric acid (50%) followed by myristic acid (22%), palmitic acid (8%), caprylic acid (7%) and capric acid (7%) (Dayrit 2015). The lauric acid contents in cow's milk (1.6%) and goat milk (5.7%) shows that the fat composition of coconut oil is unique and significantly different from common dairy milk while soy milk does not contain lauric acid (Lima et al. 2011; Lopez et al. 2019). Coconut milk also contains phospholipids, and these phospholipids contribute to the stability of coconut milk emulsion (Dave et al. 2019).

In young coconut kernel, 0.4–3.5% of starch can be found and the starch content increases with maturity (Gatchalian et al. 1993). According to Balasubramaniam 1976, polygalactomannan is another polysaccharide that can be found in the kernel. The carbohydrate content of coconut milk has been reported variedly due to different volumes of water used to extract coconut milk (Khuwijitjaru et al. 2012; Tulashie et al. 2022; Nadeeshani et al. 2015). About 1.2–2.4% carbohydrates are present in coconut milk prepared by using 3 g of coconut meat in 50 mL of water (Azlin-hasim et al. 2019).

Research has been conducted comparing the coconut milk with dairy milk to highlight the importance of coconut milk as a vegan replacement to cow's milk. (Singh et al. 2021; Kamath 2020; Tulashie et al. 2022). In addition to the vegan nature, coconut milk also shows healthy characteristics such as lower long chain saturated fat content, and absence of lactose which causes discomfort among the people with lactose intolerance. Many nutrients such as proteins, total fat and energy are high in coconut milk compared to cow's milk. However, the nutrient content for a given weight of coconut milk solution depends on the amount of water used in the preparation of coconut milk. Total fat, proteins, total sugar, and reducing sugar percentages are higher in the first extract while total phenol content is higher in the second extract (Nadeeshani et al. 2015). Coconut milk is commercially available as coconut cream and coconut powder. According to Karunasiri et al. (2020a), nutritional value of coconut milk extracted from coconut kernel slightly varied with different forms of coconut milk such as powdered, liquid and domestically prepared coconut milk.

Coconut milk also contains phenolic compounds that can act as antioxidants. The main source of phenolic compounds in coconut is coconut testa (Seneviratne et al. 2009). Phenolic compounds mainly dissolve in aqueous phase of coconut milk. The main phenolic compounds present in coconut milk are gallic acid, chlorogenic acid, *p*-hydroxybenzoic acid, caffeic acid, vanillic acid, syringic acid, and ferulic acid (Karunasiri et al. 2020a). Ultrasound assisted extraction of minerals followed by inductively coupled plasma optical spectrometry indicates that coconut milk contains calcium (5.8–131 $\mu g\ g^{-1}$), copper (0.27–1.56 $\mu g\ g^{-1}$), iron (0.76–5.52 $\mu g\ g^{-1}$), potassium (212–1781 $\mu g\ g^{-1}$), magnesium (14.9–201 $\mu g\ g^{-1}$), manganese (0.11–3.88 $\mu g\ g^{-1}$), sodium (274–625 $\mu g\ g^{-1}$), phosphorous (26–341 $\mu g\ g^{-1}$) and znic (0.74–3.2 $\mu g\ g^{-1}$) (Abdul and Iqbal 2011; Santos et al. 2014).

4.4 Health Benefits of Coconut Milk and Kernel

The health benefits of coconut milk remain almost unexplored. Therefore, the studies related to health effects are limited to a handful of publications. Evaluation of the health effects of coconut milk or coconut kernel can be considered as the same because a solution of coconut kernel (coconut milk) is prepared for the evaluation of the potential of coconut milk. Various investigations include *in vitro* chemical analysis, animal studies, human studies and *in silico* approaches. In addition, the potential nutritional properties have been suggested based on the compounds present in coconut milk (Bharti et al. 2021). Major fatty acids present in coconut milk are medium chain. Medium chain fatty acids are known to decrease serum cholesterol in mice by a mechanism involved in the reduction of bile acid reabsorption (Li et al. 2018). A study involving Wistar rats indicates that a coconut milk diet does not increase or decrease serum cholesterol levels significantly compared to a standard basal diet (Karunasiri et al. 2020a). However, coconut milk diet has increased HDL levels and decreased LDL levels compared to a soya milk diet in healthy subjects (Ekanayaka et al. 2013). In addition to lipidemic effects, coconut milk is also known to enhance antioxidant properties. The polyphenolic compounds, gallic acid, chlorogenic acid, *p*-hydroxybenzoic acid, caffeic acid, vanillic acid, syringic acid, and ferulic acid are known to display antioxidant properties (Bros and Michel 2002). Treatment of yeast cells with the phenolic antioxidants of coconut milk followed by hydrogen peroxide induced oxidative stress indicate that macromolecules such as proteins, lipids and DNA are protected against induced stress by coconut milk-based antioxidants (Karunasiri et al. 2020a). Antioxidant activities of coconut milk as evaluated by total phenol content, ferric reducing antioxidant power, and oxygen radical absorbance capacity show that coconut milk has higher values for these *in vitro* antioxidant properties compared to cow's milk and goat's milk (Alyaqoubi et al. 2015). For the production of canned coconut milk, white coconut kernel without brown testa is used to avoid any color due to brown testa. However, as the testa is the main source of antioxidants, coconut milk prepared by white coconut meat alone needs to be preserved against oxidation. BHT or α-tochopherol can be used to arrest the process of rancidity in such coconut milk samples (Pongtongkam and Chaiseri 2020). There are no reports on the comparative antioxidant properties of coconut milk prepared by white kernel alone and white kernel with coconut testa.

While saturated fats are blamed for hypercholesterolemic effects without considering the chain length of fatty acids, dietary fiber isolated from coconut kernel has displayed hypocholesterolemic effects (Rajamohan and Archana 2018). The chain length of fatty acids has been shown to be more crucial in determining the lipidemic effects than the degree of unsaturation. Therefore, hypocholesterolemic effects of coconut milk may be attributed to the desirable chain length of fatty acids of coconut oil (Senanayake et al. 2021). Coconut milk has been shown to display beneficial effects on intestinal *Lactobacillus* spp. *In silico* studies indicate that coconut milk antioxidants make at least 41 metabolic products, and these metabolites display antioxidant and anti-inflammatory activities in the gut. *Lactobacillus* spp. are protected against H_2O_2 induced and aerobic oxidative stress when they were exposed to coconut milk based antioxidants prior to the exposure to oxidative stress conditions (Wadanambi et al. 2023).

4.5 Products and Byproducts of Coconut Kernel

Main byproducts of coconut kernel are coconut milk, coconut oil (copra oil), virgin coconut oil, coconut paring oil, desiccated coconut and coconut oil meal (Fig. 4.2.) Virgin coconut oil is produced from coconut milk by centrifugation, freezing followed by centrifugation, and fermentation of coconut milk by *Lactobacillus* strains. All these processes are helpful to denature proteins and separate proteins, carbohydrates and water from the oil layer of coconut oil emulsion (Seneviratne and Jayathilaka 2016).

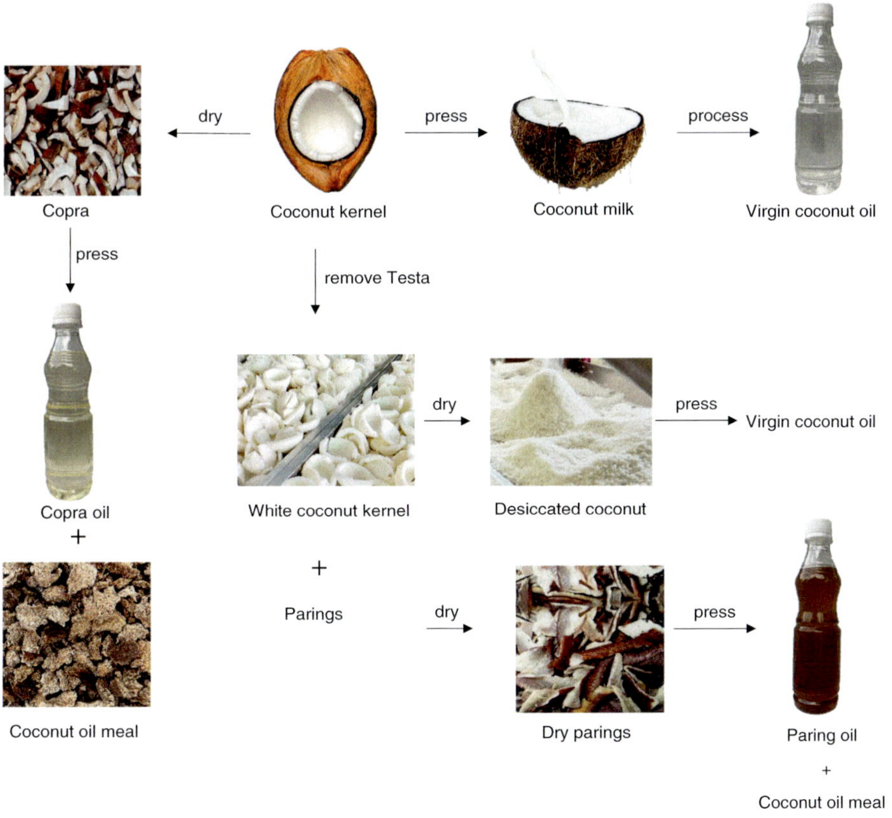

Fig. 4.2 By-products of coconut kernel

4.5.1 Virgin Coconut Oil

Virgin coconut oil is one of the major products of coconut kernel. Virgin coconut oil is prepared for commercial purposes by wet extraction methods based on coconut milk and dry extraction methods based on desiccated coconut. In both dry and wet extraction methods, temperatures are maintained below 60 °C throughout the process to preserve thermally unstable beneficial substances and to prevent any other reactions that may lead to the production of unwanted compounds. In addition to culinary applications, virgin coconut oil can be used to produce moisturizers and hair oil (Agero and Verallo-Rowell 2004). In the wet extraction of coconut oil, coconut milk extract from the coconut kernel is processed. Due to the nutritional value, purity and pleasant smell of the virgin coconut oil extracted by wet extraction, this oil is used in the production of baby oil and hair oil. Virgin coconut oil is applied on babies' skin as a thin layer to protect the skin from various diseases. As there are low free fatty acid contents in virgin coconut oil, it has a high shelf life (Chomtho et al. 2016). Several studies have been conducted on various applications of virgin coconut oil (Satheesh 2015). Virgin coconut oil with coconut fat has been used to produce ice cream with coconut aroma (Choo et al. 2010). Virgin coconut oil is used to prepare various meat and vegetable dishes. Due to its thermal stability at high temperatures, virgin coconut oil is ideal for deep frying (Marikkar et al. 2007). Due to the rich medium chain triglyceride content, coconut oil is easily metabolized to produce energy with minimum possibility of deposition (Ng et al. 2021). Virgin coconut oil and copra oil can also be used to make lip balm, shampoo, soaps and detergents due to its high triglyceride content (Sukeksi and Diana 2020; Ngan et al. 2020). VCO can also be used as hair oil. It also blocks 20% of the UV rays received by the skin (Korać and Khambholja 2011). Antimicrobial properties and medicinal properties of coconut oil have been reviewed (Kappally et al. 2015; Satheesh 2015).

4.5.2 Copra Oil

Copra oil is coconut oil prepared by the dried coconut kernel by pressing. Copra oil is still the main coconut oil consumed by many coconut producing countries. There is no special temperature control during the production of copra oil. Fresh coconut kernel can be sun-dried or kiln died to remove water from the kernel prior to the pressing. Sun-drying may take 7–14 days depending on the intensity and duration of sunlight. This drying process lowers the moisture level of coconut kernel to about 6%. At this stage, coconut kernel is called copra. The fatty acid composition is not considerably affected by the method of extraction of coconut oil. Therefore, both virgin coconut oil and copra oil have almost similar fatty acid profiles milk (Seneviratne and Jayathilaka 2016; Seneviratne and Dissanayake 2005). However, components such as phenolic compounds, vitamins etc. are different in copra oil compared to virgin coconut oil (Seneviratne et al. 2009; Seneviratne and Dissanayake

2008). Reports indicate that the vitamin and phenolic fraction is less in copra oil compared to virgin coconut oil (Nevin and Rajamohan 2006; Ramesh et al. 2020).

4.5.3 Paring Oil

Paring oil is prepared by pressing of parings including testa, removed from coconut kernel. This oil is considered as lower quality coconut oil due to commercial reasons. This oil gets oxidized faster compared to other coconut oils and the color also varies from pale yellow to light brown. Free fatty acid content is at least 3–4 times higher in paring oil compared to other coconut oils (Yalegama et al. 2015). The coconut oil extracted from paring portion with testa contains higher mono- and polyunsaturated fatty acid content and lower phenolic and vitamin E antioxidants (Appaiah et al. 2014). The presence of higher percentage of unsaturated fatty acids and the lower content of antioxidants may contribute to low oxidative stability of paring oil. Even though the commercial quality of paring coconut oil is lower, there is no evidence to support that the nutritional properties of paring coconut oil is poorer compared to virgin coconut oil or copra oil.

4.5.4 Coconut Oil Meal

Coconut oil meal is a byproduct of the extraction of coconut milk by dry method from coconut copra and desiccated coconut. It is mainly used as an animal food to feed cattle and pigs. Protein content of the oil meal is about 20% with albumin and globulin as main proteins while moisture content is about 7% (Samson et al. 1971). About 80% of the nitrogen in the coconut oil meal originates from amino acids. The main amino acids are alanine, valine, glycine, isoleucine, leucine, proline, threonine, serine, phenylalanine, aspartic acid, glutamic acid and arginine. Main minerals present in coconut oil meal are calcium, phosphorus, magnesium, potassium, zinc copper and manganese (Creswell and Brooks 1971a). Coconut oil meal up to 10% in the diet helped weight gain in pigs (Creswell and Brooks 1971b). Coconut oil meal up to 20% in the diet increases the rate of egg production in hens. However, the egg weight was depressed by feeding coconut meal (Wignjosoesastro et al. 1972). Coconut oil meal is a rich source of antioxidants with high thermal stability. The phenolic antioxidants of coconut oil meal include gallic acid, catechin, chlorogenic acid, *p*-hydroxybenzoic acid, caffeic acid, syringic acid, ferulic acid, *p*-coumaric acid, elagic acid and apigenin (Seneviratne et al. 2016). Due to the high thermal stability of the phenolic extracts of coconut oil meal, these extracts can be used to preserve baked foods and these extracts are excellent replacements of synthetic antioxidants (Senanayake et al. 2019). The shelf life of sunflower oil can also be extended by the coconut oil meal-based antioxidants. In addition to its importance as a food preservative, coconut oil meal-based antioxidants provide beneficial health effects. These antioxidants have been shown to inhibit the oxidation of lipids, as tested by thiobarbituric acid reactive substance (TBARS) assay, inhibit protein oxidation as tested by protein carbonyl assay and inhibit nicked DNA formation as tested in HEp-2 cells. The serum DPPH radical scavenging activity and the Trolox equivalent antioxidants capacity in Wistar rats further confirms the antioxidant potential of the coconut oil meal-based antioxidants (Karunasiri et al. 2020b).

4.5.5 *Coconut Milk*

The characteristics of coconut milk have been described earlier. Coconut milk is the emulsion of coconut fat, proteins and water, which can be prepared by squeezing freshly grated coconut kernel. Concentrated coconut milk is known as coconut cream. Coconut milk can be used in making dishes such as fish, meat, curries, ice cream, pudding, cocktails, jam, cookies etc. These products are commercially promoted in many countries including India, Sri Lanka, Philippines, Malaysia, Indonesia and Thailand. Indonesia is one of the major coconut milk exporters in the world (Ekanayaka et al. 2013).

4.5.6 *Coconut Cream*

Coconut cream is the viscous extract of coconut kernel partially defatted or not. Coconut cream is a commercial form of coconut milk available. Coconut cream can either be directly used or diluted with water to be used in various edible preparations. This is available in the market as bottles, cans, pouches or packets (Maghazechi et al. 2021)

4.5.7 *Coconut Skimmed Milk*

During the coconut cream preparation process, the separated supernatant solution consists of soluble compounds of coconut kernel and this dilute solution is called skimmed coconut milk. In regions where animal proteins are deficient, skimmed coconut milk can be used as a substitute for protein sources, as it contains quality protein which is suitable for the preparation of edible products or as a protein supplement (Dayrit 2015). Coconut skimmed milk production includes filtering the coconut milk produced using pared coconut kernel by using a mesh and adjusting the pH of the coconut milk to 6–7 by adding NaOH followed by pasteurization of coconut milk at 600 °C for 1 h. As the final step, solution is centrifuged to separate the high protein containing coconut skimmed milk which separated as the aqueous layer (Dayrit 2015).

4.5.8 Desiccated Coconut

Desiccated coconut is the dehydrated product of grated coconut kernel. As indicated in Fig. 4.2, desiccated coconut is prepared by drying white coconut kernel. In Asia, desiccated coconut is used for preparing various vegetable and meat dishes. It is also an ingredient in cakes, chocolates, and many other sweet foods. Coconut cake, cookies, energy bars, and ice cream are among other foods where desiccated coconut is an essential ingredient. In countries that do not produce coconut, desiccated coconut is used as a substitute for fresh grated coconut. Depending on the thickness of the grated coconut kernel, desiccated coconut can be graded (D'Aquino et al. 1991). As fresh coconut is a rich source of proteins lipids and carbohydrates, microbial contamination is a common problem at various stages of desiccated coconut production. *Staphylococcus aureus* and *Aspergillus flavus* are among the main organisms that contaminate desiccated coconut.

There are several health benefits of desiccated coconut. It contains minimal to no bad cholesterol and the fats present are healthy fats. Additionally, it contains copper, selenium, manganese and fiber that support better heart health, minimize the cancer risk and improve male fertility (D'Aquino et al. 1991). Dietary fiber of desiccated coconut promotes weight loss. When fiber combines with the fluids and transports through the digestive tract, stomach is filled for a longer period, causing loss of appetite, which results in weight loss. Additionally, it lessens the possibility of accumulating visceral abdominal fat (D'Aquino et al. 1991). Desiccated coconut has the potential to reduce the osteoporosis and arthritis as it has been proven by researchers that the fatty acids in coconuts strengthen bones and stop them from deteriorating. Diabetes patients have reduced blood manganese concentrations. Dried coconut kernel has considerable amount of manganese that can help lower the risk of developing diabetes (Kazi et al. 2008).

4.5.9 Copra

Copra is prepared from dried coconut kernel and the production process is given in Fig. 4.2. For export purposes, usually fresh coconut kernel is sun dried and oil is extracted by pressing. Lauric acid is one of the major components in this extracted oil. The quality of copra oil depends on the quality of copra used for the extraction of oil. Depending on the drying conditions, copra may get contaminated with aflatoxins and polycyclic aromatic hydrocarbons. To produce desiccated coconut, strict hygienic conditions should be maintained to avoid fungal contamination. The drying in open ovens where coconut kernel is exposed to smoke or fire is not recommended due to possible polycyclic aromatic hydrocarbon generation (Samarasinghe et al. 2023).

4.5.10 Coconut Chips

Coconut chips is a ready to eat snack. Preparation procedure can be varied depending on the flavor added to it. It is mainly prepared as salted and sweetened forms. Coconuts of 9–10 months of maturity are used to produce coconut chips. Coconut chips are a good source of dietary fiber. Once taken, it prolongs the feeling of fullness. This is due to the fact that most other snacks contain quickly absorbing carbohydrates, proteins and fats but coconut chips contain considerable quantity of fiber. Similar to coconut oil, coconut chips contain medium-chain fatty acids, a form of saturated fat that is known to burn to produce energy without the probability of deposition (Manikantan et al. 2016).

4.5.11 Coconut Butter

White coconut meat is ground into coconut butter. Coconut butter is not as smooth as other dairy products or butter varieties made from fruits. There are little flakes of coconut meat in it however the product is packed with nutrients to maintain good health (Mardiati et al. 2022). The benefits of coconut butter are similar to those of coconut oil, including helping with weight loss, increasing immunity, and many others. However, unlike coconut oil, coconut butter contains higher levels of saturated fat and dietary fiber. Coconut butter stands out next to breast milk, which is the most well-known source of lauric acid for a newborn, because of its high lauric acid content. (Wang et al. 2015). Coconut butter contains medium-chain fatty acids, which are simpler to digest. As a result, it lessens inflammation. Therefore, it makes for an excellent dietary supplement for those with osteoporosis, Crohn's disease, gallbladder illness and diabetes. Cancer can also be treated with its help (Wang et al. 2015). In addition to its many health advantages, coconut butter has the potential to moisturize the skin and hair while providing vitamins that protect the skin and hair (Wallace 2019).

4.5.12 Coconut Flour

The majority of coconut flour is produced as a by-product of the production of coconut milk and is made from dried and powdered coconut kernel. Coconut flour is white or off-white in color and it is free of gluten. Therefore, it is frequently used as a wheat flour substitute in the food industry. When making food products using coconut flour for specific diet requirements, recipes must be altered because coconut flour is thicker than wheat flour and retains more moisture. (Bawalan 2000). Coconut flour provides protein, fat and fiber. Since iron is the main mineral found in coconut flour, vegans and vegetarians can receive enough iron from it (Bawalan 2000).

4.6 Comparison of Coconut Milk and Other Plant-Based Milk

There are several types of plant-based milk in the market. Soy milk, rice, almond, hemp, pea, oats and coconut milk are some of them. Coconut milk is a rich source of saturated fatty acids when compared to other plant-based milk. Whole milk also contains considerable amount of saturated fatty acids (Sagon 2022). The amount of calcium and protein content of coconut milk and other plant-based milk is less compared to animal milk. When compared to other milk, coconut milk has a specific flavor with mild sweet taste which makes it preferable to use with coffee and cereal. (Sagon 2022). According to Kubala and Krans (2023) calories, proteins and fat content of almond milk, coconut milk, soy milk and rice milk varies. The specialty of coconut milk is that it does not contain cholesterol and it can be considered as low carb diet Even though coconut milk contains comparatively high amount of fats, they are in the form of medium chain fatty acids. The absorption of medium chain fatty acids is quicker than other fats and it has potential to metabolize into energy at more speed (Nagashree et al. 2017). As medium chain fatty acids are not stored in the fat cells, it helps to maintain the body mass index as well. Also, it has been proved that coconut fats which contain medium chain fatty acids reduce the risk of heart diseases and lower the cholesterol levels (Ekanayaka et al. 2013).

Calorie content of almond milk is low and it can be considered as a good source of Vitamin A, D and calcium. It is lactose free naturally. At the same time, it is low in protein and contains carrageenan which can trigger digestive issues in humans (Sethi et al. 2016). Some of the advantages of soymilk are it serves as a good source of calcium and vitamin A, B12 and D. It consists of a high quantity of protein similar to cow's milk. But it has low calorie level compared to whole milk and it contains low level of saturated fats (D'Adamo and Sahin 2014). However, it has been recognized that soy milk is an allergen to many adults and children. Nowadays in most of the countries, soy is produced by genetically modified plants, and it has become a concern for consumers (Zaheer and Akhtar 2017).

Oat milk is commonly consumed milk available in the market. It has a mild flavor, and it is naturally sweet. Oat milk can be used with cereals and smoothies. According to Whitehead et al. (2014), a serving of oats milk (240 mL) contains 140–170 calories, 3–5 g proteins, 20–29 g of carbohydrates and nearly 5 g of fat. Calorie amount of oat milk is similar to that of cow's milk. But it has half the amount of protein and fat found in cow's milk and twice as much as the amount of carbohydrate found in cow's milk. When compared to other plant-based milk, oat milk has high content of fibers and beta glucan, which converts into a thick gel like matrix when it passes through the gut. This beta glucan has the possibility to bind with cholesterol and reduce the absorption of cholesterol in the body. As a result, it helps to reduce the risk of high cholesterol (Othman et al. 2011). Beta glucan also increases the feeling of fullness and reduces the necessity to eat more food. Therefore, it helps to reduce the glucose level in the blood after a meal (Rebello et al. 2014). According to Onning et al. 1999, men who have consumed 750 mL of oats milk daily for 5 weeks exhibit the reduction of LDL cholesterol by 5% and total cholesterol by 3%.

Compared to soy milk, almond milk, oats milk and coconut milk, rice milk is the least allergenic to consumers (Vanga and Raghavan 2018). Rice milk has sweet taste naturally and it is a source of Vitamin A, D and calcium. However, the carbohydrate quantity of rice milk is comparatively high. Therefore, it is risky to be used by diabetic patients. The protein content of the rice milk is also very low and there is a risk of inorganic arsenic and cadmium in rice products, especially for infants and children (Zhu et al. 2008).

Coconut milk contains Vitamin A, C, D, calcium and iron and poses a low risk to consumers who are allergic to nuts. Coconut milk alone cannot provide the protein requirement of the body and hence additional protein sources must be introduced. As in almond milk, coconut milk may also contain carrageenan which causes digestive difficulties in some consumers. A proper comparison of coconut milk with other plant-based milks and cow's milk needs more nutritional data of coconut milk and physicochemical properties of any food prepared with coconut milk. Therefore, more research is needed to investigate nutritional advantages and functional properties of coconut milk (D'Amato et al. 2012).

4.7 Development of New Products from Coconut Milk

Innovations in many food or cosmetic industries based on coconut byproducts are lacking. The development of new products based on coconut kernel and various byproducts are important for the sustainability of coconut industry. Industries can pay attention to the production of new soaps, anti-dandruff shampoo, sterilizing agents, fungicides, natural fertilizer, repellents, deodorizing agents and itching medication due to the significant biochemical, phytochemical and physiochemical properties of coconut kernel (Wardah et al. 2020). Studies have emphasized the significance of incorporating stabilizers or thickeners, such as tapioca starch, in the formulation of yogurt-like products from coconut milk. The addition of tapioca starch serves to modify the viscosity, rheological properties, and syneresis (the release of liquid) of the products due to its ability to swell when hydrated. Based on sensory evaluation, preference for yogurt-like products that are firmer and more viscous when tapioca starch is added at concentrations between 1.0% and 2.0% (w/w) was found. This addition not only enhances the texture and mouthfeel of the products but also improves their overall sensory appeal, contributing to a more satisfying consumer experience (Pachekrepapol et al. 2021). Catechin fortified coconut milk was developed utilizing nanoencapsulation techniques (Ruengdech and

Siripatrawan 2021). Nanoencapsulation proved effective in preserving the antioxidant activity of catechins in high-pressure-processed coconut milk during storage. These findings indicate that catechin nano encapsulation (CaNE) have significant potential as food fortification ingredients for various food products. However, investigating the effects of CaNE fortification on consumer acceptability and examining the digestibility and release of catechins from CaNE under simulated gastrointestinal (GI) conditions are future areas of research as understanding these aspects will contribute to the development of coconut milk formulations that offer enhanced health benefits. Also addition of coconut milk and coconut sugar in the formulation of ice cream resulted in the higher levels of total phenolics and minerals in the final product. Additionally, the study provided insights into the development of non-dairy or vegan delicacies using coconut as a primary ingredient. This suggests a promising avenue for expanding the range of coconut-based products in the market, catering to the preferences of a diverse consumer base and meeting the growing demand for non-dairy alternatives (Beegum et al. 2022).

4.8 Conclusion

Coconut kernel and the products and byproducts of coconut kernel are rich sources of both micro and macro nutrients and various secondary metabolites. Therefore, many health benefits can be expected by the consumption of coconut kernel-based products such as coconut oil, coconut milk and coconut water due to their biochemical, phytochemical and physiochemical properties. High content of medium chain fatty acids in coconut oil and coconut milk, provide many advantages when compared to other plant-based milk and oils. Due to antioxidant and anti-inflammatory properties, coconut kernel products can be used as ideal ingredients for cosmetic industry, detergent industry and culinary industry. Much more research work is needed to develop coconut-based products in industries other than the food industry and cosmetic industry. Coconut producing countries have a major role to play in generating more convincing evidence on nutritional properties and related health benefits of coconut kernel products and performing research and development activities towards designing new products based on coconut kernel and its byproducts.

References

Abdul HS, Iqbal M (2011) Chemical composition of meat (kernel) and nut water of major coconut (*Cocos nucifera L.*) cultivars at coastal area of Pakistan. Pak J Bot 43:357–363

Adoyo GO, Sila DN, Onyango AN (2021) Physico-chemical properties of kernel from coconut (*Cocos nucifera L.*) varieties grown at the Kenyan Coast. Acad J 15(8):313–321

Agero AL, Verallo-Rowell VM (2004) A randomized double-blind controlled trial comparing extra virgin coconut oil with mineral oil as a moisturizer for mild to moderate xerosis. Dermatitis 15(3):109–116. https://doi.org/10.2310/6620.2004.04006

Alyaqoubi S, Abdullah AM, Samudi M, Abdullah N, Addai ZR, Musa KH (2015) Study of antioxidant activity and physicochemical properties of coconut milk (Pati santan) in Malaysia. J Chem Pharm Res 7(4):967–973
Appaiah P, Sunil L, Kumar PK, Krishna AG (2014) Composition of coconut testa, coconut kernel and its oil. J Am Oil Chem Soc 91:917–924
Arumughan C, Balachandran C, Sundaresan A (1993) Development of a process for coconut cream on commercial scale. J Food Sci Technol 30:408–412
Azlin-hasim S, Siang QL, Yusof F, Zaino LMK, Yusof HM (2019) Chemical composition and potential adulterants in coconut milk sold in Kuala Lumpur. Malaysian Appl Biol 48(3):27–34
Balasubramaniam K (1976) Polysaccharides of the kernel of maturing and matured coconuts. J Food Sci 41(6):1370–1373
Bawalan DD (2000) The economics of production, utilization and marketing of coconut flour from coconut milk residue. Coconut Res Dev J 16(1):34
Beegum PPS, Nair JP, Manikantan MR et al (2022) Effect of coconut milk, tender coconut and coconut sugar on the physico-chemical and sensory attributes in ice cream. J Food Sci Technol 59:2605–2616. https://doi.org/10.1007/s13197-021-05279-y
Bharti BK, Badshah J, Beniwal BS (2021) A review on comparison between bovine milk and plant-based coconut milk. Pharma Innov J 10(3):374–378
Bros W, Michel C (2002) Chemistry of the antioxidant effect of polyphenols. Ann N Y Acad Sci 957:57–69
Chakraborty P (1985) Functional properties of coconut protein isolate obtained by ultrafiltration. J Food Sci Technol Mysore 22:248–254
Child R (1974) Coconuts, 2nd edn. Longmans/Green & Co, London
Chomtho K, Suteerojntrakool O, Chomtho S (2016) Effectiveness of medium chain triglyceride ketogenic diet in Thai children with intractable epilepsy. J Med Assoc Thail 99(2):159–165
Choo SY, Leong SK, Lu FSH (2010) Physicochemical and sensory properties of icecream formulated with virgin coconut oil. Food Sci Technol Int 16(6):531–541
Creswell DC, Brooks CC (1971a) Composition, apparent digestibility and energy evaluation of coconut oil and coconut meal. J Anim Sci 33(2):366–369
Creswell DC, Brooks CC (1971b) Effect of coconut meal on coturnix quail and of coconut meal and coconut oil on performance, carcass measurements and fat composition in swine. J Anim Sci 33(2):370–375. https://doi.org/10.2527/jas1971.332370x
D'Adamo CR, Sahin A (2014) Soy foods and supplementation: a review of commonly perceived health benefits and risks. Altern Ther Health Med 20(1):39–51
D'Amato A, Fasoli E, Righetti PG (2012) Harry Belafonte and the secret proteome of coconut milk. J Proteome 75(3):914–920. https://doi.org/10.1016/j.jprot.2011.10.009
D'Aquino M, Benedetti PC, Di Felice M, Gentili V, Tomassi G, Maiorino M, Ursini F (1991) Effect of fish oil and coconut oil on antioxidant defense system and lipid peroxidation in rat liver. Free Radic Res Commun 12(13):147–152. https://doi.org/10.3109/10715769109145779
Dave AC, Ye A, Singh H (2019) Structural and interfacial characteristics of oil bodies in coconuts (*Cocos nucifera L.*). Food Chem 276:129–139
Dayrit FM (2015) The properties of lauric acid and their significance in coconut oil. J Am Oil Chem Soc 92:1–15. https://doi.org/10.1007/s11746-014-2562-7
De Leon SY, Delores MI (2004) 'Coconut': processing fruits. In: Barrett DM, Somogyi L, Ramaswamy HS (eds) Science and technology, 2nd edn. CRC Press, Boca Raton, pp 707–737
Dendy DAV, Timmins WH (1973) Development of wet coconut process assigned to extract protein and oil from fresh coconut. TPI, Bengaluru
Ekanayaka RA, Ekanayaka NK, Perera B, De Silva PG (2013) Impact of a traditional dietary supplement with coconut milk and soya milk on the lipid profile in normal free-living subjects. J Nutr Metab 2013:481068. https://doi.org/10.1155/2013/481068
Garcia R, Arocena R, Laurena A, Tecson-Mendoza E (2005) 11S and 7S globulins of coconut (*Cocos nucifera L.*): purification and characterization. J Agric Food Chem 53:1734–1739

Gatchalian MM, De Leon SY, Yano T (1993) Comparative profiles of young coconut (*Cocos nucifera, L.*) from fresh and stored nuts. Food Qual Prefer 4(4):193–200
Goh YI, Koren G (2008) Folic acid in pregnancy and fetal outcomes. J Obstet 2008(28):3–13
Gonzales O, Tanchuco R (1977) Chemical composition and functional properties of coconut protein isolate (CPI). Philippine J Coconut Stud 11:21–30
Gonzalez ON (1990) 'Coconut milk, coconut-based beverages, coconut proteins': coconut as food. PCRDF, Quezon City
Grimwood BE, Ashman F (1975) Coconut palm products: their processing in developing countries. Food and Agriculture Organization, Rome
Grisingha SN (1991) Production of coconut butter. MS dissertation, Kasetsart University
Gunetileke K, Laurentius S (1974) Conditions for the separation of oil and protein from coconut milk emulsion. J Food Sci 39(2):230–233
Hagenmaier RN, Carter CM, Mattil KF (1973) Aqueous processing of fresh coconuts for recovery of oil and coconut skim milk. J Food Sci 38:516–518
Hagenmaier R, Mattil KF, Cater CM (1974) Dehydrated coconut skim milk as a food product: composition and functionality. J Food Sci 39(1):196–199
Hagenmaier R, Lopitakwong R, Verasestakul S (1975) Nutritive value and food uses of coconut skim milk solids. J Food Sci 40(6):1324–1325
Jackson JC, Gordon A, Wizzard G, McCook K, Rolle R (2004) Changes in chemical composition of coconut (*Cocos nucifera*) water during maturation of the fruit. J Sci Food Agric 84(9):1049–1052. https://doi.org/10.1002/jsfa.1783
Jayalekshmy A, Arummaghan C, Naraynan S, Mathew AG (1986) Changes in the chemical composition of coconut water during maturation. J Food Sci Technol 23:203–207
Kamath R (2020) Formulation of vegan health beverage using coconut milk and fortifying it with flaxseed oil. Bombay Technol 67(1):e151201. https://doi.org/10.36664/bt/2020/v67i1/151201
Kannaian UPN, Edwin JB, Rajagopal V, Shankar SN, Srinivasan B (2020) Phytochemical composition and antioxidant activity of coconut cotyledon. Heliyon 6(2):e03411
Kappally S, Shirwaikar A, Shirwaikar A (2015) Coconut oil—review of potential applications. Hygeia J Drugs Med 7(2):34–41
Karunasiri AN, Gunawardane M, Senanayake CM, Jayathilaka N, Seneviratne KN (2020a) Antioxidant and nutritional properties of domestic and commercial coconut milk preparations. Int J Food Sci 2020:3489605. https://doi.org/10.1155/2020/3489605
Karunasiri AN, Senanayake CM, Hapugaswatta H, Jayathilaka N, Seneviratne KN (2020b) Protective effect of coconut oil meal phenolic antioxidants against macromolecular damage: in vitro and in vivo study. J Chem 2020:3503165. https://doi.org/10.1155/2020/3503165
Kazi TG, Afridi HI, Kazi N, Jamali MK, Arain MB, Jalbani N, Kandhro GA (2008) Copper, chromium, manganese, iron, nickel, and zinc levels in biological samples of diabetes mellitus patients. Biol Trace Elem Res 122(1):1–18. https://doi.org/10.1007/s12011-007-8062-y
Khuwijitjaru P, Watsanit K, Adachi S (2012) Carbohydrate content and composition of product from subcritical water treatment of coconut meal. J Ind Eng Chem 8(1):225–229
Kobayashi H, Morisaki N, Tago Y, Hashimoto Y, Iwasaki S, Kawachi E, Nagata R, Shudo K (1997) Structural identification of a major cytokinin in coconut milk as 14-O-(3-O-[β-Dgalactopyranosyl-(1→2)-α-D-galactopyranosyl-(1→3)-α-L-arabinofuranosyl]-4-O-(α-L-arabinofuranosyl)-β-D-galactopyranosyl)-trans-zeatin riboside. Chem Pharma Bull (Tokyo) 1997(45):260–264
Korać RR, Khambholja KM (2011) Potential of herbs in skin protection from ultraviolet radiation. Pharmacogn Rev 5:164–173
Kubala J, Krans B (2023) Comparing milks: almond, dairy, soy, rice and coconut. Healthline. https://www.healthline.com/health/milk-almond-cow-soy-rice
Kwon KS, Bae D, Park KH, Rhee KC (1996a) Aqueous extraction and membrane techniques improve coconut protein concentrate functionality. J Food Sci 61:753–756
Kwon K, Park KH, Rhee KC (1996b) Fractionation and characterization of proteins from coconut (*Cocos nucifera L.*). J Agric Food Chem 44(7):1741–1745

Li H, Liu Y, Zhang X, Xu Q, Zhang Y, Xue C, Guo C (2018) Medium-chain fatty acids decrease serum cholesterol via reduction of intestinal bile acid reabsorption in C57BL/6J mice. Nutr Metab 15(2018):37

Lima LDS, Oliveira RL, Bagaldo AR, Neto AFG, Ribeiro VVDM, Lanna DPD (2011) Composition and fatty acid profile of milk from cows on pasture subjected to licuri oil supplement. Rev Bras Zootec 40(12):2858–2865

Lopez A, Vasconi M, Moretti VM, Bellagamba F (2019) Fatty acid profile in goat milk from high- and low-input conventional and organic systems. Animals 9(7):452

Maghazechi A, Nafchi AM, Tan TC, Seow EK, Easa AM (2021) Rheological characterization of coconut cream emulsion using steady-state shear and time-dependent modeling. J Food Eng 306:110642

Mahayothee B, Koomyart I, Khuwijitjaru P, Siriwongwilaichat P, Nagle M, Müller J (2016) Phenolic compounds, antioxidant activity, and medium chain fatty acids profiles of coconut water and meat at different maturity stages. Int J Food Prop 19:2041–2051

Manikantan MR, Mathew AC, Madhavan K, Arumuganathan T, Arivalagan M, Shameena Beegum PP, Hebbar KB (2016) Coconut chips-entrepreneurship driven ICAR-CPCRI technology for healthy alternative nonfried snack food. Technical bulletin No. 107. ICAR-Central Plantation Crops Research Institute, Kasaragod

Manivannan A, Bhardwaj R, Padmanabhan S, Suneja P, Hebbar KB, Kanade SR (2018) Biochemical and nutritional characterization of coconut (Cocos nucifera L.) haustorium. Food Chem 238:153–159

Mardiati E, Rikawarastuti R, Wiradona I (2022) The effect of dental paste from coconut butter as a replacement to toothpaste on reducing debris index and plaque index in class 3 to 5 students in elementary school. Open Access Macedonian J Med Sci 10:184–189

Marikkar JMN, Jayasundarav JMMA, Prasadika SAH, Jayasinghe CVL, Premakumara GAS (2007) Assessment of the stability of virgin coconut oil during deep-frying. Coconut Res Dev J 22:34–41

Molina MR, Lachance PA (1973) Studies on the utilization of coconut meal a new enzymic-chemical method for fiber free protein extraction of defatted coconut flour. J Food Sci 38(4):607–610

Nadeeshani R, Wijayaratna UN, Prasadani WC, Ekanayake S, Seneviratne KN, Jayathilaka N (2015) Comparison of the basic nutritional characteristics of the first extract and second extract of coconut milk. Int J Innov Res Sci Eng Technol 4:9516–9521. https://doi.org/10.15680/IJIRSET.2015.0410003

Nagashree RS, Manjunath NK, Indu M, Ramesh M, Venugopal V, Sreedhar P, Pavithra N, Nagendra HR (2017) Effect of a diet enriched with fresh coconut saturated fats on plasma lipids and erythrocyte fatty acid composition in normal adults. J Am Coll Nutr 36(5):330–334. https://doi.org/10.1080/07315724.2017.1280713

Nevin KG, Rajamohan T (2006) Virgin coconut oil supplemented diet increases the antioxidant status in rats. Food Chem 99:260–266

Ng YJ, Tham PE, Khoo KS, Cheng CK, Chew KW, Show PL (2021) A comprehensive review on the techniques for coconut oil extraction and its application. Bioprocess Biosyst Eng 44(9):1807–1818. https://doi.org/10.1007/s00449-021-02577-9

Ngan T, Hien T, Nhan L, Cang M, Danh P, Phuc N, Bach L (2020) Development and evaluation of shampoo products based on coconut oil source from Ben Tre Province (Vietnam). IOP Conf Ser Mater Sci Eng 959:012026

Ohler JG (1984) Coconut, tree of life. Food and Agriculture Organization of the United Nations, Rome

Ohler JG (1999) Modern coconut management: palm cultivation and products. Intermediate Technology Publications, Rome

Onning G, Wallmark A, Persson M, Akesson B, Elmståhl S, Oste R (1999) Consumption of oat milk for 5 weeks lowers serum cholesterol and LDL cholesterol in free-living men with moderate hypercholesterolemia. Ann Nutr Metab 43(5):301–309. https://doi.org/10.1159/000012798

Othman RA, Moghadasian MH, Jones PJ (2011) Cholesterol-lowering effects of oat β-glucan. Nutr Rev 69(6):299–309. https://doi.org/10.1111/j.1753-4887.2011.00401.x

Pachekrepapol U, Kokhuenkhan Y, Ongsawat J (2021) Formulation of yogurt-like product from coconut milk and evaluation of physicochemical, rheological, and sensory properties. Int J Gastron Food Sci 25:100393

Patil U, Benjakul S (2017) Characteristics of albumin and globulin from coconut meat and their role in emulsion stability without and with proteolysis. Food Hydrocoll 69:220–228

Phonphoem W, Sinthuvanich C, Aramrak A, Sirichiewsakul S, Arikit S, Yokthongwattana C (2022) Nutritional profiles, phytochemical analysis, antioxidant activity and DNA damage protection of Makapuno derived from Thai aromatic coconut. Foods 11(23):3912

Pongtongkam P, Chaiseri S (2020) Effect of antioxidants on reduction of lipid oxidation in canned coconut milk. Agric Nat Resour 54:423–430

Pue AG, Rivu R, Sundarrao K, Kaluwin C, Singh K (1992) Preliminary studies on changes in coconut water during maturation of the fruit. Sci New Guinea 18:81–84

Purseglove JW (1972) Tropical crops, monocotyledons, vol 2. Wiley, London

Rajamohan T, Archana U (2018) Nutrition and health aspects of coconut. In: Krishnakumar V, Thampan P, Nair M (eds) The coconut palm (Cocos nucifera L.)—research and development perspectives. Springer, Singapore, pp 757–777. https://doi.org/10.1007/978-981-13-2754-4_15

Ramesh SV, Pandiselvam R, Thushara R, Manikantan MR, Hebbar KB, Beegum S, Mathew AC, Neenu S, Shil S (2020) Engineering intervention for production of virgin coconut oil by hot process and multivariate analysis of quality attributes of virgin coconut oil extracted by various methods. J Food Process Eng 43(6):e13395

Rebello CJ, Chu YF, Johnson WD, Martin CK, Han H, Bordenave N, Shi Y, O'Shea M, Greenway FL (2014) The role of meal viscosity and oat β-glucan characteristics in human appetite control: a randomized crossover trial. Nutr J 13:49. https://doi.org/10.1186/1475-2891-13-49

Rethinam P, Krishnakumar V (2002) Coconut water: a promising natural health drink-distribution, processing and nutritional benefits. Springer, Cham. https://doi.org/10.1007/978-3-031-107139

Ruengdech A, Siripatrawan U (2021) Application of catechin nanoencapsulation with enhanced antioxidant activity in high pressure processed catechin-fortified coconut milk. LWT 140:110594

Sagon C (2022) Coconut milk, almond milk or soy milk? AARP. https://www.aarp.org/health/healthy-living/info-2017/coconut-almond-soy-milk-cs.html

Samarasinghe HGAS, Samaranayake UC, Dharmaprema GADBS (2023) Exploring the quality and safety issues in the coconut oil processing industry in Sri Lanka: a review. J Sci Univ Kelaniya 16(2):63–76

Samson SJAS, Khaund RN, Cater CM, Mattil KF (1971) Extractability of coconut proteins. J Food Sci 36(5):725–728. https://doi.org/10.1111/j.1365-2621.1971.tb03289.x)

Santos ACMB, Carvalho LSB, Lima DC, Leão DJ, Teixeira LSG, Korn MGA (2014) Determination of micronutrient minerals in coconut milk by ICP OES after ultrasound-assisted extraction procedure. J Food Compos Anal 34(1):75–80. https://doi.org/10.1016/j.jfca.2014.02.008

Satheesh N (2015) Review on production and potential applications of virgin coconut oil. Annals Food Sci Technol 16(1):115–126

Senanayake CM, Algama CH, Wimalasekara RL, Weerakoon WNMTDN, Jayathilaka N, Seneviratne KN (2019) Improvement of oxidative stability and microbial shelf life of vanilla cake by coconut oil meal and sesame oil meal phenolic extracts. J Food Qual 2019:1263629. https://doi.org/10.1155/2019/1263629

Senanayake CM, Hapugaswatta H, Samarawickrama GR, Jayathilaka N, Seneviratne KN (2021) Effect of chain length and saturation of the fatty acids in dietary triglycerides on lipid metabolism in Wistar rats. J Food Biochem 45(4):e13664. https://doi.org/10.1111/jfbc.13664

Seneviratne KN, Dissanayake DMS (2005) Effect of method of extraction on the quality of coconut oil. J Sci Univ Kelaniya Sri Lanka 2:63–72

Seneviratne KN, Dissanayake DMS (2008) Variation of phenolic content in coconut oil extracted by two conventional methods. Int J food Sci Technol 43:597–602

Seneviratne K, Jayathilaka N (2016) Coconut oil: chemistry and nutrition. Lakva Publishers, Battaramulla

Seneviratne KN, Hapuarachchi CD, Ekanayake S (2009) Comparison of the phenolic-dependent antioxidant properties of coconut oil extracted under cold and hot conditions. Food Chem 114(4):1444–1449. https://doi.org/10.1016/j.foodchem.2008.11.038

Seneviratne KN, Prasadani WC, Jayawardena B (2016) Phenolic extracts of coconut oil cake: a potential alternative for synthetic antioxidants. Food Sci Technol Campinas 36(4):591–597

Sethi S, Tyagi SK, Anurag RK (2016) Plant-based milk alternatives an emerging segment of functional beverages: a review. J Food Sci Technol 53(9):3408–3423. https://doi.org/10.1007/s13197-016-2328-3

Singh SG, Vij R, Katoch S (2021) Comparison of dairy milk with vegan milk of different types available in India. Pharma Innov J 10(11):24–29

Sukeksi L, Diana V (2020) Preparation and characterization of coconut oil based soap with kaolin as filler. J Phys Conf Ser 1542:012046. https://doi.org/10.1088/1742-6596/1542/1/012046

Thungkao P (1988) Application of emulsifiers and gums for the stabilization of canned coconut milk. Master's thesis, Department of Food Science and Technology, Kasetsart University, Bangkok

Timmins WH, Kramer EC (1977) The canning of coconut cream. Philippines J Coconut Stud 2:15–25

Tulashie SK, Amenakpor J, Atisey S, Odai R, Akpari EEA (2022) Production of coconut milk: a sustainable alternative plant-based milk. Case Stud Chem Environ Eng 6:2022. https://doi.org/10.1016/j.cscee.2022.100206

Vanga SK, Raghavan V (2018) How well do plant based alternatives fare nutritionally compared to cow's milk? J Food Sci Technol 55(1):10–20. https://doi.org/10.1007/s13197-017-2915-y

Wadanambi PM, Seneviratne KN, Jayathilaka N (2023) *In silico* evaluation of coconut milk phenolic antioxidants and their inhibition of oxidative stress in intestinal *Lactobacillus* spp. *in vitro*. Chem Pap 77:2611–2624. https://doi.org/10.1007/s11696-022-02650-x

Wallace TC (2019) Health effects of coconut oil—a narrative review of current evidence. J Am Coll Nutr 38(2):97–107

Wang J, Wang X, Li J, Chen Y, Yang W, Zhang L (2015) Effects of dietary coconut oil as a medium-chain fatty acid source on performance, carcass composition and serum lipids in male broilers. Asian Australas J Anim Sci 28(2):223–230. https://doi.org/10.5713/ajas.14.0328

Wardah S, Djatna T, Marimin M, Yani M (2020) New product development in coconut-based agro-industry: current research progress and challenges. Earth Environ Sci 472:012053. https://doi.org/10.1088/1755-1315/472/1/012053

Whitehead A, Beck EJ, Tosh S, Wolever TM (2014) Cholesterol-lowering effects of oat β-glucan: a meta-analysis of randomized controlled trials. Am J Clin Nutr 100(6):1413–1421. https://doi.org/10.3945/ajcn.114.086108

Wignjosoesastro N, Brooks CC, Herrick RB (1972) The effect of coconut meal and coconut oil in poultry rations on the performance of laying hens. Poult Sci 51(4):126–1132

Yalegama C, Sovis M, Dissanayake D (2015) Effect of antioxidant and heat treatment on the free fatty acids formation of differently processed coconut oil. COCOS 21:43–52

Yong JW, Ge L, Ng YF, Tan SN (2009) The chemical composition and biological properties of coconut (*Cocos nucifera L.*) water. Molecules 14(12):5144–5164. https://doi.org/10.3390/molecules14125144

Zaheer K, Akhtar MH (2017) An updated review of dietary isoflavones: nutrition, processing, bioavailability and impacts on human health. Crit Rev Food Sci Nutr 57(6):1280–1293. https://doi.org/10.1080/10408398.2014.989958

Zhu YG, Williams PN, Meharg AA (2008) Exposure to inorganic arsenic from rice: a global health issue? Environ Pollut (Barking Essex: 1987) 154(2):169–171. https://doi.org/10.1016/j.envpol.2008.03.015

Chapter 5
Coconut Tender and Mature Nut Water: The Tropical Refreshing and Nutritive Drink

V. Krishnakumar

Abstract Coconut water, derived from the *Cocos nucifera* L. has evolved from a traditional tropical beverage to a globally recognized natural functional drink. Its composition, rich in sugars, minerals, vitamins, amino acids, and phytohormones, contributes to its popularity and perceived health benefits. Quality parameters like water-to-nut ratio and total soluble solids are crucial in determining the suitability of coconut varieties for water production, with dwarf varieties often being preferred for their flavor profile. Scientific research continues to uncover the health and medicinal properties of coconut water, expanding its potential beyond hydration. Its use in plant tissue culture and micropropagation highlights its versatility, stemming from its unique chemical composition. This chapter aims to provide a comprehensive overview of coconut water's biochemical composition, health benefits, and various derived products, shedding light on its diverse applications and value.

Keywords Coconut water · Tender coconut water · Maturity indices · Functional drink · Coconut water-based products

5.1 Introduction

Coconut water (CW) refers to the clear water within the endosperm or kernel of the of 7–8 months old tender fruit prior to the formation of solid endosperm (Yong et al. 2009). The tender coconut water (TCW) is the nutritious, sweet beverage of tropics obtained from the immature nuts of coconut. CW has garnered much attention in the rapidly evolving functional foods sector catering to the development of products enriched with nutritional contents. The natural CW has a calorific value of 17–19 100 g^{-1} (Salgueiro and Nunes 2008). The CW mainly comprises water (95%) and carbohydrates (4%) whereas protein and fat contents are low (less than 1%). CW

V. Krishnakumar (✉)
ICAR-Central Plantation Crops Research Institute (ICAR-CPCRI), Regional Station, Kayamkulam, Kerala, India

S. V. Ramesh, S. Praveen (eds.), *Coconut-Based Nutrition and Nutraceutical Perspectives*, https://doi.org/10.1007/978-981-97-3976-9_5

also contains small quantities of vitamins and minerals contributing to less than 10% of daily RDA values.

During the developmental stage of the nut, it was observed that nuts at 7–8 months of maturity are characterized by high total sugars in water, with the sugar content gradually decreasing thereafter (Burns et al. 2020; Prades et al. 2012a; Priya and Ramaswamy 2014). Hence, coconut water extracted from nuts in their early stages of maturity (such as tender, young, or immature coconuts) is regarded as a revitalizing beverage (Prades et al. 2012b; Tan et al. 2014a). This is attributed to its sensory appeal, nutritional content, and potential health benefits (Kumar et al. 2021). During the initial stages of its development, coconut water typically contains around 2% total solids. This concentration gradually rises as the coconut matures, peaking around the 7th month, just before the solid endosperm forms, and then decreases again thereafter.

Coconut water (CW) is described as a slightly cloudy to transparent liquid, lacking colour, and possessing a unique flavour that is sweet with a subtle acidity (Borse et al. 2007). Its pH typically falls within the range of 4.2 to 6.0. The nutrients present in CW originate from the seed's apoplasm (the area surrounding the cell wall) and are transported internally via plasmodesmata into the endosperm. CW is abundant in electrolytes, vitamins, minerals, cytokinins, and proteins, making it renowned for its diverse medicinal properties. CW is commonly consumed by directly extracting it from the inner part of coconuts (Steiner and Desser 2008; Marikkar and Madhrapperuma 2012). Additionally, it serves as a rehydrating beverage post vigorous physical activity, as highlighted by Saat et al. (2002). However, due to its perishable nature, exposure to atmospheric oxygen leads to decreased enzyme activity and increases the risk of external microbial contamination. Consequently, this can alter CW's characteristic properties, including its nutritive value, taste, and colour.

The terms Coconut Water (CW), Tender Coconut Water (TCW), and Green Coconut Water (GCW) are often used interchangeably to refer to the liquid endosperm of coconuts. However, they do showcase differences primarily related to maturity and coconut variety. TCW typically refers to the water collected from coconuts that are 7–8 months mature, known for its sweetness and sometimes referred to as Young Coconut Water (Tetra Pack 2019). Mature Coconut Water (MCW) or simply Coconut Water (CW) is obtained from nuts aged 10–13 months, while GCW specifically comes from a variety known as green dwarf or green coconut (Dwiloka et al. 2020). Nevertheless, there are instances where TCW and GCW are used interchangeably.

While both TCW and MCW hold nutritional significance, it is primarily the fresh TCW from young nuts that is favoured by consumers as a health drink. This preference extends to both direct consumption after extraction from tender nuts and consumption after processing into various packaged beverages (Mahayothee et al. 2016). Notably, MCW is often not preferred as a refreshing beverage due to its less appealing taste. Consequently, there exists a general belief among consumers that TCW is nutritionally rich and contains mostly health-protective nutrients.

5.2 Global Demand for Coconut Water

CW is widely regarded as a natural energy booster due to its antioxidant content and other nutritional properties, making it an ideal choice for replenishing lost energy during sports and strenuous activities. It has also gained popularity as a convenient ready-to-drink (RTD) healthy beverage, often seen as a healthier alternative to carbonated drinks and processed juices. In fact, CW has become the fastest-growing beverage category not only in the USA but also in other countries. Major multinational companies like Vita Coco®, Zico®, O.N.E.®, and Coca-Cola (ZICO) have capitalized on this trend by being early entrants into the TCW market, positioning CW as a natural sports drink. Consequently, their sales have seen significant growth, reaching up to US $30 million in the late 2000s. Today, CW is available in a variety of flavours such as pineapple, mango, lime, matcha tea, and many more, catering to diverse consumer preferences.

The global market for organic CW is poised to be driven by its numerous health benefits. Additionally, CW's characteristics such as antioxidant content, enhanced taste, and diverse micronutrients may lead consumers to prefer it over conventional soft drinks. Reports highlighting the beauty benefits of daily CW consumption, along with its popularity in yoga institutes and health clubs, are expected to create opportunities for companies in the organic CW market. Major regions for organic CW consumption include Latin America, North America, Asia-Pacific, Europe, Japan, the Middle East, and Africa. Consumption of CW is particularly high in tropical countries like Sri Lanka, India, Thailand, and Brazil, where large-scale coconut cultivation is prevalent. In the UK alone, organic CW consumption stands at approximately 25–26 million liters. The global organic CW market size is projected to reach nearly US$9.25 billion by 2029, with a compound annual growth rate (CAGR) of 15.89% during the forecast period. The increasing demand for CW-based products, including pasteurized TCW, sparkling CW, flavored CW, and pure CW vinegar, has spurred the growth of the coconut-based beverage industry.

5.3 Composition of Tender Nut Water

5.3.1 Sugars

In MCW, the primary sugars are sucrose, sorbitol, glucose, and fructose (Ogundiya 1991). Additionally, minor sugars such as galactose, xylose, and mannose are present, while tartaric, citric, and malic acids are the predominant organic acids, according to Deb Mandal and Mandal (2011). Campbell-Falck et al. (2000) further highlighted that the main sugars responsible for the sweet taste in CW are fructose, glucose, and sucrose. The sugar content in CW typically follows a decreasing order of fructose > glucose > sucrose. The sucrose content varies with the maturity of the nuts, with the order being OMC > MC > IMC, as observed by Magda (1992).

Initially, during the early stages of nut growth, only invert sugars are present, reaching a maximum concentration by the 5th and 6th month of maturity. Subsequently, the sucrose level rises, although the total sugar concentration declines rapidly until it reaches approximately 2.0 g/100 mL. In fully mature nuts, sucrose typically constitutes around 50.0% of the total sugar content, while the concentration of reducing sugars (glucose and fructose) reaches around 5.0% when CW is fully formed. Ajibogun and Oboma (2013) reported higher glucose content in TCW compared to MCW. The sugar content of green sea CW from 7-month-old nuts was reported as 280 mg/100 mL for sucrose, 2378 mg/100 mL for glucose, and 2400 mg/100 mL for fructose (Rosa and Abreu 2000).

Apshara et al. (2007) observed that coconut cultivar and stage of maturity influence the sugar content in CW. In all three stages of nut development (i.e., 6, 7, and 8 months), the mean total sugar content was higher in the COD cultivar, with the COD × WCT hybrid recording the highest value. The maturity of nuts also affects Brix (soluble solids content), pH, and total sugar levels in different coconut cultivars. The total sugar levels increase from the 5th to the 7th month, reaching a maximum in various cultivars. In the Green Dwarf coconut variety, Kwiatkowski et al. (2008) reported a decrease in total sugar and reducing sugar content from the 6th to the 9th month of maturity. Anselme et al. (2018) found that monosaccharides present in sugar made from TCW followed the order fructose > glucose > mannose, with traces of galactose. Sugars from EGD, MYD, and PB121+ cultivars were slightly sweeter due to higher sucrose content compared to PB113+. The percentage of total sugar and total reducing sugar in TCW and MCW was reported as 4.8% and 3.1%, and 4.0% and 2.0%, respectively (Sandhya and Rajamohan 2008). Coconut water from 6-month-old nuts contained 5.23 g/100 g of total sugars, with sucrose, glucose, and fructose at 0.06, 2.61, and 2.55, respectively (Yong et al. 2009).

In the early stages of nut maturity, coconut water primarily contains glucose and fructose, with reducing sugars being the predominant sugars until the nut matures at around 8 months, after which non-reducing sugars become more prevalent. The variation in total sugars of MCW from various varieties and origins ranged from 1.8 to 4.4 g/100 mL (Prades et al. 2012a). Tan et al. (2014a) observed that the composition and physico-chemical properties of coconut water are influenced by the maturity stage of nuts. The Total Soluble Solids (TSS), indicating the sweetness of coconut water, was highest in MCW (from 8 to 9 months old nuts) compared to immature coconut (IMC) (5–6 months) or over-mature coconut (OMC) water (>12 months). Appaiah et al. (2015) observed that the total sugars content remained almost similar at 4.2, 3.9, and 4.6 g/100 g at different stages of maturity, while there was a slight increase in total solids content depending on the maturity, i.e., TCW1 (3.4), TCW2 (3.7), and MCW (4.3). Aroucha et al. (2015) found that the Green Dwarf coconut cultivar exhibited better physico-chemical composition than Red Dwarf, and nuts harvested at 8th months had higher fructose content than nuts of 7 months maturity.

5.3.2 *Vitamins*

CW serves as a potential source of vitamin C (ascorbic acid) and the vitamin B complex, with its physico-chemical composition varying according to the stage of maturation, variations between varieties, and soil components (Khan et al. 2003; Medeiros and Medeiros 2012). Thampan and Rethinam (2004) reported the presence of nicotinic acid (0.64 μg mL^{-1}) and pantothenic acid (0.52 μg mL^{-1}) in CW. It contains water-soluble vitamins, particularly vitamins B such as Biotin, Niacin, Folic acid, and vitamins C (Deb Mandal and Mandal 2011; Shenkin 2006; Vigliar et al. 2006). Yong et al. (2009) observed trace amounts of Thiamine (B1) and 0.0001 mg/100 mL of Riboflavin (B2) in TCW from 6-month-old nuts. Additionally, CW contains folate (vitamin B9), with Green sea-CW from 7-month-old nuts containing 1.2 mg/100 mL of vitamin C (Rosa and Abreu 2000). Mantena et al. (2003) reported the ascorbic acid content of CW (from 7 to 9 months old nuts) to be 2.2–3.7 mg/100 mL. Freshly harvested CW was found to contain 2.0 mg/100 mL of vitamin C by Dignan et al. (2004) and 1.89 mg/100 mL by Martial-Didier et al. (2017). Sandhya and Rajamohan (2008) reported higher vitamin C content for TCW than MCW (25 mg dL^{-1} and 15 mg dL^{-1}, respectively). The total ascorbic acid content of CW from 6-month-old nuts was found to be 0.0741 mg/100 mL (Yong et al. 2009). Santos et al. (2013) reported vitamin C content in coconuts of four varieties to range from 11.30 to 25.80 μg/mL. Unpasteurized CW from MGD had the highest ascorbic acid content (30.18 μg/mL), while pasteurization at 90 °C for 5 min decreased it to 1.65 μg/mL. Similarly, pasteurization also decreased MYD's content from 19.10 to 3.59 μg/mL. The maturity of nuts and the location of cultivation influence the vitamin C content of CW, with Fowoyo and Alamu (2018) observing the highest and lowest contents (5.56 and 2.20 mg/kg) for MCW and TCW from the Adankolo Market.

5.3.3 *Amino Acids*

CW is abundant in amino acids such as alanine, arginine, cysteine, histidine, lysine, tryptophan, tyrosine, and serine (Deb Mandal and Mandal 2011; Vigliar et al. 2006; Yong et al. 2009). Among the 11 amino acids identified and quantified in TCW, serine, glycine, histidine, tyrosine, phenylalanine, isoleucine, and leucine recorded values greater than 5 mg/500 mL. Sandhya and Rajamohan (2006) noted that L-arginine constituted the major fraction of Free Amino Acids (FAAs), with its content in TCW being 30 mg%. Twishsri et al. (2014) observed significant differences in the contents of aspartic acid, cystine, and serine among other essential amino acids. These differences were noted in the contents of histidine, isoleucine, methionine, and phenylalanine as well. The contents followed the order: 12-month-old nuts of Nam Hom × Kathi hybrid >7-month-old nuts of Maphrao Nam Hom >11-month-old nuts of Maphrao Nam Hom. Besides esters and phenols, Biswas et al. (2020) characterized the presence of pentosyl methyl groups and Free Amino Acids (FAAs) in TCW. Nasution et al. (2020) reported the arginine content (mg/100 mL) of CW from fresh mature nuts, canned CW, and fresh aromatic nuts to be 2.02, 1.85, and 3.14, respectively. Both tall and aromatic varieties of coconut water contained arginine in their composition. Wei et al. (2022) characterized 18 types of amino acids in fresh CW, with high contents of alanine, proline, and phenylalanine, while the total amino acid content reached 588.2 mg/L.

5.3.4 Polyphenols

Phenolic content contributes significantly to the complex flavour profile of CW, with its concentration decreasing as the nut matures. Chang and Wu (2011) reported the presence of (+)-catechin and (−)-epicatechin in CW, with concentrations of 0.344 μg mL^{-1} and 0.242 μg mL^{-1}, respectively. Phenolics are crucial phytochemicals with various bioactive properties, including antioxidant activity (Mahayothee et al. 2016). Catechin and salicylic acid are among the phenolic components found in CW samples, while gallic, caffeic, salicylic, and p-coumaric acids are found in the coconut meat. Green CW (from 9-month-old nuts) was observed to have a lower total phenolic content (TPC as mg GAE per liter) compared to MCW from 12-month-old nuts, with values of 46.03 and 69.16, respectively (Arzeta-Ríos et al. 2020). Wei et al. (2022) identified a total of 37 polyphenol compounds in fresh CW, including 19 flavonoids, 7 anthocyanins, 2 benzaldehydes, and 9 phenolic acids. Among them, chlorogenic acid, procyanidin, L-epicatechin, cinnamic acid, synapic acid, and baicalein were found to be abundant. While coconut water (CW) remains inside the nut, it is considered sterile and stable (Yong et al. 2009). However, upon extraction and exposure to air, certain reactions occur, primarily oxidation facilitated by enzymes such as Polyphenol oxidase (PPO) and Peroxidase (POD), which are naturally present in the CW (da Fonseca et al. 2009a). PPO and POD are the main browning enzymes, leading to changes in the sensory and nutritional quality of Tender Coconut Water (TCW) (Duarte et al. 2002). Campos et al. (1996) noted that both enzymes were present and active in green CW, with their optimal activity occurring at pH 6.0 and 5.5, and at temperatures of 25 °C and 35 °C, respectively. Abreu and Faria (2007) reported the activities of PPO and POD (U per ml) for Green Dwarf CW as 2.33 and 12.2, respectively, while according to Aliberti et al. (2009), the range of activities for CW from green coconuts (U per ml) are 0.1–34.8 and 0.1–6.2.

5.3.5 Antimicrobial Peptides (AMPs)

Antimicrobial peptides (AMPs) are increasingly recognized as a promising class of antibiotics due to their various beneficial properties, including their amphipathic structures, cationic nature, and low likelihood of inducing microbial resistance (Biswaro et al. 2018). Over the years, numerous novel AMPs with promising therapeutic properties have been discovered. These peptides are small in size, consisting of amino acid polymers, and demonstrate efficacy against a wide range of microorganisms (Cruz et al. 2014). One such example is Coconut antimicrobial peptide (CnAMP), a naturally occurring bioactive peptide derived from green coconut water. CnAMP holds potential as an effective agent against microbial pathogens, contributing to the growing interest in utilizing natural sources for the development of antimicrobial therapies. Wang and Ng (2005) identified four peptides in TCW, including a 10 kDa peptide with antifungal activity. Mandal et al. (2009) further investigated and purified novel antimicrobial peptides (Cn-AMPs) weighing over 3 kDa from TCW. They identified peptides named Cn-AMP1, Cn-AMP2, and Cn-AMP3, which exhibited high efficiency against both pathogenic Gram-positive and Gram-negative bacteria (*E. coli, B. subtilis, P. aeruginosa, S. aureus*), with Cn-AMP1 showing the highest activity. Interestingly, the three-dimensional structures of these isolated peptides did not bear any resemblance to existing protein structures. Santana et al. (2015) elucidated the structure of Cn-AMP1, a disulfide-free peptide isolated from green coconut water. Additionally, Prabhu et al. (2014) found that Cn-AMP2, an anionic host defense peptide from green coconut water, possessed anti-proliferative activity against the 1321 N1 and U87MG human glioma cell lines. Anaya et al. (2020) investigated the cellular uptake of the coconut water antimicrobial peptide Cn-AMP1 in LS180 and Caco-2 cells. They found that this peptide did not interfere with P-glycoprotein (P-gp) expression and activity, suggesting that it did not alter the bioavailability of xenobiotics. These findings highlighted the potential of Cn-AMP1 as a novel antimicrobial compound.

5.3.6 Aromatics

TCW contains a minor fraction of aromatic compounds, contributing to its characteristic aroma (Prades et al. 2012a). Various organic acids such as malic, succinic, citric, acetic, and tartaric acids influence the taste of TCW, while volatile compounds contribute to its aroma. Jirovetz et al. (2003) identified 30 compounds in MCW, with nonanal (14.2%), nonanol (11.2%), heptanal (8.2%), ethyl octanoate (6.2%), heptanol (5.3%), and 2-nonanol (5.1%) being the most abundant. Additionally, da Fonseca et al. (2009b) detected alcohols, ketones, thiols, carboxylic acids, phenols, and esters with short carbon chains in the essential oil of TCW. Among these compounds, ester n-propyl ethanoate likely contributes to the flavor of TCW. The fragrant substance 2-acetyl-1-pyrroline (2-AP) imparts the unique aroma characteristic of Thai Aromatic Coconut, which is the primary coconut cultivar for young TCW consumption in Thailand (Luckanatinvong and Sornkeaw 2011). Krisanapook et al. (2016) investigated the synthesis of 2-AP throughout nut development and factors influencing fragrance control. It was observed that the presence of 2-AP in both CW and solid endosperm at the 6th month of growth, with its concentration increasing as the nut matured. Interestingly, the amount of 2-AP was higher in the kernel than in CW. Jaroonchon et al. (2017) discovered the presence of 2-AP in CW and coconut meat at the 2nd and 5th months of growth, respectively. However, 2-AP content in CW (47 ng g^{-1}fw) was detectable only when the nut matured to 6 months, and it increased with maturity, reaching a maximum of 2036 ng g^{-1} fw at 9 months of growth. Although the content of 2-AP was highest at the 9th month of aromatic CW and meat, the ideal stage for consuming aromatic coconut is when the nuts are 6½ to 7 months old. At this stage, the meat texture is optimal, and CW exhibits the best smell and taste.

5.3.7 *Electrolytes*

CW is a rich source of potassium (K), sodium (Na), and other trace minerals like calcium (Ca) and magnesium (Mg), which help restore electrolyte balance in the body. This makes it an ideal post-workout drink. The concentration of these electrolytes in CW creates an osmotic pressure similar to that found in the body, without affecting plasma coagulation, thereby aiding in hydration (Petroianu et al. 2004). Specifically, CW contains natural electrolytes at millimolar concentrations, including Ca (6.6 m mL^{-1}), K (77.3 m mL^{-1}), and Na (2.2 m mL^{-1}), along with sugars that can help overcome dehydration in athletes.

The levels of K and Mg ions in CW exceed those found in extracellular fluids (ECF), making it an excellent source of electrolytes. Additionally, CW serves as a significant source of Ca for the body, potentially preventing nutritional rickets in infants. Other essential minerals such as iron (Fe), zinc (Zn), and manganese (Mn) are also present in appreciable amounts in CW. Despite minerals constituting only 0.4–1% of the liquid volume in a coconut, they play a crucial role in maintaining its isotonic properties. The mineral content of CW varies throughout the nut maturation process. According to Aragao et al. (2001a), K remains the most abundant electrolyte throughout maturation, while sodium (Na) experiences an increase. Calcium (Ca), magnesium (Mg), chloride (Cl^-), iron (Fe), and copper (Cu) levels remain stable during maturation, with sulfur (S) showing a gradual increase. These changes are primarily attributed to biochemical processes responsible for transforming the liquid endosperm into solid endosperm (Aragao et al. 2001b). Several studies have highlighted K as the most significant mineral element in CW (Richter et al. 2005; Uphade et al. 2008). Rosa and Abreu (2000) reported K to be the highest mineral content (156.86 mg 100 g^{-1}), followed by calcium (Ca) (17.10 mg 100 g^{-1}) in Green sea-CW from nuts aged 7 months. The differences in mineral composition between TCW and MCW are mainly attributed to variations in K, chloride (Cl^-), iron (Fe), and sulfur (S) content (Thampan and Rethinam 2004), although Santoso et al. (1996) observed differences mainly in K, copper (Cu), and sodium (Na) content. Chidambaram et al. (2013) noted that TCW is characterized by high levels of K+ among cations and Cl^- among anions, with an acidic to neutral pH and high electrical conductivity. The K content (mg 100 mL^{-1}) varies with nut maturity, being 198.7 and 215.8 at 7th and 9th months of maturity, respectively (Priya and Ramaswamy 2014). As the solid albumen forms and hardens, the volume of CW decreases, leading to a concentration of ions like K^+ and Cl^- in the kernel, causing significant variations in their concentration during TCW maturation. Additionally, comparisons of CW composition have shown notable differences in phosphorus (P), sulfur (S), and chloride (Cl−) content.

The high potassium content makes CW an ideal natural hydration beverage, serving as an excellent alternative to commercialized isotonic drinks. Halim et al. (2018) found MCW to possess higher ergogenic properties compared to TCW due to its elevated content of functional electrolytes. CW from MYD × Tagnanan Tall is identified as particularly ideal for developing a natural ergogenic drink due to its high K and Na contents. Trace elements, required by the body in small quantities for normal growth and development, are also present in CW. These essential elements, in the form of low-molecular-weight stable complexes, are known for their bioavailability. CW samples from various origins exhibit particularly high concentrations of iron (Fe), nickel (Ni), copper (Cu), zinc (Zn), and manganese (Mn), especially in samples from the Ivory Coast. Alchoubassi et al. (2021) reported total element concentrations (ppm) ranging from 0.2 to 2.7 for Fe, 0.3 to 1 for Cu, 3 to 14 for Mn, and 0.5 to 2.0 for Zn, with variations based on nut origin and maturity.

5.3.8 *Enzymes*

Enzymes such as phosphatase, catalase, dehydrogenase, diastase, peroxidase, polyphenol oxidase, and RNA polymerases have been identified in CW, as reported by Deb Mandal and Mandal (2011), Jayakumar et al. (2015), Yong et al. (2009), and Prades et al. (2012a). Additionally, CW contains oxido reductase enzymes, including polyphenol oxidase (PPO) and peroxidase (POD). The enzymatic activity is highest in nuts aged 5–7 months and diminishes with ripening (Rosa and Abreu 2000). While these enzymes serve specific and vital functions within the nut, upon exposure to atmospheric air, they can initiate undesired reactions, particularly leading to the development of pink discoloration.

5.3.9 Phytohormones

CW has been identified as containing indole-3-acetic acid (IAA), the primary auxin in plants, as highlighted by Ma et al. (2008). The IAA content in green TCW was reported as 150.6 nM, while in MCW, it ranged from 0.25 ± 0.03 to 1.46 ± 0.13 μg mL^{-1} (Wu and Hu 2009). Additionally, Tan et al. (2014b) estimated the concentration ($\times 10^{-3}$ μM) of various phytohormones in CW, revealing values of 198.2, 15.3, 49.6, and 0.1 for indole-3-acetic acid, abscisic acid, gibberellic acid, and zeatin, respectively. Moreover, CW stands out as the richest natural dietary source of cytokinins. Extensive studies have uncovered many previously uncharacterized coconut cytokinins (Ge et al. 2008; Ma et al. 2008). Lazim et al. (2015) observed that variety and nut maturity influenced the content of cytokinins in CW. Among the MGD and MYD varieties, MGD exhibited the highest cytokinin content, measured at 3.2841 μM. Trans-zeatin riboside emerged as the major cytokinin compound in both varieties. Total cytokinin concentration peaked during the immature stage (120–200 days) for the MYD variety, while for MGD, it was high during the mature (220–300 days) and over mature (beyond 320 days) stages.

5.4 Composition of Mature Coconut Water

The water obtained from coconuts aged 10 to 13 months, termed as MCW, generally exhibits differences compared to the water from younger coconuts. In MCW, sugar levels and total phenolic contents tend to be lower than in the water from tender or young coconuts. Conversely, MCW typically has higher protein levels and pH values compared to the water from younger coconuts. It's interesting to note how the composition and properties of coconut water change as the nuts mature. The decrease in quantity of coconut water and the increase in crude fat content during ripening can indeed impact its flavour negatively. Additionally, the differences in salt, protein, and sugar content between MCW and TCW highlight how these factors influence the overall characteristics and taste of the water obtained from coconuts at different stages of maturity (Zhang et al. 2018a, b; Fowoyo and Alamu 2018). Adjusting the processing methods and adding specific components like amino acids can potentially mitigate these changes and improve the quality and shelf life of MCW. These insights are valuable for understanding how coconut water can be utilized and optimized for various applications based on its age and composition (Awua et al. 2011; Nasution et al. 2019). Tanqueco et al. (2007) and Prades et al. (2012a) highlight the variability in total sugar and total phenolic content in MCW across different coconut varieties and origins. In MCW from various varieties, the total sugar content ranged from 1.8 to 4.4 g/100 mL, indicating significant differences based on genetic and environmental factors. Furthermore, Tanqueco et al. (2007) observed that the total free sugar content varied among different coconut varieties, with Aromatic Dwarf exhibiting the highest total free sugar content, followed by Laguna Tall and San Ramon Tall. This variation in sugar content can influence the sweetness and overall flavor profile of MCW from different coconut varieties. Similarly, the total phenolic content in MCW also showed variability across coconut varieties, with Laguna Tall exhibiting the highest phenolic content, followed by Aromatic Dwarf and San Ramon Tall. Phenolic compounds contribute to the antioxidant properties and flavor profile of coconut water, and their levels can be influenced by genetic factors and environmental conditions. Additionally, Tan et al. (2014a) highlighted the influence of nut maturity stage on the composition and physico-chemical properties of coconut water. The Total Soluble Solids (TSS), an indicator of sweetness, was highest in MCW from 8 to 9 months old nuts compared to immature (5–6 months old nuts) or overmature (>12 months old nuts) coconuts. Overall, these findings underscore the importance of considering factors such as coconut variety, origin, and nut maturity stage in understanding the variability in the composition and quality of MCW. Studies have revealed variations in the total phenolics content (TPC) and enzymatic activity of PPO and peroxidase POD in CW at different stages of nut maturity (Tan et al. 2014a). Specifically, the TPC in CW was highest in immature coconuts (IMC) to MC and overmature coconuts (OMC), indicating a decrease in phenolic content as the coconut matures. This decrease in phenolic content is accompanied by a reduction in the enzymatic activity of PPO and POD as the coconut matures.

Furthermore, the vitamin C content in CW was found to vary with nut maturity, with CW from 10-month-old mature nuts exhibiting lower vitamin C content compared to CW from 6-month-old mature nuts. This suggests that the vitamin C content of CW may decline as the coconut matures (Sandhya and Rajamohan 2008). Additionally, the protein content was higher in MCW compared to TCW, indicating differences in nutritional composition between the two (Keng et al. 2017). Moreover, the alcohol content in fermented MCW and TCW was directly related to their sugar content, with higher sugar content resulting in higher alcohol content (Akpomie et al. 2020). Finally, CW from 9-month-old nuts had a lower TPC compared to CW from 12-month-old nuts, and they also differed in their antioxidant capacity as measured by the ABTS radical scavenging assay. These findings highlight the impact of nut maturity on the nutritional composition and antioxidant properties of CW (Arzeta-Ríos et al. 2020).

5.5 Health Benefits of Coconut Water

CW is a nutritional powerhouse, boasting a diverse array of vitamins, minerals, phytohormones, enzymes, and antioxidant compounds. These components play vital roles in human health and are associated with various biological activities and pharmacological effects. CW's rich phytochemical composition includes β-sitosterol, a phytoestrogen known for its diverse health benefits. β-sitosterol has been linked to the prevention of osteoporosis and the acceleration of wound healing. Additionally, CW contains cytokinins like kinetin and trans-zeatin, which exhibit anti-aging effects on human fibroblast cells and possess anti-carcinogenic and anti-thrombotic properties. Trans-zeatin, a significant cytokinin in CW, has shown potential inhibitory effects on acetylcholinesterase (AChE), suggesting a role in the treatment of Alzheimer's disease (AD) and related dysfunctions. Furthermore, research suggests that cytokinins isolated from CW may have anti-cancer properties, sparking interest in their therapeutic potential. Beyond cytokinins and β-sitosterol, CW boasts an array of medicinal properties, including detoxification, antimicrobial, antibacterial, and anti-inflammatory effects. It's also revered for its rejuvenating and diuretic properties. CW has been traditionally used to address gastric dysfunction, dysentery, and child malnutrition, and it may offer some control over hypertension. Studies in experimental animals have revealed that CW possesses hepatoprotective, hypolipidemic, and anti-hypertensive properties. Additionally, in induced diabetic rats, CW has demonstrated hypoglycemic, anti-thrombotic, and antioxidant activities, further underscoring its potential as a therapeutic agent for various health conditions. CW is renowned for its numerous health benefits, including its ability to alleviate symptoms of an upset stomach by soothing the stomach lining and addressing issues like nausea, bloating, and loss of appetite. Regular consumption of TCW helps correct electrolyte imbalances, making it an ideal post-workout drink that also promotes bowel regularity and aids in weight management. Moreover, TCW has been shown to increase hemoglobin levels and serve as an antidote for certain poisons. Its components, such as polysaccharides, lectins, proteins, and peptides, stimulate the immune system and are beneficial in treating conditions like anemia and reducing hemolytic anemia. TCW also plays a role in balancing blood sugar levels by increasing insulin production and regulating blood glycogen levels. Additionally, it contains active chemicals that may help control HIV infection. In medical settings, CW has been used as a short-term intravenous hydration fluid due to its sterility and osmolarity similar to human plasma (Adetayo et al. 2015; Dissanayake 2017). When administered intravenously, precautions are taken to account for its high potassium content, especially if the coconut shell remains intact. CW's high potassium content also makes it valuable for oral rehydration therapy and in managing conditions like hypertension and anxiety (Campbell-Falck et al. 2000). Furthermore, it has been beneficial in the management of diseases such as myocardial infarction. Beyond its direct medical applications, CW exhibits strong antioxidant activity, contributing to its overall health-promoting properties. It is also occasionally fermented to extend its shelf life and enhance its probiotic content, offering additional health benefits (Bandalan and Galvez 2016).

5.5.1 Anti-microbial

The antimicrobial properties of CW extend beyond its phenolic compounds to include peptides with anti-fungal activity (Effong et al. 2010; Fan et al. 2017). For instance, a 10 kDa peptide isolated from CW demonstrated significant anti-fungal effects against various pathogens, including *Fusarium oxysporum, Mycosphaerella arachidicola*, and *Physalospora piricola* (Wang and Ng 2005). Research has identified antimicrobial peptides in CW with inhibitory properties against both Gram-positive and Gram-negative human pathogens. These peptides, which are lower than 3 kDa in size, have been purified and characterized from TCW (Mandal et al. 2009; Nasimuddin et al. 2016). Additionally, TCW has demonstrated a strong dose-dependent anti-fungal effect against Candida albicans, with the highest inhibitory effect observed at a concentration of 1000 μg mL^{-1} (Cholan et al. 2017). Furthermore, TCW exhibits high antimicrobial activity against gastrointestinal pathogens compared to MCW. This difference is attributed to the potency of antimicrobial compounds present in TCW, such as lauric acid and peptides, which decrease substantially as the coconut matures. These findings underscore the potential of TCW as a natural antimicrobial agent with efficacy against a broad spectrum of pathogens (Fowoyo and Alamu 2018).

5.5.2 Anti-bacterial

Nasimuddin et al. (2016) has reported the antibacterial effect of CW against *Candida albicans* and *Klebsiella pneumoniae*. However, Baharvand et al. (2021) found that the antibacterial effect of CW on *Aggregatibacter actinomycetemcomitans* was weak. Additionally, Rohaeti et al. (2018) investigated CW-based cellulose composites and found that composites containing cellulose-glycerol-chitosan-silver nanoparticles exhibited the highest antibacterial activity against *Staphylococcus aureus*, while composites of cellulose-glycerol-silver nanoparticles showed the highest activity against *Escherichia coli* and *Candida albicans*. Furthermore, the presence of *Lactobacillus* sp. enhances the antibacterial activity of fermented CW, as demonstrated by Goderska and Czarnecki (2007). Kantachote et al. (2017) found that MCW fermented with *Lactobacillus plantarum* DW12 strain inhibited the growth of various organisms, with *Vibrio parahaemolyticus* being the most inhibited. Similarly, Wijewardena and Amarakoon (2020) reported that fermentation of CW with *Lactobacillus acidophilus* DSM 20079 and *Lactobacillus plantarum* enhanced its antibacterial activity, with *Lactobacillus acidophilus* DSM 20079 showing the highest activity against target pathogens after 48 h of incubation. Unfermented CW did not exhibit any inhibitory effects on the target pathogens.

5.5.3 Anti-inflammatory Effect

The anti-inflammatory potential of CW is attributed to its ability to inhibit prostaglandin production, thereby reducing inflammation and pain. Its rich nutritional composition enables it to treat inflammation both internally and externally. Ajeigbe et al. (2011) found that CW reduced nociception and inflammation in a duration-dependent manner, suggesting its potential as an anti-nociceptive and anti-inflammatory agent. This effect is likely mediated by CW's unique combination of sugars, vitamins, minerals, amino acids, and cytokinin acids. Furthermore, Lakshmanan et al. (2020) demonstrated that TCW reduces proinflammatory gene expression and hepatocyte injury caused by elevated inflammatory cytokines and nitric oxide production. Additionally, Rao and Najam (2016) reported that TCW exhibits a higher anti-inflammatory effect compared to MCW, indicating the potential of CW to mitigate inflammation and associated health issues.

5.5.4 Anti-hypertensive Effect

The significant decrease in blood pressure (BP) and the occurrence of frequent urination after consuming CW indicate its potential diuretic effects without causing electrolyte disorder. The ability of TCW to create a favorable metabolic environment and its antioxidant activity make it an ideal choice for treating clinical conditions associated with hypertension. According to research by Alleyne et al. (2005), regular consumption of CW along with mauby bark syrup controlled hypertension effectively. CW contributed to improved and controlled hypertension by reducing mean systolic and diastolic pressure. Farapti et al. (2013) observed that consuming TCW from 6 to 8-month-old nuts of hybrid coconuts, which had a potassium content of 1789 ± 116.7 mg L^{-1}, at a dosage of 300 mL twice daily for 14 consecutive days, tended to decrease systolic BP, although not diastolic BP. Similarly, Gullapalli et al. (2013) reported that consuming fresh TCW at a dosage of 300 mL/day for 1½ months resulted in a reduction of 10.5 mmHg in systolic BP and 6.8 mmHg in diastolic BP among patients. The high potassium content in TCW causes vasodilation and improves endothelial function, contributing to its beneficial effects on blood pressure regulation.

5.5.5 Hepatoprotective Effect

TCW administered at a dosage of 6 mL/100 g of body weight exhibited hepatoprotective and antioxidant effects in female Sprague Dawley rats intoxicated with CCl_4, as demonstrated by Loki and Rajamohan (2003). Similarly, Okere et al. (2011) found that administering CW at a dosage of 100 mL/kg of body weight for 2 weeks reduced hyperbilirubinemia in alloxan-induced diabetic rats, with lowered serum levels of AST and ALT confirming its hepatoprotective properties. Manna et al. (2014) reported that TCW from 6 to 7-month-old nuts, along with its active phytoconstituent shikimic acid, reversed hydrogen peroxide-induced oxidative damage in hepatocytes. Moreover, Offor et al. (2014) observed dose-dependent significant reductions in the activities of liver enzymes such as AST, ALT, and ALP in albino rats following CW administration, highlighting its hepatoprotective effect.

Various other studies have also reported the beneficial hepatoprotective effects of TCW, including those conducted by Bispo et al. (2017), Mordi et al. (2015), Ndubuka et al. (2015), Nair and Rajamohan (2014), Okafor et al. (2016a), and Okafor et al. (2016b).

5.5.6 Cardioprotective Effect

TCW, being a significant source of free amino acids like L-arginine, is reported to exert cardioprotective effects (Appaiah et al. 2015; Pattigadapa et al. 2011). Various reports suggest that TCW has a beneficial impact on cardiovascular health by reducing serum levels of total cholesterol, LDL, VLDL, and triglycerides. While epidemiological studies propose that high levels of HDL can mitigate cardiovascular diseases like ischemic stroke and MI, the effect of TCW on HDL levels remains controversial (Anurag and Rajamohan 2003; Sandhya and Rajamohan 2006). Anurag and Rajamohan (2003) demonstrated that feeding Sprague-Dawley male albino rats TCW at a dosage of 4 mL/100 g of body weight per day for 45 days protected them from MI induction, leading to improved mitochondrial enzyme activities and reduced mitochondrial lipid peroxidation. Similarly, Sandhya and Rajamohan (2006) reported the cardioprotective effects of MCW or TCW administration in cholesterol-fed rats. They observed that feeding CW for 45 days lowered serum levels of total cholesterol, VLDL + LDL cholesterol, and triglycerides while increasing HDL cholesterol levels. Further supporting evidence came from Tangpong et al. (2008) and Radenahmad et al. (2016), who confirmed the beneficial effects of TCW on lipid profiles by increasing HDL cholesterol without affecting total cholesterol, LDL cholesterol, or triglyceride levels, while also noting no adverse effects on liver and renal functions in rats.

5.5.7 Diuretic Properties

Consuming CW offers several benefits for urinary health. Its natural electrolytes, including potassium (K) and magnesium (Mg), can have a mild diuretic effect, helping to increase urine output and potentially reduce the risk of bladder infections. Additionally, CW contains potassium citrate, which prevents calcium from forming stones in the urinary tract, thus helping to prevent kidney stone formation. Studies by Spencer (2007), Bhagya et al. (2012), and Shubhashree et al. (2014) have highlighted the role of potassium in CW in increasing plasma potassium levels, which may contribute to its anti-hypertensive effects and act as a K-sparing natriuretic. Furthermore, research by Patel et al. (2018a, b) found that consuming TCW at a rate of 2 L/day for 4 days increased urinary citrate, potassium, and chloride levels in individuals without a history of kidney stones. This indicates that CW can enhance urinary excretion and promote the elimination of potentially harmful substances.

Moreover, a study by Wei et al. (2022) demonstrated that CW significantly increased urine excretion and the excretion of sodium (Na) and chloride ions, further supporting its potential as a diuretic and its ability to promote urinary health.

5.5.8 Antioxidant Property

The antioxidant properties of CW have been extensively studied by various researchers, highlighting its potential in combating oxidative stress and related conditions (da Fonseca et al. 2009b; Yong et al. 2009). Loki and Rajamohan (2003) have demonstrated that TCW administration in rodent models can lead to the recovery of antioxidant enzyme levels, such as superoxide dismutase (SOD) and catalase, while decreasing lipid peroxidation, indicating its antioxidant action. The antioxidant potential of CW is attributed to its unique composition, including micronutrients, kinetin, shikimic acid, quinic acid, ascorbic acid, flavonoids, and phenolic compounds (Deb Mandal and Mandal 2011; Ololade et al. 2017). These compounds contribute to CW's total antioxidant capacity, which has been reported to be significant (Ololade et al. 2017). Furthermore, the high content of L-arginine in TCW may play a role in reducing free radical generation, increasing antioxidant activity, and inhibiting lipid peroxidation (Zulaikhah et al. 2015). Studies by Bhagya et al. (2012) and Manna et al. (2014) have shown that CW can decrease free radical activity and improve oxidative stress-related conditions, such as insulin resistance and liver damage. Research by Rao and Najam (2016) and Reddy et al. (2018) further supports the antioxidant effects of TCW, demonstrating its ability to increase antioxidant enzyme levels and decrease lipid peroxidation. More specifically, Reddy et al. 2018 reported the beneficial effect of consumption of TCW by the workers suffering from mercury contamination. Additionally, studies by Agbafor et al. (2015), Kumar et al. (2018), Ndubuka et al. (2015), Rodsamran and Sothornvit (2018), and Vishakh et al. (2014) have contributed to the understanding of CW's antioxidant properties, reflecting the growing interest in natural products and their nutraceutical potential.

5.5.9 Anti-diabetic Effect

The research on the therapeutic effects of CW in managing diabetes is quite extensive and promising. Studies by Preetha et al. (2012), Pinto et al. (2015), and Uddin et al. (2019) have demonstrated that both MCW and TCW have antidiabetic effects, leading to decreased blood glucose levels, improved long-term blood sugar control, and reduction in factors associated with diabetes such as frequent urination, weight loss, and abnormal lipid profiles. Furthermore, research by Ehsayed et al. (2020), Nova et al. (2020), and Zhang et al. (2020) has highlighted the ability of CW to attenuate oxidative stress, inhibit lipid peroxidation, and protect against diabetic complications such as diabetic retinopathy. The protective effects of CW on kidney tissues and its ability to improve renal parameters in diabetic rats have also been demonstrated by Alatawi and Alshubaily (2021).

Studies by Dai et al. (2021) and Zulaikhah et al. (2021) further support the anti-diabetic properties of TCW, showing reductions in blood glucose levels and inflammatory markers in diabetic rats. However, the effect of CW on weight change in diabetic conditions appears to be inconclusive based on the findings of Dai et al. (2021). Overall, the research suggests that CW has promising therapeutic potential in managing diabetes and its associated complications, offering a natural and potentially effective approach to diabetes management.

5.5.10 Hypolipidemic Effect

The research findings from Sandhya and Rajamohan (2008) and Thomas et al. (2017) provide compelling evidence of the hypolipidemic effects of TCW supplementation in animal models. Sandhya and Rajamohan (2008) demonstrated that TCW supplementation in rats fed a fat-cholesterol enriched diet led to a reduction in lipid levels, including total cholesterol, LDL, and triglycerides. Interestingly, the hypolipidemic effect observed with TCW supplementation was comparable to that of lovastatin, a commonly prescribed medication for lowering cholesterol levels. Furthermore, TCW supplementation was associated with increased hepatic bile acid and fecal bile acids and neutral sterols, indicating its potential role in promoting lipid metabolism and excretion. Similarly, Thomas et al. (2017) reported that administration of TCW to male Wistar rats fed a high-fat diet resulted in significant reductions in total cholesterol, LDL cholesterol, and triglyceride levels, while also increasing HDL cholesterol levels.

5.6 Major Value Added Products of Coconut Water

The diverse nutritional profile and functional properties of CW make it a versatile ingredient for enriching a wide range of food and beverage products.

5.6.1 Nata de coco

Nata de coco, also known as coconut gel, originated in the Philippines in 1949 and is made through the fermentation of MCW by *Acetobacter xylinum*, now known as *Gluconacetobacter xylinus* (Nugroho and Aji 2015; Suwannapinunt et al. 2007). It is a chewy, translucent, jelly-like food product that comes in various textures, ranging from very soft and chewy to rather hard. The colour of nata de coco can vary from creamy white to yellow. Chemically, the main fiber component in nata de coco is cellulose, specifically bacterial cellulose (BC). The structure of bacterial cellulose (BC) consists of glucose monomers and lacks hemicellulose, lignin, or pectin (Dayal and Catchmark 2016). This composition contributes to the unique texture and properties of nata de coco. Traditionally, nata de coco is produced in rectangular sheets with a thickness of approximately 1–2 cm. Nata de coco is commonly consumed as a candy or mixed with beverages. Its versatility allows it to be used in a variety of culinary applications, adding texture and flavor to desserts, drinks, and other dishes. The production of nata de coco, or coconut gel, can be influenced by various factors such as the microbial consortium used in fermentation, the immobilization of bacteria, and the composition of the fermentation media. Lakshminarayan (2015) introduced a new technique that utilized a consortium of bacteria and a yeast strain to optimize the production of nata de coco. This approach likely aimed to enhance the fermentation process and increase the yield of nata de coco. Nugroho and Aji (2015) experimented with immobilized *Gluconacetobacter xylinus* to produce nata de coco from MCW. They observed that the average time for nata production was 11 days, with an average thickness of 0.8 cm. Immobilization of the bacteria may have facilitated better control over the fermentation process and improved the consistency of the product. Andasuryani et al. (2017) found that cellulose from nata de coco produced using different fermentation media, such as MCW, coconut milk, and coconut skim, exhibited variations in shape. This suggests that the composition of the fermentation media can influence the structure and characteristics of nata de coco. Indrianingsih et al. (2017) proposed optimal conditions for producing BC films from MCW, recommending a 5% carbon source, pH 5, and a 7-day incubation period. These conditions likely contribute to the efficient production of high-quality BC films with desirable properties for various applications.

Drying plays a crucial role in determining the structure, performance, and application of nata de coco, with dried nata being more preferred due to its convenience and portability. Zhang et al. (2011) compared different drying methods and found that freeze drying resulted in a product with the highest crystallinity, swelling ability, and tensile strengths. Nata de coco, when cut into cubes and immersed in syrup of sugar, can be used as a sweet candy dessert. Additionally, it finds application in various food items such as drinks, puddings, ice cream, pickles, nut salads, and cocktails. Its versatility allows it to be used as a low-calorie additive, thickener, stabilizer, and texture modifier in food applications (Chawla et al. 2009). Azeredo et al. (2019) utilized nata de coco as a raw food material for preparing desserts, additives for drinks, sauces, stuffings, and garnishes for dishes, highlighting its culinary versatility. Furthermore, Rahmayanti et al. (2019) demonstrated the use of dried nata de coco to extend the shelf life of nuts, indicating its potential as a food ingredient with preservative properties. By converting MCW into nata de coco, which is primarily composed of cellulose, it can be further processed into cellulose diacetate, offering added value to its original nature. Membranes fabricated from cellulose diacetate derived from MCW are highly competitive compared to traditional pulps, offering higher membrane permeability (Radiman and Yuliani 2008). Furthermore, MCW serves as a cost-effective and dual carbon source for bacterial cellulose (BC) production by microorganisms like *Gluconacetobacter persimmonis*

(Hungund et al. 2013). BC derived from nata de coco has a unique structure that has led to the development of various non-food applications including biocompatible wound dressings, drug delivery systems, nanomaterials, biodegradable composites, and electronic devices (Treesuppharat et al. 2017).

For instance, carboxymethyl-nata can be used for nut coating, while hydrogel composites derived from nata de coco show promise in drug delivery systems. Moreover, nata de coco has been identified as an efficient green adsorbent for heavy metal cations (Nguyen et al. 2023). Beyond its industrial applications, nata de coco has been associated with various health benefits. It is primarily composed of cellulose, an insoluble fiber, which promotes bowel movements and aids in weight management by promoting feelings of fullness (Tallei et al. 2022). Its low calorie and fat content make it suitable for inclusion in weight-loss diets. Additionally, nata de coco is a good source of vitamin C, essential for a healthy immune system. In many Asian countries, nata de coco has become a popular dessert after meals, enjoyed by people of all ages.

5.6.2 Vinegar

CW serves as an excellent carbohydrate source for the production of fermented beverages and vinegar. Two main technologies have been developed for vinegar production from MCW: the slow process and the quick generation process (Markose and Poduval 1999). The slow process is suitable for cottage-level production, utilizing relatively inexpensive equipment, while the quick generation process is more appropriate for large-scale manufacturing. To produce CW vinegar, the filtered coconut water undergoes an alcoholic fermentation followed by acetification at ambient temperature. Initially, the sugar content is adjusted by adding refined sugar, as raw CW typically has a low sugar content (about 3% w/v). During industrial production, up to 10% (w/v) sugar may be added to enhance fermentation (Yong et al. 2009). The acetification process typically takes about a week, during which acetic acid concentration gradually increases. The final product usually contains between 3% and 4% (v/v) acetic acid (Sanchez 1990). Optimal conditions for fermentation, including inoculum type, pH, total soluble solids (TSS), and nutrient concentration, have been studied to maximize ethanol yield (Shanika and Wansapala 2018). Overall, CW vinegar production offers a sustainable and economically viable method for utilizing coconut water while producing a valuable end product. Naturally fermented CW vinegar is not only flavorful but also packed with essential minerals such as calcium (Ca), iron (Fe), magnesium (Mg), phosphorus (P), potassium (K), sodium (Na), and vitamins like beta-carotene. Primarily used to enhance and preserve foods, CW vinegar is a popular ingredient in salad dressings and marinades.

One of the notable health benefits of CW vinegar is its potential to lower blood sugar levels, attributed to its main component, acetic acid. Additionally, CW vinegar consumption has been associated with weight loss due to its ability to slow down the rate of bowel movement, leading to increased feelings of fullness. Moreover, CW vinegar possesses various health-promoting properties, including anti-inflammatory and antimicrobial effects. Studies have shown that vinegar, including CW vinegar, exhibits bioactivities such as antibacterial, anti-obesity, anti-insulin resistance, and anti-tumor effects (Seo et al. 2014). Specifically, the acetic acid, gallic acid, and vanillic acid contents in CW vinegar contribute to its anti-obesity, hypolipidemic, and anti-inflammatory effects, reducing the risk of obesity and promoting overall health (Mohamad et al. 2017; Mohamad et al. 2019). Furthermore, research on freeze-dried CW vinegar has demonstrated dose-dependent anti-tumor effects in murine 4T1 breast cancer cells, highlighting its potential as a natural therapeutic agent against cancer. Overall, CW vinegar not only adds flavor to dishes but also offers a range of health benefits, making it a valuable addition to a balanced diet and lifestyle.

5.6.3 Exopolysaccharides

Exopolysaccharides (EPSs) are valuable metabolites produced by various microorganisms, including lactic acid bacteria (LAB), and they serve as essential thickening and stabilizing agents in the food industry, enhancing food quality. Shivakumar and Vijayendra (2006) and Survase et al. (2007) have explored the utilization of CW as a cost-effective carbon source for EPS production by microorganisms achieving promising yields of EPS: 11.50 g L^{-1} of water-insoluble EPS and 4.01 g L^{-1} of water-soluble EPS after 72 and 96 h of fermentation, respectively, using CW and *Agrobacterium* sp. Seesuriyachan et al. (2011) investigated the fermentation of 100% MCW by *Lactobacillus confusus* TISTR 1498 and found that with a pH of 5.5, agitation speed at 50 rpm, and an initial sucrose concentration of 100 g L^{-1}, the EPS yield increased significantly up to 38.2 g L^{-1} within 24 h. Similarly, studies by Goveas et al. (2021) and Guo et al. (2022) highlight the potential of utilizing CW and MCW as substrates for EPS production, demonstrating their versatility and effectiveness in supporting microbial growth and EPS synthesis. The produced EPS can serve as a valuable biomaterial with various applications, including as a thickening and stabilizing agent in drinks, cosmetics, and pharmaceutical formulations.

5.6.4 Coconut Water Kefir

Coconut water kefir (CWK) offers a refreshing and health-promoting beverage option made by fermenting coconut water with kefir granules containing beneficial lactic acid bacteria (LAB) and yeast. This fermentation process results in a slightly sour, sweet, and fizzy drink reminiscent of champagne, with added probiotics and enzymes beneficial for gut health. Studies by Limbad et al. (2015) and Dwiloka et al. (2020) have shown that CWK has a low level of sourness, a pleasant sour aroma, and high viscosity, making it an enjoyable beverage with potential health benefits. Limbad et al. (2020) provided a recipe for preparing CWK, and fermented the constituents for up to 48 h at 30 °C. This fermentation period allows for the development of desired flavors and textures while ensuring the retention of beneficial microbial cultures. Furthermore, studies by Limbad et al. (2023) and Aziz et al. (2023) highlight the potential of CWK as a functional food product due to its high total phenolic content (TPC), antioxidant activity, and sensorial acceptance. MCWK (fermented coconut water kefir) demonstrated even greater potential, with higher TPC and antioxidant activities compared to unfermented coconut water. Overall, CWK offers a convenient way to incorporate the benefits of coconut water and probiotics into one's diet, providing a sugar-free option suitable for various dietary preferences and health conditions. Its versatility also extends to its potential use as a starter culture in other fermented food products, further enhancing its value in promoting overall health and well-being.

5.6.5 Gama-Aminobutyric Acid

Gamma-aminobutyric acid (GABA) is a valuable compound found in coconut water, particularly in fermented MCW, with potential therapeutic benefits. Studies by Rahman et al. (2018), Ganesh et al. (2023), and Lazim et al. (2023) have demonstrated the ability of certain microbial strains, such as *Lactobacillus acidophilus* and *L. plantarum*, to increase GABA content during fermentation of coconut water. This increase in GABA levels is attributed to the fermentation process, which promotes the conversion of precursor amino acids, such as glutamic acid, into GABA. Ganesh et al. (2023) suggested that compounds like zeatin present in coconut water may inhibit GABA transaminase, the enzyme responsible for GABA degradation, leading to an accumulation of GABA. Lazim et al. (2023) identified optimal fermentation conditions for maximizing GABA yield, highlighting the potential of fermented coconut water as a functional beverage for managing conditions like hypertension and Parkinson's disease. These findings underscore the potential of fermented coconut water as a source of GABA, which has been associated with stress-alleviating properties and may offer therapeutic benefits for various health conditions.

5.6.6 Carbon Dots

Carbon dots (CDs) have garnered significant interest in various fields due to their unique properties and potential applications. Researchers have explored different methods to synthesize CDs from coconut water (CW), a readily available and sustainable source of carbon (Purbia and Paria 2016; Manoharan et al. 2020; Preethi et al. 2021; Nugroho et al. 2022). Moreover, Jayan et al. (2021) developed a green synthetic approach to synthesize CDs with tunable fluorescence activity from TCW, showcasing the potential for eco-friendly CD production. Jayan and Jayan (2023) reported the synthesis of fluorescent graphene quantum dots from TCW, expanding the repertoire of CD synthesis techniques from this renewable resource. Overall, these studies underscore the versatility of CW as a carbon source for synthesizing CDs with diverse properties and functionalities, opening up new avenues for their utilization in bio-imaging, sensing, and other applications.

5.6.7 Mannosylerythritol Lipids

The production of mannosylerythritol lipids (MELs) using coconut water as a carbon source shows promising results. Prasad et al. (2018) demonstrated a method involving the centrifugation and sterilization of coconut water before inoculating it with *Pseudozyma antarctica* JCM10317, resulting in the production of MEL-A. Similarly, Madihalli et al. (2020) achieved a significant yield of MELs using coconut water, with a higher proportion of MEL-A compared to conventional carbon sources like glycerol. The MEL-A obtained from coconut water showed improved physicochemical properties, including enhanced emulsifying and antioxidant activities, as well as a lower critical micellar concentration. These findings highlight the potential of coconut water as a sustainable and effective substrate for the production of bioactive compounds like MELs.

5.6.8 Bacterial Cellulose

Bacterial cellulose (BC) derived from CW holds immense promise as a versatile biomaterial with various advantageous properties. Studies have highlighted optimal conditions for BC synthesis from CW, showcasing its potential for diverse applications (Indrianingsih et al. 2017). Irham et al. (2020) explored the use of CW supplemented with *Curcuma longa* and *Ziziphus mauritiana* extracts for BC production, showcasing the potential for enhancing BC properties through natural additives. Additionally, Lin et al. (2022) found a significant increase in BC yield with pre-fermentation, with *Saccharomyces cerevisiae* SC7 leading to a notable 165% increase compared to using fresh CW alone. Moreover, Nurfajriani et al. (2021) demonstrated the feasibility of producing BC using *A. xylinum* with CW as the medium, further expanding the repertoire of BC synthesis methods utilizing CW. Overall, these studies underscore the potential of CW-derived BC as a valuable biomaterial, offering a renewable and sustainable alternative with promising applications in various fields, including biomedicine, tissue engineering, and packaging.

5.6.9 Probiotics

Probiotic fermentation of CW presents an innovative approach to developing functional beverages with probiotic benefits, offering consumers a novel combination of hydration and probiotic support. CW's natural isotonic properties, including rehydration and electrolyte replacement, make it an excellent base for probiotic drinks. Several studies have explored the development of probiotic beverages using CW, demonstrating its potential in this field. Research by Haniyah and Purwan (2023) highlighted the potential of fermenting TCW with *Lactobacillus casei* to produce a probiotic drink capable of supporting digestive tract health and boosting immunity. The choice and quantity of sugars used during fermentation can influence the chemical properties of probiotic drinks. For instance, the addition of brown sugar was found to impact total acidity, pH, and antioxidant activity in probiotic drinks (Nisa and Purwani 2023). However, the addition of brown sugar to young CW probiotic drinks did not significantly affect the total LAB count, indicating the feasibility of incorporating sweeteners without compromising probiotic content. Overall, these studies underscore the potential of CW as a substrate for probiotic fermentation, offering a versatile platform for the development of functional beverages that promote both hydration and gut health. Continued research in this area can further optimize probiotic drink formulations and enhance their health-promoting properties.

5.6.10 Sports Drink/Rehydration Drink

CW is gaining recognition as a natural sports drink due to its inherent composition of electrolytes, minerals, vitamins, complex carbohydrates, and protein. With its optimal replenishment and rehydration properties, CW is being promoted as a suitable beverage for consumption before, during, or after workouts. Its natural ratio of electrolytes, minerals, and vitamins, combined with lower acidity and no added sugar, make it an ideal option for athletes and fitness enthusiasts. One of the key electrolytes found in CW is potassium (K), which plays a crucial role in enhancing rehydration by replacing intracellular water post-exercise. Additionally, CW naturally contains magnesium (Mg), calcium (Ca), and phosphorus (P), providing added rehydration benefits compared to traditional sports drinks, which often lack these nutrients. While CW contains all major electrolytes, its sodium (Na) content is relatively lower than that of most sports drinks. To address this, some studies have explored enriching CW with sodium to enhance its rehydration effectiveness. Research by Ismail et al. (2007) found that Na-enriched CW was as effective as a commercial sports drink for whole-body rehydration after exercise-induced dehydration, with less nausea and stomach upset reported. In the field of sports nutrition, CW has been shown to provide hydrating effects comparable to carbohydrate-electrolyte sports drinks. Various formulations of CW-based sports drinks have been developed, incorporating additional ingredients like honey, salt, and sugar to optimize hydration and performance. Moreover, CW may have clinical applications as an oral rehydration medium, particularly in cases of severe dehydration due to conditions like diarrhea. Studies have indicated that CW could effectively replace fluid loss from the gastrointestinal tract and restore plasma volume after exercise-induced dehydration. Overall, CW offers a natural and effective alternative to traditional sports drinks, providing athletes with the hydration and electrolyte balance needed to support performance and recovery. Further research in this area may uncover additional benefits and applications of CW in sports nutrition and hydration.

5.7 Conclusions and Future Directions

The increasing focus on health and wellness worldwide has fueled the demand for CW due to its array of essential nutrients such as potassium (K), magnesium (Mg), and calcium (Ca). These minerals play crucial roles in the body's functions, making CW more than just a hydrating option. Its lower caloric content compared to sugary beverages and artificial sports drinks also makes it an attractive choice for weight-conscious individuals. Furthermore, numerous scientific studies support the health benefits of CW, enhancing its credibility and encouraging broader adoption.

However, one significant drawback of CW is its short shelf-life and susceptibility to microbial contamination with prolonged exposure. To address these challenges, producers are offering frozen organic CW, extending its shelf life and enabling transportation to regions where fresh coconuts are not readily available. Packaging innovations, such as tetra packs, cans, plastic bottles, and powdered forms, are also improving accessibility and convenience for consumers.

The discovery of various nutraceutical and medicinal properties of TCW (tender coconut water) indicates its potential to improve human health further. Further research is needed to better understand the functions and properties of TCW components, such as kinetin and kinetin riboside, and their stability. This knowledge can lead to the development of innovative, nutritionally rich products and applications in fields like nanotechnology and biocatalysis.

While many animal studies have demonstrated the medicinal properties of CW, there is a need for more clinical studies involving humans to validate these findings. Future research should explore the impact of various CW processing technologies on bioavailability and overall health outcomes in human populations. Sensory and consumer evaluations will also help gauge the market potential of innovative CW products. Overall, continued research and development efforts are essential to unlock the full potential of CW for human health and well-being.

References

Abreu LF, Faria JAF (2007) Infuencia da temperatura e do acidoascorbicosobreaesta-bilidadefsico-quimica e atividadeenzima-tica da agua de coco (*Cocos nucifera* L.) acondicionada assepticamente, Cienc. Food Sci Technol (Campinas) 27(2):226–232. https://doi.org/10.1590/S0101-20612007000200003

Adetayo A, Oluwakemi A, Yinus O (2015) Comparative analysis of water in tender and matured coconut nuts and use as oral rehydration solution. Chem Mater Res 7(2):7–10

Agbafor SO, Elom ME, Ogbanshi AO, Oko AJ, Uraku VUO, Nwankwo BA, Ale, Obiudu KI (2015) Antioxidant property and cardiovascular effects of coconut (Cocos nucifera) water. Int J Biochem Res Rev 5(4):259–263

Ajibogun OA, Oboma YI (2013) Biochemical composition of coconut water: Nigeria species. Int J Med Bio Med Sci 1(1):1–4

Akpomie OO, Akponah E, Ehwarieme AD, Paul RE (2020) Antimicrobial activity of coconut water, oil and palm kernel oils extracted from coconut and palm kernel on some plasmid mediated multi-drug resistant organisms associated with food spoilage. Afr J Microbiol Res 14(7):366–373. https://doi.org/10.5897/AJMR2020.9363

Alatawi KA, Alshubaily FA (2021) Coconut products alleviate hyperglycaemic, hyperlipidimic and nephropathy indices in streptozotocin-induced diabetic Wistar rats. Saudi J Biol Sci 28:4224–4231. https://doi.org/10.1016/j.sjbs.2021.06.060

Alchoubassi G, Kińska K, Bierla K, Lobinski R, Szpunar J (2021) Speciation of essential nutrient trace elements in coconut water. Food Chem 339:127680. https://doi.org/10.1016/j.foodchem.2020.127680

Aliberti NCM, da Silva RMS, Gut JAW, Tadini CC (2009) Thermal inactivation of polyphenol oxidase and peroxidase in green coconut (*Cocos nucifera*) water. Int J Food Sci Tech 44(12):2662–2668. https://doi.org/10.1111/j.1365-2621.2009.02100.x

Alleyne T, Roache S, Thomas C, Shirley A (2005) The control of hypertension by use of coconut water and mauby: two tropical food drinks. West Indian Med J 54(1):3–8. https://doi.org/10.1590/S0043-31442005000100002

Anaya K, Podszun M, Franco OL, Gadelha CAA, Frank J (2020) The coconut water antimicrobial peptide CnAMP1 is taken up into intestinal cells but does not alter p-glycoprotein expression and activity. Plant Foods Hum Nutri 75:396–403. https://doi.org/10.1007/s11130-020-00826-y

Andasuryani KA, Rahmi ID, Derosya V (2017) Characteristics of nata de coco of three types coconut fermentation media. Res J Pharm Biol Chem Sci 8(2):658–664

Anselme AL, Louis KKJ, Albarin GG, Roger BK, Didier YS (2018) Physicochemical coconut water assessment and of the microbiological quality of its sugar extracted of five coconuts ecotypes at the Marc Delorme Station, Côte d'Ivoire. Int J Appl Biol Pharm Tech 9(1):24–31. https://doi.org/10.21276/Ijabpt

Anurag P, Rajamohan T (2003) Cardioprotective effects of tender coconut water in experimental myocardial infarction. Plant Food Hum Nutr 58(3):1–12. https://doi.org/10.1023/B:QUAL.0000040363.64356.05

Appaiah P, Sunil L, Prasanth Kumar PK, Gopala Krishna AG (2015) Physicochemical characteristics and stability aspects of coconut water and kernel at different stages of maturity. J Food Sci Technol 52(8):5196–5203. https://doi.org/10.1007/s13197-014-1559-4

Apshara SE, Arunachalam V, Jayabose C, Kumaran PM (2007) Evaluation of coconut hybrids for tender nut purpose. Indian J Hortic 64(3):320–323

Aragao WM, Isberner IV, Cruz EMO (2001a) Água-de-coco. Embrapa CPATC/Tabuleiros Costeiros, Aracaju

Aragao WM, Cruz EMO, Helvecio JS (2001b) Caracterizaçãomorfológica do fruto e química da água de coco emcultivares de coqueiroanão. Agrotrópica 13(2):49–58

Aroucha EMM, Paiva CA, Alves Júnior AR, Araújo NO, Silva AC, Aroucha Filho JC (2015) Característicasfísico-químicas de água-de-coco de diferentescultivaresemfunção do estádio de

maturação. In: Congresso Brasileiro de Processamentomínimo e Póscolheita de frutas, fores e hortaliças (CD ROM), Maio de 2015
Arzeta-Ríos AJ, Ramírez DG, Trejo BR, Moncada MCY, Prada HZ (2020) Microwave heating effect on total phenolics and antioxidant activity of green and mature coconut water. Int J Food Eng 16(12):20190378. https://doi.org/10.1515/ijfe-2019-0378
Awua AK, Doe ED, Agyare R (2011) Exploring the influence of sterilisation and storage on some physicochemical properties of coconut (*Cocos nucifera* L.) water. Bio Med Central Res Notes 4:451–454
Azeredo HMC, Barud H, Farinas CS, Vasconcellos VM, Claro AM (2019) Bacterial cellulose as a raw material for food and food packaging applications. Front Sustain Food Syst 3:7. https://doi.org/10.3389/fsufs.2019.00007
Aziz NS, Chin ZK, Razali MNS, Sofian-Seng NS, Kasim KF (2023) Development of mature coconut (*Cocos nucifera* L.) probiotic beverage: physicochemical characteristics, microbial count, antioxidant activity, and sensory acceptance. Int Food Res J 30(1):119–129. https://doi.org/10.47836/ifrj.30.1.09
Baharvand M, Shokri M, Hassani S, Mirzaei H, Mahdian M (2021) Antibacterial effect of coconut water and coconut oil on *Aggregatibacter actinomycetemcomitans*. J Res Dent Maxillofac Sci 6(3):40–45
Bandalan EB, Galvez LA (2016) Optimization of coconut water beverage fermented with lactobacillus acidophilus. Ann Trop Res 38(1):196–202. https://doi.org/10.32945/atr38117.2016
Bhagya D, Prema L, Rajamohan T (2012) Therapeutic effect of tender coconut water on oxidative stress in fructose fed insulin resistant hypertensive rats. Asian Pac J Trop Med 5(4):270–276. https://doi.org/10.1016/S1995-7645(12)60038-8
Bispo VS, Dantas LS, Filho CAB, Pinto IFD, Silva RPD, Otsuka FAM, Santos RB, Santos AC, Trindade HR (2017) Reduction of the DNA damages, hepatoprotective effect and antioxidant potential of the coconut water, ascorbic and caffeic acids in oxidative stress mediated by ethanol. An Acad Bras Cienc 89(2):1095–1109. https://doi.org/10.1590/0001-3765201720
Biswaro LS, da Costa Sousa MG, Rezende TMB, Dias SC, Franco OL (2018) Antimicrobial peptides and nanotechnology, recent advances and challenges. Front Microbiol 9:1–14. https://doi.org/10.3389/fmicb.2018.00855
Biswas K, Mohanta YK, Kumar VB, Hashem A, Abd_Allah EF, Mohanta D, Mohanta TK (2020) Nutritional assessment study and role of green silver nanoparticles in shelf-life of coconut endosperm to develop as functional food. Saudi J Bio Sci 27(1):1280–1288. https://doi.org/10.1016/j.sjbs.2020.01.011
Borse BB, Rao LJM, Ramalakshmi K, Raghavan B (2007) Chemical composition of volatiles from coconut sap (neera) and effect of processing. Food Chem 101:877–880
Burns DT, Johnston EL, Walker MJK (2020) Authenticity and the potability of coconut water—a critical review. J AOAC Int 103(3):800–806. https://doi.org/10.1093/jaocint/qsz008
Campbell-Falck D, Falck TT, Tutuo TMN, Clem K (2000) The intravenous use of coconut water. Am J Emerg Med 18(1):108–111. https://doi.org/10.1016/s0735-6757(00)90062-7
Campos CF, Souza PE, Coelho JV, Gloria MBA (1996) Chemical composition, enzyme activity and effect of enzyme inactivation on flavor quality of green coconut water. J Food Process Preserv 20(6):487–500. https://doi.org/10.1111/j.1745-4549.1996.tb00761.x
Chang C, Wu RT (2011) Quantification of (+)-catechin and (−)-epicatechin in coconut water by LC–MS. Food Chem 126:710–717. https://doi.org/10.1016/j.foodchem.2010.11.034
Chawla PR, Bajaj IB, Survase SA, Singhal RS (2009) Microbial cellulose: fermentative production and applications. Food Tech Biotech 47(2):107–124
Chidambaram S, Singaraja C, Prasanna MV, Ganesan M, Sundararajan M (2013) Chemistry of tender coconut water from the Cuddalore coastal region in Tamil Nadu, India. Nat Resour Res 22(2):91–101. https://doi.org/10.1007/s11053-013-9203-y
Cholan PK, Manipal S, Rajmohan KR (2017) Assessment of the anti- fungal activity of green coconut water (*Cocos nucifera* L.) on *Candida albicans*, an in-vitro study. J Pharm Sci Res 9(2):251–254

Cruz J, Guzmán FC, Fernández-Lafuente R, Torres R (2014) Antimicrobial peptides: promising compounds against pathogenic microorganisms. Curr Med Chem 21(20):2299–2232. https://doi.org/10.2174/0929867321666140217110155

da Fonseca AM, Monte FJQ, de Oliveira MCF, de Mattos MC, Cordell R, Braz-Fliho GA, TLG L (2009a) Coconut water (*Cocos nucifera* L.)—a new biocatalyst system for organic synthesis. J Mol Catal B Enzym 57(1–4):78–82. https://doi.org/10.1016/j.molcatb.2008.06.022

da Fonseca AM, Bizerra AMC, da Souza JSN, Monte FJQ, de Oliveira MCF, de Mattos MC, Cordell GA, Braz-Filho R, Lemos TLG (2009b) Constituents and antioxidant activity of two varieties of coconut water (*Cocos nucifera* L.). Rev Bras 19(1):193–198. https://doi.org/10.1590/S0102-695X2009000200002

Deb Mandal M, Mandal S (2011) Coconut Cocos nucifera L.: Arecaceae: in health promotion and disease prevention. Asian Pacific Journal of Tropical Medicine. 4(3):241–247

Dai Y, Peng L, Zhang X, Wu Q, Yao J, Xing Q, Zheng Y, Huang X, Chen S, Xie Q (2021) Effects of coconut water on blood sugar and retina of rats with diabetes. Peer J 9:e10667. https://doi.org/10.7717/peerj.10667

Dayal MS, Catchmark JM (2016) Mechanical and structural property analysis of bacterial cellulose composites. Carbohydr Polym 144:447–453. https://doi.org/10.1016/j.carbpol.2016.02.055

Dignan C, Burlingame B, Kumar S, Aalbersberg W (2004) The Pacific Islands food composition tables, 2nd edn. FAO, Rome

Dissanayake A (2017) Health benefits of coconut oil, coconut sugar and coconut water consumption. Indian Coconut J 60(1):16–20

Duarte ACP, Coelho MAZ, Leite SGF (2002) Identification of Peroxidase and Tyrosinase in Green Coconut Water Identificación De Peroxidasa Y Tirosinasa En Jugo De Coco Verde Identificación De Peroxidasa E Tirosinasa En Xugo De Coco Verde. CYTA-Journal of Food 3(5):266–270

Dwiloka B, Rizqiati H, Setiani BE (2020) Physicochemical and sensory characteristics of green coconut (*Cocos nucifera* L.) water kefir. Int J Food Stud 9(2):346–359. https://doi.org/10.7455/ijfs/9.2.2020.a7

Effong GS, Ebong PE, Eyong EU, Uwah AJ, Ekong UE (2010) Amelioration of chloramphenicol induced toxicity in rats by coconut water. J Appl Sci Res 6(4):331–335

Ehsayed HH, Sobhi HM, Kassem MS (2020) Coconut liquid as dietary interventions for hyperglycemic rats. Plant Arch 20(Suppl 1):3395–3403

Fan X, Wagner K, Sokorai KJB, Ngo H (2017) Inactivation of Gram-positive bacteria by novel phenolic branched-chain fatty acids. J Food Prot 80(1):6–14. https://doi.org/10.4315/0362-028X.JFP-16-080

Farapti, Sayogo S, Siregar P (2013) Effect of tender coconut water on systolic and diastolic blood pressure in prehypertensive women. Health Sci J Indones 4(2):64–68

Fowoyo P, Alamu J (2018) Nutritional composition and antimicrobial acidity of coconut water against selected gastrointestinal pathogens. Int J Micro Biol Appl 5(1):1–8

Ganesh L, Deepa B, Manikkoth S, Nadh AG (2023) Anxiolytic activity of coconut water by GABA modulation as evidenced by pharmacological experiments and molecular docking studies. Res J Pharm Technol 16(8):3544–3548. https://doi.org/10.52711/0974-360X.2023.00585

Ge L, Yong JWH, Tan SN, Hua L, Ong ES (2008) Analyses of gibberellins in coconut (*Cocos nucifera* L.) water by partial filling micellar electrokinetic chromatography mass spectrometry with reversal of electroosmotic flow. Electrophoresis 29(10):2126–2134. https://doi.org/10.1016/j.chroma.2006.08.027

Goderska K, Czarnecki Z (2007) Characterization of selected strains from *Lactobacillus acidophilus* and *Bifdobacterium bifdum*. Afr J Micro Biol Res 1(6):65–78

Goveas LC, Ashwath KS, Nazerath BR, Dsouza O, Ullekh UA, Muddappa VS (2021) Development of coconut water-based exopolysaccharide rich functional beverage by fermentation with probiotic *Lactobacillus plantarum* SVP2. Biocat Agric Biotechnol 34:102030. https://doi.org/10.1016/j.bcab.2021.102030

Gullapalli HS, Tekade AP, Gullapalli NH (2013) Effect of supplementation of tender coconut water on blood pressure of primary hypertensive subjects. Int J Med Res Health Sci 2(2):172–176

Guo Y, Li W, Chen H, Chen W, Zhang M, Zhong Q, Chen W (2022) Optimization and rheological study of an exopolysaccharide obtained from fermented mature coconut water with *Lipomyces starkeyi*. Foods 11:999. https://doi.org/10.3390/foods11070999

Halim HH, Dee EW, Dek MSP, Hamid AA, Ngalim A, Saari N, Jaafar AH (2018) Ergogenic attributes of young and mature coconut (*Cocos nucifera* L.) water based on physical properties, sugars and electrolytes contents. Int J Food Prop 21(1):2378–2389. https://doi.org/10.1080/10942912.2018.1522329

Haniyah F, Purwan E (2023) The effect of brown sugar addition on total acid, pH, and antioxidant activity of young coconut water (*Cocos nucifera* L.) probiotic drinks. In: Ichsan B, Nursanto D, Firmansyh SM, Porusia M, Hudiyawati D, Perdana SS (eds) Proceedings of the international conference on health and well-being (ICHWB 2022). Atlantis Press, Dordrecht, pp 120–132. https://doi.org/10.2991/978-94-6463-184-5_12

Hungund B, Prabhu S, Shetty C, Acharya S, Prabhu V, Gupta SG (2013) Production of bacterial cellulose from *Gluconacetobacter persimmonis* GH-2 using dual and cheaper carbon sources. J Microb Biochem Technol 5(2):31–33. https://doi.org/10.4172/1948-5948.1000095

Indrianingsih AW, Rosyida VT, Jatmiko TH, Prasetyo DJ, Poeloengasih CD, Apriyana W, Nisa K, Nurhayati S, Hernawan DC, Pratiwi D, Suwanto A, Ratih D (2017) Preliminary study on biosynthesis and characterization of bacteria cellulose films from coconut water. IOP Conf Ser Earth Environ Sci 101:012010. https://doi.org/10.1088/1755-1315/101/1/012010

Irham WH, Tamrin, Marpaung L, Marpongahtun (2020) Characterization of bacterial cellulose from coconut water supplemented *Curcuma longa* L and *Ziziphus mauritiana* extract. AIP Conf Proc 2267:020056. https://doi.org/10.1063/5.0023953

Ismail I, Singh R, Sirisinghe RG (2007) Rehydration with sodium-enriched coconut water after exercise-induced dehydration. Southeast Asian J Trop Med Public Health 38(4):769–785

Jaroonchon N, Krisanappok K, Imsabi W (2017) The development of 2 acetyl-1-pyrroline (2-AP) in Thai aromatic coconut. Songklanakarin J Sci Technol 39(2):179–183. https://doi.org/10.14456/sjst-psu.2017.21

Jayakumar K, Rajasekaran S, Nagarajan M, Vijayarengan P (2015) Bioactive enzyme activity and medicinal properties of tender coconut (*Cocos nucifera* L.). Intl J Modern Biochem 4(1):10–14

Jayan JS, Jayan SS (2023) Synthesis of fluorescent graphene quantum dots from tender coconut water. https://doi.org/10.2139/ssrn.4362687

Jayan SS, Jayan JS, Sneha B, Abha K (2021) Facile synthesis of carbon dots using tender coconut water for the fluorescence detection of heavy metal ions. Mater Today Proc 43(6):3821–3825. https://doi.org/10.1016/j.matpr.2020.11.417

Yong JWH, Ge L, Ng YF, Tan SN (2009) The chemical composition and biological properties of coconut (*Cocos nucifera* L.) water. Molecules 14:5144–5164. https://doi.org/10.3390/molecules14125144

Jirovetz L, Buchbauer G, Ngassoum MB (2003) Solid-phase-microextraction-headspace aroma compounds of coconut (*Cocos nucifera* L.) milk and meat from Cameroon. Ernährung Nutr 27:300–303

Kantachote D, Ratanaburee A, Hayisama W, Sukhoom A, Nunkaew T (2017) The use of potential probiotic *Lactobacillus plantarum* DW12 for producing a novel functional beverage from mature coconut water. J Funct Foods 32:401–408. https://doi.org/10.1016/j.jff.2017.03.018

Keng SK, Easaa AM, Muhamedb AMC, Ooib CH, Chew TT (2017) Composition and physicochemical properties of fresh and freeze-concentrated coconut (*Cocos nucifera*) water. J Agrobiotech 8(1):13–24

Khan MN, Rehman M, Khan KW (2003) A study of chemical composition of *Cocos nucifera* L. (coconut) water and its usefulness as rehydration fluid. Pakistan J Bot Karachi 35(5):925–930

Krisanapook K, Jaroonchon N, Imsabai W (2016) Physiological traits and 2-acetyl-1-pyrroline development of aromatic coconut nut. Acta Hortic 1129:79–84. https://doi.org/10.17660/ActaHortic.2016.1129.11

Kumar S, Manna K, Das A (2018) Tender coconut water attenuates heat stress-induced testicular damage through modulation of the NF-κB and Nrf2 pathways. Food Funct 9(10):5463–5479. https://doi.org/10.1039/c8fo01207e

Kumar M, Saini SS, Agarwal PK, Roy P, Sircar D (2021) Nutritional and metabolomics characterization of the coconut water at different nut developmental stages. J Food Compos Anal 96:103738. https://doi.org/10.1016/j.jfca.2020.103738

Kwiatkowski A, Clemente E, Scarcelli A, Vida JB (2008) Quality of coconut water 'in natura'belonging to Green Dwarf fruit variety in different stages of development, in plantation on the northwest area of Parana, Brazil. Journal of Food, Agriculture and Environment 6(1):102–105

Lakshmanan J, Zhang B, Wright KT, Jaganathan V, Schultz DJ, Klinge CM, Harbrecht BG (2020) Tender coconut water suppresses hepatic inflammation by activating AKT and JNK signaling pathways in an in vitro model of sepsis. J Funct Foods 64:103637. https://doi.org/10.1016/j.jff.2019.103637

Lakshminarayan NG (2015) Nata-de-coco production. https://www.linkedin.com/pulse/nata-de-coco-production-n-g-lakshminarayan

Lazim MIM, Badruzaman NA, Peng KS, Long K (2015) Quantification of cytokinins in coconut water from different maturation stages of Malaysia's coconut (*Cocos nucifera* L.) varieties. J Food Process Technol 6:515. https://doi.org/10.4172/2157-7110.1000515

Lazim MIM, Mohamad S, Rahman IA, Koh SP, Manan MA, Asri MAM (2023) Optimization of process parameters for GABA and L-DOPA production on fermented coconut drink. Food Res 6(4):102–108. https://doi.org/10.26656/fr.2017.6(S4).012

Limbad MJ, Gutierrez-Maddox MJ, Hamid N (2015) Coconut water: an essential health drink in both natural and fermented forms. In: Owen JP (ed) Nut and pomace extracts: biological activity, potential applications and beneficial health effects. Nova Science, New York, pp 145–156

Limbad M, Maddox NG, Hamid N, Kantono K (2020) Sensory and physicochemical characterization of sourdough bread prepared with a coconut water kefir starter. Foods 9(9):1165. https://doi.org/10.3390/foods9091165

Limbad M, Maddox GN, Hamid N, Kantono K, Liu T, Young T (2023) Microbial and physicochemical transformations during fermentation of coconut water kefir beverage. Appl Sci 13:7257. https://doi.org/10.3390/app13127257

Lin X, Song Z, Jiang H, Hao Y, Hu X, Liu S, Li C (2022) Production of bacterial cellulose in the medium with yeasts pre-fermented coconut water or with addition of selected amino acids. Foods 11:3627. https://doi.org/10.3390/foods11223627

Loki AL, Rajamohan T (2003) Hepatoprotective and antioxidant effect of tender coconut water on carbon tetrachloride induced liver injury in rats. Indian J Biochem Biophys 40(5):354–357

Luckanatinvong V, Sornkeaw P (2011) Quality of blanched aromatic coconut for export. Agric Sci J 42(1):147–150

Ma Z, Ge L, Lee ASY, Yong JWH, Tan SN, Ong ES (2008) Simultaneous analysis of different classes of phytohormones in coconut (*Cocos nucifera* L.) water using high-performance liquid chromatography and liquid chromatography-tandem mass spectrometry after solid-phase extraction. Anal Chim Acta 610(2):274–281. https://doi.org/10.1016/j.aca.2008.01.045

Madihalli C, Sudhakar H, Doble M (2020) Production and investigation of the physico-chemical properties of MEL-A from glycerol and coconut water. World J Micro Biol Bio Tech 36(6):88. https://doi.org/10.1007/s11274-020-02857-8

Magda RR (1992) Coco-soft drink: health beverage from coconut water. Food Market Tech 6(6):22–23

Mahayothee B, Koomyart I, Khuwijitjaru P, Siriwongwilaichat P, Nagle M, Müller J (2016) Phenolic compounds, antioxidant activity, and medium chain fatty acids profiles of coconut water and meat at different maturity stages. Int J Food Properties 19(9):2041–2051. https://doi.org/10.1080/10942912.2015.1099042

Mandal SM, Dey S, Mandal M, Sarkar S, Maria-Neto S, Franco OL (2009) Identification and structural insights of three novel antimicrobial peptides isolated from green coconut water. Peptides 30(4):633–637. https://doi.org/10.1016/j.peptides.2008.12.001

Manna K, Khan A, Das D, Kesh SB, Das U, Ghosh S, Dey RS, Saha KD, Chakraborty A, Chattopadhyay S, Dey S, Chattopadhyay D (2014) Protective effect of coconut water concentrates and its active component shikimic acid against hydroperoxide mediated oxidative stress through suppression of NF-κB and activation of Nrf2 pathway. J Ethnopharmacol 155(1):132–146. https://doi.org/10.1016/j.jep.2014.04.046

Manoharan P, Dhanabalan SC, Alagan M, Muthuvijayan S, Ponraj JS, Somasundaram CK (2020) Facile synthesis and characterisation of green luminescent carbon nanodots prepared from tender coconut water using the acid-assisted ultrasonic route. Micro Nano Lett 15(13):920–924. https://doi.org/10.1049/mnl.2020.0101

Mantena S, Jagadish, Badduri SR, Siripurapu KB, Unnikrishnan MK (2003) In vitro evaluation of antioxidant properties of *Cocos nucifera* Linn. water. Nahrung 47(2):126–131. https://doi.org/10.1002/food.200390023

Marikkar JMN, Madhrapperuma WS (2012) Coconut. In: Siddiq M, Ahmed A, Lobo MG, Ozadali F (eds) Tropical and subtropical nuts: post-harvest physiology, processing and packaging. Wiley, Ames, pp 159–178

Markose VT, Poduval S (1999) Vinegar from waste coconut water. Coco Info Int 6(1):15–16

Martial-Didier AK, Siméon BK, Fatou C, Parfait JKNE, Kablan T (2017) Effects of storage temperature on physicochemical parameters of coconut (*Cocos nucifera* var. dwarf of Guinea Equatorial) water. Intl J Sci Eng Res 8(12):1745–1749

Medeiros VFLP, Medeiros AC (2012) O usoterapêutico da água de coco. (Therapeutic use of coconut water). J Surg Clin Res 3(2):75–83. https://doi.org/10.20398/jscr.v3i2.3570

Mohamad NE, Yeap SK, Beh BK, Romli MF, TeoYWK SSA, Adzni S, Long K, Alitheen NB (2017) Comparison of in vivo toxicity, antioxidant and immunomodulatory activities of coconut juice, nipah juice and pine-apple vinegar. J Sci Food Agr 98(2):534–540. https://doi.org/10.1002/jsfa.8491

Mohamad NE, Yeap SK, Abu N, Lim KL, Zamberi NR, Nordin N, Sharifuddin SA, Long K, Alitheen NB (2019) In vitro and in vivo antitumour effects of coconut water vinegar on 4T1 breast cancer cells. Food Nutr Res 63:1616. https://doi.org/10.29219/fnr.v63.1616

Mordi JC, Euzuegbu U, Opajobi AO, Ojieh AE (2015) Hepatoprotective effects of palm oil and coconut water in the serum of Wistar rats exposed to cadmium chloride contaminated diet. Biokemistri 27(2):79–84

Nair SVG, Rajamohan T (2014) The role of coconut water on nicotine-induced reproductive dysfunction in experimental male rat model. Food Nutr Sci 5(12):1121–1130. https://doi.org/10.4236/fns.2014.512122

Nasimuddin S, Rajan PD, Sumathi G (2016) A study of in vitro antimicrobial activity of coconut water and coconut oil on gram-positive and gram-negative bacteria. World J Pharm Res 5(8):696–700. https://doi.org/10.20959/wjpr20168-6695

Nasution Z, Jirapakkul W, Lorjaroenphon Y (2019) Aroma compound profile of mature coconut water from tall variety through thermal treatment. J Food Meas Charact 13:277–286. https://doi.org/10.1007/s11694-018-9942-x

Nasution Z, Jirapakkul W, Tongkhao K, Chanput W (2020) The effect of coconut water on adipocyte differentiation and lipid accumulation in 3T3-L1 cells. J Nutr Sci Vitaminol (Tokyo) 66(Supplement):S343–S348. https://doi.org/10.3177/jnsv.66.S343

Ndubuka GI, Okafor WC, Jervas E, Chidi IS, Udoka OC, Williams OI (2015) Protective effect of immature coconut water on hepatocytes against carbon tetrachloride-induced liver damage in Wister rats. Int J Sci Res 4(12):1427–1431

Nguyen HMH, Pham CD, Nguyen KD, Tran ATT, Le NTH, Ho PH, Le HV (2023) Bacterial cellulose-based material from coconut water as efficient green adsorbent for heavy metal cations. Chem Eng Technol 46:2547–2559. https://doi.org/10.1002/ceat.202300033

Nisa KS, Purwani E (2023) The effect of brown sugar addition on total lactic acid bacteria (LAB) and total dissolved solids (TDS) of young coconut water (*Cocos nucifera* L.) probiotic drinks. In: Ichsan B, Nursanto D, Firmansyh SM, Porusia M, Hudiyawati D, Perdana SS (eds) Proceedings of the international conference on health and well-being (ICHWB 2022). Atlantis Press, Dordrecht, pp 133–142. https://doi.org/10.2991/978-94-6463-184-5_13

Nova FS, Chasani S, Hussanna A, Zulaikhah ST (2020) Tender coconut water inhibits the process of lipid peroxidation, reduce glucose levels, and increase plasma insulin in pregnant diabetic rats. Pharm J 12(1):162–167. https://doi.org/10.5530/pj.2020.12.24

Nugroho DA, Aji P (2015) Characterization of nata de coco produced by fermentation of immobilized Acetobacter xylinum. Agric Agric Sci Proc 3:278–282

Nugroho D, Keawprom C, Chanthai S, Oh WC, Benchawattananon R (2022) Highly sensitive fingerprint detection under UV light on non-porous surface using starch-powder based luminol-doped carbon dots (N-CDs) from tender coconut water as a green carbon source. Nanomaterials 12:400. https://doi.org/10.3390/nano12030400

Nurfajriani N, Pulungan AN, Yusuf M, Bukit N (2021) Preparation and characterization of bacterial cellulose from culturation of *Acetobacter xylinum* in coconut water media. J Phys 1811:012070. https://doi.org/10.1088/1742-6596/1811/1/012070

Offor CE, Adetarami O, Nwali BU, Igwenyi IO, Afukwa CA (2014) Effect of *Cocos nucifera* water on liver enzymes. Middle East J Sci Res 21(5):844–847. https://doi.org/10.5829/idosi.mejsr.2014.21.05.8496

Ogundiya MO (1991) Glucose content of nut water in four varieties of coconut palm (*Cocos nucifera*). J Sci Food Agric 56:399–402

Okafor WC, Ndubuka GI, Jervas E, Chidi IS, Udoka OC, Ikechukwu O, William (2016a) Effects of immature coconut water on the hepato cytoarchitecture against carbon tetrachloride-induced liver damage in Wistar rats. IOSR J Dent Med Sci 15(07):60–65. https://doi.org/10.9790/0853-150716065

Okafor CW, Ekezie J, Ndubuka GI, Ndubuisi T (2016b) Immature coconut water: a renal protective agent in Wistar rats. Int J Anat Appl Physiol 2(2):26–31. https://doi.org/10.19070/2572-7451-160004

Okere OS, Adejo GO, Okoli BJ (2011) Hepatoprotective properties of crude water and oil extracts of coconut (*Cocos nucifera*) in alloxan-induced diabetic rats. Tunis J Med Plants Nat Prod 5:70–76

Ololade ZS, Kuyooro SE, Ogunmola OO, Oyelese OJ (2017) Physicochemical, volatile organic composition, phenolic, flavonoid and ascorbic acid contents, antioxidant, anti-arthritic and anti-inflammatory properties of *Cocos nucifera* juice. Glob J Med Res B Pharm Drug Discov Toxicol Med 17(2):43–49

Patel R, Asplin J, Granja I, Jiang P, Osann K, Landman J, Clayman R (2018a) Can coconut water consumption potentially prevent kidney stones? J Urol 199(4):384–385. https://doi.org/10.1016/j.juro.2018.02.965

Patel RM, Jiang P, Asplin J, Granja I, Capretz T, Osann K, Okhunov Z, Landman J, Clayman RV (2018b) Coconut water: an unexpected source of urinary citrate. Bio Med Res Int 2018:3061742. https://doi.org/10.1155/2018/3061742

Pattigadapa HS, Ramesh M, Praneeth SCH, Bhaskar RU, Lakshman G, Ankaiah M, Balu NJ (2011) Cardiotonic activity of coconut water. Recent Res Sci Tech 3(4):155–157

Petroianu GA, Kosanovic M, Shehatta IS, Mahgoub B, Saleh A, Maleck WH (2004) Green coconut water for intravenous use: trace and minor element content. J Trace Elem Exp Med 17(4):273–282. https://doi.org/10.1002/jtra.20010

Pinto IFD, Silva RP, Filho ABC, Dantas LS, Bispo VS, Matos IA, Otsuka FAM, Santos AC, Matos HR (2015) Study of antiglycation, hypoglycemic, and nephroprotective activities of the Green Dwarf variety coconut water (*Cocos nucifera* L.) in alloxan-induced diabetic rats. J Med Food 18(7):802–809. https://doi.org/10.1089/jmf.2014.0046

Prabhu S, Dennison SR, Mura M, Lea RW, Snape TJ, Harris F (2014) Cn-AMP2 from green coconut water is an anionic anticancer peptide. J Pept Sci 20(12):909–915. https://doi.org/10.1002/psc.2684

Prades A, Dornier M, Diop N, Pain JP (2012a) Coconut water uses, composition and properties: a review. Nuts 67(2):87–107. https://doi.org/10.1051/nuts/2012002

Prades A, RRA A, Dornier M, Pain JP, Boulanger R (2012b) Characterisation of the volatile profile of coconut water from five varieties using an optimised HS-SPME-GC analysis. J Sci Food Agric 92(12):2471–2478. https://doi.org/10.1002/jsfa.5655

Prasad C, Harshal S, Dobe M (2018) A process for reducing cloud point in hydrocarbon fuels using nanostructured mannosylerythritol lipids and method of producing the same. Patent Application ID: 771/CHE/2015

Preetha PP, Devi VG, Rajamohan T (2012) Hypoglycemic and antioxidant potential of coconut water in experimental diabetes. Food Funct 3(7):753–757. https://doi.org/10.1039/c2fo30066d

Preethi M, Viswanathan C, Ponpandian N (2021) A green path to extract carbon quantum dots by coconut water: another fluorescent probe towards Fe^{3+} ions. Particuology 58:251–258. https://doi.org/10.1016/j.partic.2021.03.019

Priya SR, Ramaswamy L (2014) Tender coconut water—natures elixir to mankind. Int J Recent Sci Res 5(8):1485–1490

Purbia R, Paria S (2016) A simple turn on fluorescent sensor for the selective detection of thiamine using coconut water derived luminescent carbon dots. Biosens Bioelectron 79:467–475. https://doi.org/10.1016/j.bios.2015.12.087

Radenahmad N, Sawangjaroen K, Mitranun W, Sayoh I (2016) Beneficial effects of young coconut juice feeding on lipid and renal metabolism in ovariectomized rats: novel preliminary finding. Songklanagarin J Sci Technol 38(1):57–65

Radiman C, Yuliani G (2008) Coconut water as a potential resource for cellulose acetate membrane preparation. Polym Int 57(3):502–508. https://doi.org/10.1002/pi.2374

Rahman IA, Lazim MIM, Mohamad S, Peng KS, Othaman MA, Manan MA, Asri MAM (2018) The influence of lactobacilli in gaba and amino acid profile of fermented mature coconut water. Open Food Sci J 10:8–15. https://doi.org/10.2174/1874256401810010008

Rahmayanti HD, Amalia N, Yuliza E, Sustini E, Abdullah M (2019) Dried nata de coco for extend the shelf life of nuts. IOP Conf Ser Mater Sci Eng 622:012010. https://doi.org/10.1088/1757-899X/622/1/012010

Rao SS, Najam R (2016) Coconut water of different maturity stages ameliorates inflammatory processes in model of inflammation. J Intercult Ethnopharmacol 5(3):244–249. https://doi.org/10.5455/jice.20160402120142

Reddy P, Kumar KMR, Lakshmi MT, Kiran SR (2018) Tender coconut water uses, health benefits, good nutritive value and antioxidant capacity. Indian J Public Health Res Dev 9(4):184. https://doi.org/10.5958/0976-5506.2018.00280.2

Richter EM, de Jesus DP, Muñoz RAA, do Lago CL, Angnes L (2005) Determination of anions, cations, and sugars in coconut water by capillary electrophoresis. J Braz Chem Soc 16(6A):1134–1139. https://doi.org/10.1590/S0103-50532005000700008

Rodsamran P, Sothornvit R (2018) Bioactive coconut protein concentrate films incorporated with antioxidant extract of mature coconut water. Food Hydrocoll 79:243–252. https://doi.org/10.1016/j.foodhyd.2017.12.037

Rohaeti E, Fx EWL, Rakhmawati A (2018) Mechanical properties and antibacterial activity of cellulose composite based coconut water with addition glycerol, chitosan, and silver nanoparticle. Orient J Chem 34(3):1341–1349

Rosa MF, Abreu FAP (2000) Água de Coco: Métodos de Conservação Fortaleza: EMBRAPA – SPI, Document no. 37, June 2000. p 40 Rosa and Abreu 2000

Saat M, Singh R, Sirisinghe RG, Nawawi M (2002) Rehydration after exercise with fresh young coconut water, carbohydrate-electrolyte beverage and plain water. J Physiol Anthropol Appl Hum Sci 21(2):93–104. https://doi.org/10.2114/jpa.21.93

Salgueiro CCM, Nunes JF (2008) Powder coconut water (PCW®) on biotechnological processes. Journal of Biotechnology 136:S101–S102

Sanchez PC (1990) Vinegar. In: Coconut as food. Philippine Coconut Research and Development Foundation, Manila, pp 151–161

Sandhya VG, Rajamohan T (2006) Beneficial effects of coconut water feeding on lipid metabolism in cholesterol fed rats. J Med Food 9(3):400–407. https://doi.org/10.1089/jmf.2006.9.400

Sandhya VG, Rajamohan T (2008) Comparative evaluation of the hypolipidemic effects of coconut water and lovastatin in rats fed fat cholesterol enriched diet. Food Chem Toxicol 46:3586–3592. https://doi.org/10.1016/j.fct.2008.08.030

Santana MJ, de Oliveira AL, Queiroz LHK Jr, Mandal SM, Matos CO, Dias RO, Franco OL, Liao LM (2015) Structural insights into Cn-AMP1, a short disulfide-free multifunctional peptide from green coconut water. FEBS Lett 589(5):639–644. https://doi.org/10.1016/j.febslet.2015.01.029

Santoso U, Kubo K, Ota T, Tadokoro T, Maekawa A (1996) Nutrient composition of kopyor coconuts (Cocos nucifera L.). Food chemistry 57(2):299–304

Santos JL, Bispo VS, Filho AB, Pinto IFD, Dantas LS, Vasconcelos DF, Abreu F, Melo DA, Matos IA, Freitas FP, Gomes OF, Medeiros MHG, Matos HR (2013) Evaluation of chemical constituents and antioxidant activity of coconut water (*Cocos nucifera* L.) and caffeic acid in cell culture. An Acad Bras Cienc 85(4):1235–1247. https://doi.org/10.1590/0001-37652013105312

Seesuriyachan P, Kuntiya A, Hanmoungjai P, Techapun C (2011) Exopolysaccharide production by *Lactobacillus confusus* TISTR 1498 using coconut water as an alternative carbon source: the effect of peptone, yeast extract and beef extract. Songklanakarin J Sci Technol 33:379–387

Seo KI, Lee J, Choi RY, Lee HI, Lee JH, Jeong YK, Kim MJ, Lee MK (2014) Anti-obesity and anti-insulin resistance effects of tomato vinegar beverage in diet-induced obese mice. Food Funct 5:1579–1586

Shanika HKV, Wansapala MAJ (2018) Optimization of submerged batch fermented coconut water vinegar production process. Int J Sci Res 7(1):1849–1858

Shenkin A (2006) The key role of micronutrients. Clin Nutr 25(1):1–13. https://doi.org/10.1016/j.clnu.2005.11.006

Shivakumar S, Vijayendra SV (2006) Production of exopolysaccharides by Agrobacterium sp. CFR-24 using coconut water—a by-product of food industry. Lett Appl Microbiol 42(5):477–482. https://doi.org/10.1111/j.1472-765X.2006.01881.x

Shubhashree MN, Venkateshwarlu G, Doddamani SH (2014) Therapeutic and nutritional values of Narikelodaka (tender coconut water)—a review. Res J Pharmacogn Phytochem 6(4):195–201

Spencer DA (2007) Urinary stones: principles of ambulatory medicine, 7th edn. Lippincott Williams and Wilkins, Philadelphia, pp 754–766

Steiner I, Desser A (2008) Coconut water—composition, properties and processing. Ernähr 32:513–516

Survase SA, Saudagar PS, Singhal RS (2007) Use of complex media for the production of scleroglucan by *Sclerotium rolfsii* MTCC 2156. Bioresour Technol 98:1509–1512. https://doi.org/10.1016/j.biortech.2006.05.022

Suwannapinunt N, Burakorn J, Thaenthanee S (2007) Effect of culture conditions on bacterial BC (BC) production from Acetobacter xylinum TISTR976 and physical properties of BC parchment paper. J Sci Tech 14:357–365

Tallei TE, Marfuah S, Abas AH, Abram AADP, Pasappa N, Anggini PS, Soegoto AS, Wali F, Emran TB (2022) Nata as a source of dietary fiber with numerous health benefits. J Adv Biotechnol Exp Ther 5(1):189–197. https://doi.org/10.5455/jabet.2022.d107

Tan TC, Cheng LH, Bhat R, Rusul G, Easa AM (2014a) Composition, physicochemical properties and thermal inactivation kinetic of polyphenol oxidase and peroxidase from coconut water obtained from immature, mature and overly-mature coconut. Food Chem 142:121–128. https://doi.org/10.1016/j.foodchem.2013.07.040

Tan SN, Yong JWH, Ge L (2014b) Analyses of phytohormones in coconut (*Cocos nucifera* L.) water using capillary electrophoresis-tandem mass spectrometry. Chromatographia 1:211–226. https://doi.org/10.3390/chromatography1040211

Tangpong J, Nasrisuk T, Suangyaya W, Jantamattukan W (2008) Phytoestrogen of young coconut juice reduced hyperlipidemia and lipid peroxidation in over weight rats. Oxidants and antioxidants in Biol. Oxygen Club of California. Book of Abstracts, 12–15 Mar 2008, Santa Barbara, CA

Tanqueco RE, Rodriguez FM, Laude RP, Crueno ME (2007) Total free sugars, oil and total phenolics content of stored coconut (*Cocos nucifera* L.) water. Philipp J Sci 136(2):103–108

Tetra Pak (2019) The chemistry of coconut water. In: Coconut handbook. https://coconuthandbook.tetrapak.com/chapter/chemistry-coconut-water. Tetra Pak South East Asia Pte Ltd, Coconut Knowledge Centre, 19 Gul Lane, Singapore 629414

Thampan PK, Rethinam P (2004) Coconut products for health and medicine. Indian Coconut J 35:6–15

Thomas SZ, Pertiwi D, Bagus SA, Nuri S, Jelita BEM, Alfza NS (2017) Effect of tender coconut water on blood lipid levels in high fat diet fed male rats. J Krishna Inst Med Sci Univ 6(2):63–68

Treesuppharat W, Rojanapanthu P, Siangsanoh C (2017) Synthesis and characterization of bacterial cellulose and gelatin-based hydrogel composites for drug-delivery systems. Biotechnol Rep (Amsterdam, Netherlands) 15:84–91. https://doi.org/10.1016/j.btre.2017.07.002

Twishsri W, Runheem P, Usathit S, Watanayothin S, Naka P (2014) Study on fatty acid composition and amino acid content of coconut endosperm of selected coconut cultivars in Thailand. Acta Hort 1024:427–432. https://doi.org/10.17660/ActaHortic.2014.1024.59

Uddin S, Ali I, Hassan M, Hamayun L, Ali U, Saud S, Khan I, Ahmad W, Shah AB, Zeb A, Khan AA (2019) Therapeutic applications of coconut water mitigates diabetes mellitus in Oryctolagus cuniculus (Rabbit). Biomed J Sci Tech Res 16(4):12214–12219. https://doi.org/10.26717/BJSTR.2019.16.002884

Uphade BK, Shelke SS, Thorat DG (2008) Studies on some physico-chemical characteristics of coconut water near sugar and chemical factory, Kopergaon (MS). Int J Chem Sci 6(4):2052–2054

Vigliar R, Sdepanian VL, Fagundes-Neto U (2006) Perflbioquímico da água de coco de coqueiros de regiãonãolitorânea. J Pediatr 82(4):308–312. https://doi.org/10.2223/JPED.1508

Vishakh RS, Moodithaya S, Kumari (2014) Evaluation of antioxidant property of West Coast Tall variety tender coconut water and synthetic Trans–Zeatin–an in-vitro study. J Pharmacogn Phytochem 3(3):155–159

Wang HX, Ng TB (2005) An antifungal peptide from the coconut. Peptides 26(12):2392–2396. https://doi.org/10.1016/j.peptides.2005.05.009

Wei J, Zhao M, Meng K, Xia G, Pan Y, Li C, Zhang W (2022) The diuretic effects of coconut water by suppressing aquaporin and renin–angiotensin–aldosterone system in saline-loaded rats. Front Nutr 9:930506. https://doi.org/10.3389/fnut.2022.930506

Wijewardena HDARR, Amarakoon R (2020) Antibacterial activity of fermented coconut water produced by *Lactobacillus acidophilus* DSM 20079 and Lactobacillus plantarum. Int J Sci Res Innov Tech 7(1):54–62

Wu Y, Hu B (2009) Simultaneous determination of several phytohormones in natural coconut juice by hollow fiber-based liquid- liquid-liquid microextraction-high performance liquid chromatography. J Chromatogr A 1216(45):7657–7663. https://doi.org/10.1016/j.chroma.2009.09.008

Zhang C, Wang L, Zhao J, Zhu P (2011) Effect of drying methods on structure and mechanical properties of bacterial cellulose films. Adv Mater Res 239–242:2667–2670. https://doi.org/10.4028/www.scientifc.net/AMR.239-242.2667

Zhang G, Chen W, Chen W, Chen H (2018a) Improving the quality of matured coconut (*Cocos nucifera* Linn.) water by low alcoholic fermentation with *Saccharomyces cerevisiae*: antioxidant and volatile compounds. J Food Sci Technol 55(3):964–976. https://doi.org/10.1007/s13197-017-3004-y

Zhang G, Li X, Chen W, Chen P, Jin X, Chen W, Chen H (2018b) Organic acid content, antioxidant capacity, and fermentation kinetics of matured coconut (*Cocos nucifera*) water fermented by Saccharomyces cerevisiae D254. Int J Food Eng 14(3):20170331. https://doi.org/10.1515/ijfe-2017-0331

Zhang X, Peng L, Dai Y, Sheng X, Chen S, Xie Q (2020) Effects of coconut water on retina in diabetic rats. Evid Based Complement Alternat Med 2020:9450634. https://doi.org/10.1155/2020/9450634

Zulaikhah ST, Anies, Suwondo A, Santosa (2015) Effect of tender coconut water on antioxidant enzymatic superoxide dismutase (SOD), catalase (CAT), glutathione peroxidase (GPx) and lipid peroxidation in mercury exposure workers. Int J Sci Res 4(12):517–524

Zulaikhah ST, Wahyuwibowo J, Suharto MN, Enggartiasto BH, Ortanto MIR, Pratama AA (2021) Effect of tender coconut water (TCW) on TNF-α, IL-1 and IL-6 in Streptozotocin (STZ) and Nicotinamid (NA) induced diabetic rats. Pharm J 13(2):500–505. https://doi.org/10.5530/pj.2021.13.63

Chapter 6
Coconut Protein Concentrate: An Invaluable Food Supplement

Sai Prasanna N, Yumnan Nandan, Murugesan Selvakumar, Nilesh Choudhary, and K. S. M. S. Raghavarao

Abstract Plant proteins play a crucial role in human nutrition and health. Coconut, known as the most economical fruit worldwide, serves as a valuable source of oil and protein. Coconut proteins are highly nutritive, showcasing a well-balanced amino acid profile and good digestibility. Notably, coconut proteins possess medicinal properties, including hypolipidemic, cardioprotective, anti-diabetic, and antioxidant effects. These attributes contribute to human health and enhance the immune system. Plant-based protein ingredients have garnered significant attention for functional food formulations, offering improved nutritional value appreciated by both consumers and the food industry. Consequently, there is a growing interest in coconut protein powder and coconut whey powder for functional food applications. This chapter aims to explore coconut sources as alternatives to plant-based protein ingredients, discussing various isolation methods for coconut proteins and elucidating their functional and health benefits.

Keywords Plant-based proteins · Coconut proteins · Anti-diabetic · Functional ingredients · Nutritional quality

6.1 Introduction

Coconut (*Cocos nucifera* L.) belongs to the Arecaceae (Palmae) family and is cultivated worldwide especially in Indonesia, the Philippines, East Africa, the Caribbean and South Asian countries. Indonesia, India, Brazil, and Sri Lanka are the major countries producing coconut globally. (Sujatha and Deepa Balakrishnan 2023). Global production of coconut is about 66.67 million tons (Kumar et al. 2021). India is the third largest coconut producer in the world, next to Indonesia and the

S. Prasanna N · Y. Nandan · M. Selvakumar · N. Choudhary · K. S. M. S. Raghavarao (✉)
Department of Chemical Engineering, Indian Institute of Technology Tirupati, Tirupati, Andhra Pradesh, India
e-mail: nilesh@iittp.ac.in; raghava@iittp.ac.in

S. V. Ramesh, S. Praveen (eds.), *Coconut-Based Nutrition and Nutraceutical Perspectives*, https://doi.org/10.1007/978-981-97-3976-9_6

Philippines, with a total annual production of 20.73 million tons as per International Coconut Community (ICC) Statistical Year Book 2021. Southern Indian states, particularly, Andhra Pradesh, Karnataka, Kerala, and Tamil Nadu produce approximately 80–90% of total country's production (Kumar et al. 2021), while Kerala state alone contributes to 36.5% of total coconut production (Anoop et al. 2023; Mangalasseri and Singh 2023).

The coconut fruit comprises an outer fibrous coat, an inner hard shell, a white kernel or endosperm, and the inner cavity is filled with coconut water. According to Divya et al. (2023), the coconut fruit consists of the kernel (51.7%), water (9.8%), and shell (38.5%). There are various coconut products, such as virgin coconut oil, coconut gratings, coconut milk, coconut water, desiccated coconut, etc. These products exhibit commendable nutritional, medicinal, and biological properties, making them valuable for applications in nutraceuticals, cosmetics, and the food industry.

The rapid growth of the population and the changing dietary habits necessitate a consideration of the importance of human health through a nutritious diet. Consequently, there has been a steady increase in the demand for nutraceuticals, including dietary supplements and functional foods that offer good nutritional value to promote human health and immunity. This demand has intensified, particularly in the aftermath of the COVID-19 pandemic and other lifestyle-related disorders. Proteins play a crucial role as an essential component of a healthy diet, supporting the development and maintenance of cellular activities in the human body. The awareness of the potential detrimental effects of consuming meat has led to an increasing need for natural proteins as an alternative to animal proteins. Plant proteins, known for being clean and environmentally friendly, have gained significant attention in the development of functional foods. Due to its high nutritional content, coconut proteins (CP) have emerged as a novel and underutilized form of plant-based protein, containing 71–77% essential amino acids within a well-balanced amino acid profile (Sorde and Ananthanarayan 2019; Patil and Benjakul 2018). Coconut protein concentrate (CPC) is garnering considerable research interest as a nutraceutical and functional ingredient. This chapter presents the sources of coconut protein, various isolation methods, and their functional or biological properties in this context.

6.2 Sources of Coconut Protein

White coconut kernel is the main source of oil and protein. The biochemical composition of the coconut kernel is protein (3.33 g/100 g), total fat (33.49 g/100 g), and dietary fibre (9 g/100 g) (Divya et al. 2023).

Defatted coconut flour: Coconut milk obtained from wet kernel is composed of more than 30% fat, 3% protein and 55% water (Neela and Prasad, 2017). During the wet processing of coconut for virgin coconut oil (VCO) production, approximately 200 million tons of coconut cake is produced worldwide as a primary by-product (Li et al. 2018) and the coconut cake is fat-free and reported to be rich in dietary fibre (40 g/100 g) and protein (13.3 g/100 g) (Divya et al. 2023). Depending on the process used to produce coconut milk and VCO, defatted coconut cake or flour has been reported to have a protein content ranging from 4% to 25% (Divya et al. 2023).

Coconut Whey: Three phases, i.e., cream, coconut skim milk, and insoluble protein are formed in coconut milk during VCO production process (Naik et al. 2012; Raghavendra and Raghavarao 2011). The total protein content in coconut skim milk and insoluble solid residues is reported to be 29.9% and 16.0%, respectively (Thaiphanit and Anprung 2016). The coconut skim milk and insoluble protein together form aqueous coconut whey (CW) which is underutilized and discarded as waste into the environment (Naik et al. 2014). CW contains high protein content (~45.9%) and is not denatured (Thaiphanit and Anprung 2016). Thus, CW serves as an alternate source of vegetable or plant protein (Santhi et al. 2020). Currently, efforts are being made to efficiently recover coconut proteins from waste streams and by-products at VCO processing industries. Indeed, the recovery and utilization of coconut protein not only enhance the nutritional value of coconut products but also contribute to value addition and promote sustainability in the food system and environment.

6.3 Fractions of Coconut Protein

Proteins can be classified based on various criteria such as their solubility, amino acid composition, molecular weight, or functional properties. Based on the solubility and amino acid (AAs) composition, there are five different fractions of coconut proteins (CPs): glutelin-1 (soluble in acetic acid), glutelin-2 (soluble in diluted NaOH), prolamin (soluble in isopropanol), and albumin (soluble in water) (Lestari et al. 2021; Patil and Benjakul 2018). In general, coconut kernels are abundant in water and salt-soluble proteins (Yalegama et al. 2024). Wang et al. (2023) isolated protein fractions from coconut kernels and found that the albumin, globulin, gliadin, and glutelin fractions of CPs constitute 44.4%, 34.7%, 6.1%, and 13.2%, respectively. However, the composition of protein fractions in defatted coconut flour is globulin (61.9%), albumin (30.6%), glutelin (4.1%), prolamins (1.1%), and insoluble nitrogen (1.8%) (Rasyid et al. 1992). Patil and Benjakul (2017) delineated the composition of CPs fractions that were isolated from the defatted coconut kernel. It comprises prolamin (2%), glutelin-1 (10%), glutelin-2 (4%), albumin (19%) and globulin (36%). Globulin fraction in coconut protein isolated from defatted coconut cake was reported to be 36–40.1% (Briceño-Islas et al. 2023). The quantity of CPs fraction in coconut kernel varies according to variety, maturation, farming methods, and environmental conditions (Patil and Benjakul 2018).

Molecular weight of coconut protein fractions are in the range of 18 to 52 kDa for albumin, <60 kDa for globulin, 17 to 56 kDa for prolamin, and 14 to 100 kDa for glutein −1 (Li et al. 2018; Patil and Benjakul 2018). The majority of protein (about 65%) found in the coconut endosperm is called cocosin. It has a hexameric, quaternary structure with a MW ranging from 300 to 360 kDa, and 55 kDa for each subunit (Briceño-Islas et al. 2023; Patil and Benjakul 2017).

6.4 Nutritional Quality of Coconut Protein

6.4.1 *Amino Acid Composition*

The WHO/FAO-recommended essential amino acid composition, as well as the amino acids' purity, digestibility, and bioavailability, determine the nutritional value of CPs. The amino acid composition of coconut kernel and CPs are mentioned in Table 6.1. The primary fractions of CPs are albumin and globulin, which together contain the amino acids glutamine and glutamic acid. These two fractions account for 21 and 40 g/100 g of total protein, respectively (Li et al. 2018; Patil and Benjakul 2018). The major fraction of CPs is globulin, and its AA profile closely resembles that of coconut kernel flour as shown in Table 6.1. Aspartic acid, glutamic acid, arginine, and lysine are among the highly charged AAs found in high concentrations in the globulin portions of CPs. The percentage of AAs with polar side chains is greater in the albumin fraction (Patil and Benjakul 2018). In comparison to the

Table 6.1 Amino acid composition in coconut kernel (Onsaard et al. 2006), defatted coconut kernel (Patil and Benjakul 2017), coconut protein powder (Thaiphanit and Anprung 2016) and concentrated coconut powder (Ng et al. 2015)

Amino acids	Coconut kernel (% of total nitrogen)	Defatted coconut kernel (g/100 g protein)		Coconut protein powder (g/100 g)	Concentrated coconut protein powder (g/100 g protein)
		Albumin	Globulin		
Arginine	31.0	16.53	14.88	12.22	14.2
Lysine	4.8	6.26	5.005	3.35	3.74
Leucine	4.4	5.131	7.23	4.77	3.17
Valine	4.1	3.89	5.47	3.32	2.99
Isoleucine	2.9	2.44	3.54	2.05	2.07
Threonine	2.7	3.17	3.40	2.76	2.50
Phenylalanine	2.5	3.45	5.19	4.31	3.86
Histidine	2.4	2.40	2.82	2.29	1.80
Methionine	1.1	1.40	1.94	1.55	1.80
Cysteine	1.0	0.00	0.01	1.63	–
Tryptophan	0.8	–	–	1.38	–
Alanine	–	5.99	4.46	3.65	2.19
Aspartic acid	–	8.02	9.20	8.65	8.95
Glutamic acid	–	24.07	19.66	21.67	21.50
Glycine	–	4.42	4.96	3.91	3.55
Proline	–	5.45	3.86	3.37	3.60
Serine	–	4.76	5.00	4.11	2.04
Tyrosine	–	2.55	3.30	2.11	1.80

albumin fraction, the globulin fraction of CPs has a lower quantity of glutamic acid, lysine, and arginine, but a larger concentration of essential AAs like valine and phenylalanine (Kwon et al. 1996). Overall, albumin fraction of CPs is rich in lysine, while globulin fraction is deficient in methionine (Yalegama et al. 2024). Thus, the composition of AAs is responsible for the variations in the albumin and globulin fractions in CPs (Patil and Benjakul 2018).

Arginine, an essential AA for humans, is abundantly present in all coconut protein sources, and by-products (Morris 2006). Arginine content of 17.90 mg/100 g was reported in albumin fraction of CPs (Kwon et al. 1996), while 42.70 mg/100 g in protein crude extract (Lachance and Molina 1974) whereas the least amount (1.6 g/100 g) of arginine is reported in residual cake obtained after coconut milk extraction (Gunetileke and Laurentius 1974). Most plant proteins have low concentrations of essential AAs such as methionine, lysine, and tryptophan, but CPs contain these essential AAs (Krajcovicova-Kudlackova et al. 2005). The coconut skim milk obtained as a by-product during VCO production is dehydrated for CPs and freeze-dried. From Table 6.1, it can be observed that concentrated CP powders contain higher concentrations of AAs, especially Arginine (12.22 g/100 g), Glutamic acid (21.67 g/100 g), Aspartic acid (8.65 g/100 g), Leucine (4.77 g/100 g), Lysine (3.35 g/100 g) and Valine (3.33 g/100 g) which are in accordance of dietary requirements for adult as suggested FAO/WHO (Thaiphanit and Anprung 2016).

6.4.2 *Digestibility*

Coconut Proteins (CPs) contain essential AAs with good digestibility (Lachance and Molina 1974). Mepba and Achinewhu (2003) isolated CPC from whole coconut meal by alkaline extraction and isoelectric precipitation method. In the vitamin-free casein diet of albino rats, the protein digestibility was 88.75%, 89.30%, and 94.02% for whole coconut meal, defatted coconut meal, and full-fat coconut proteins, respectively. Mohd-Razali et al. (2020) reported the digestibility (by trypsin and pepsin) of coconut proteins derived from fermented coconut residues by *Aspergillus awamori* as 36.54–3.22% and 15–23%.

6.5 Isolation Methods of Coconut Protein

Isolation methods play a crucial role in determining the structure, and functionality of plant-based proteins. Based on the protein concentration, plant proteins are classified as protein flour (less than 65% protein), protein concentrate (between 65% and 90% protein), and protein isolate (more than 90% protein) (Kumar et al. 2021). The methods employed for the isolation of coconut proteins are discussed briefly in this section (Fig. 6.1).

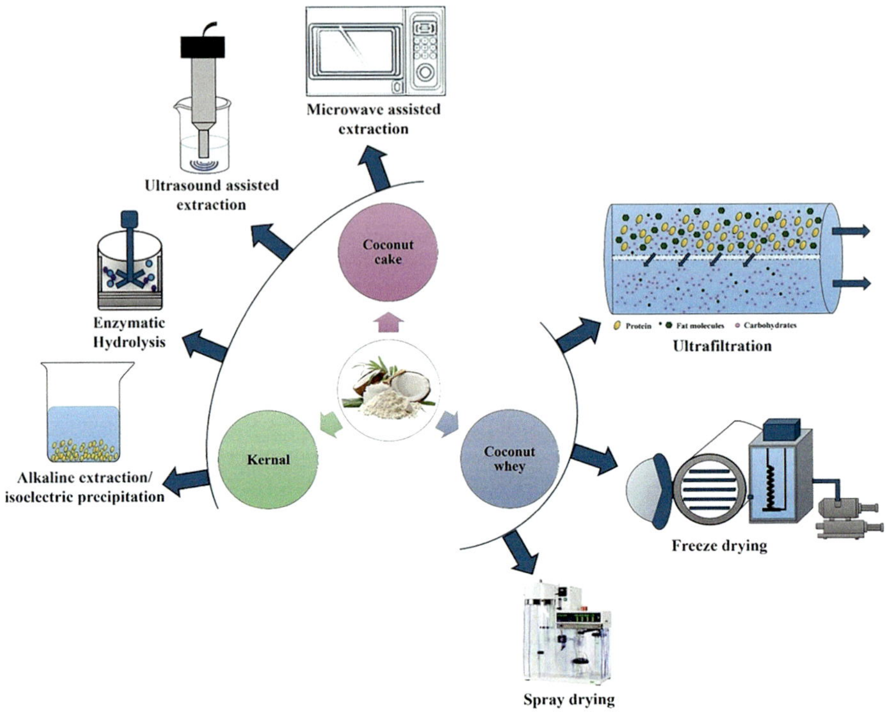

Fig. 6.1 Various methods of production of coconut proteins. Various techniques being used in the production of coconut proteins are depicted

6.5.1 Alkaline Extraction-Isoelectric Precipitation Method

This method, which involves the interplay of pH and solubility, is commonly used for isolating proteins from plant sources. Plant proteins in an alkaline medium (completely net negative charge) influence the electrostatic interactions with water, thus increasing their solubility. After the solubilization of proteins in an alkaline medium, the precipitation is performed to recover the dissolved proteins. One such method is the isoelectric precipitation, which balances the negative and positive charges of proteins at isoelectric point. It influences the repulsive electrostatic force, causing complex formation, aggregation, and finally precipitation of proteins (Cruz-Solis et al. 2023). CPs have a maximum precipitation at an isoelectric pH of 3.9–4.0 (Thaiphanit and Anprung 2016). CPs obtained through this method are dialyzed and freeze dried for concentrated CPs. The yield of CPs obtained through this method is mentioned in Table 6.2. The CPs isolated through this method were later purified through advanced chromatographic (gel filtration, ion-exchange, anion exchange, SDS- PAGE) techniques and membrane filtration processes.

Though this method is simple and inexpensive, the protein yields obtained are low (Chambal et al. 2013). The high alkaline conditions causes significant protein

Table 6.2 Summary of protein content and yield of coconut proteins isolated from various methods

Coconut source	Methodology	Conditions	Salient findings	References
Coconut pressed cake	Isoelectric precipitation method	• Cake mixed with water and pH adjusted to 11 with 0.7 M saturated Na_3PO_4 solution. Extracted with continuous stirring (250–300 rpm) at 50 °C for 1 h and centrifuged (3600 g, 20 °C, 20 min) for coconut protein supernatant	Protein content and yield obtained are ~30% (w/w) and (71%) respectively	Chambal et al. (2012)
Coconut cake	Isoelectric precipitation method	• Cake mixed with distilled water (1:12) and adjusted to pH 11 using 0.7 M Na_3PO_4	Protein content in CPP reported as 22.38 ± 0.94 and 7.21 ± 0.23 g/100 g respectively from coconut cakes pressed for milk and oil	Rodsamran and Sothornvit (2018a,b)
		• This suspension stirred at 50 °C for 1 h and centrifuged (12,000 g, 0 °C for 30 min) for supernatant		
		• This supernatant adjusted to pH 4 using 0.3 HCl and stirred at room temperature for 30 min, later centrifuged thrice and freeze-dried		
Coconut whey	Ultrafiltration (dead-end filtration) followed by spray drying	• Poly-ethersulfone membrane (MWCO—300 kDa, pore size—47 mm)	• Protein retention at TMP, 2 bar (86%) and 3 bar (87%), but slightly reduced at 4 bar (83%)	Vijayasanthi et al. (2020)
		• Spray drying conditions (flow rate—30 mL/min, nozzle diameter—2 mm, air pressure—3 bar, feed temperature—25 ± 1 °C)	• 83 wt.% protein retained and 84% sugar removed from CW through UF	

(continued)

Table 6.2 (continued)

Coconut source	Methodology	Conditions	Salient findings	References
Coconut milk	Ultrafiltration	• Coconut milk added with phosphate buffer (pH 7.5) and centrifuged (8000 rpm, 4 °C, 15 min) to remove the saturated fat	• Developed functionalized Polyethersulfone UF membrane (flat sheet type) with natural deep eutectic solvents for selective purification of coconut globulin at TMP (2 bar)	Balaraman et al. (2022)
		• Obtained skim milk was precipitated (0.1 M acetic acid and pH 4.3) and centrifuged for supernatant (coconut whey isolate) adjusted with phosphate buffer (pH 8) for coconut globulin precipitates	• Total protein content in coconut globulin through hybrid UF reported to be 7.2 mg/mL of source with yield of 53% and purity (42-fold)	
			• Coconut globulins purified with anion exchange chromatography increased purity (93-fold) and yield (68.4%)	
Coconut kernel	Ultrasound assisted extraction (UAE)	• Ground coconut pulp and water in the ratio 1:5 for coconut milk and homogenized (150 W, 23 ± 1 °C, 60 s) followed by UAE	• Protein yield in UAS treated samples reported as 49.6–86.1%	Martínez-Padilla et al. (2022)
		• Ultrasound extraction conditions: Probe (40 mm dia.), power (200 W), frequency (24 kHz), amplitude (80%), intensity (6.85 W/cm^2), energy (0.573 kW/kg) and time (2.5 min)		
		• Later ultrasound treated milk precipitated at pH 4, then separated for cream and precipitate Obtained cream solidified at 4 °C and defatted for protein precipitate.		

Coconut Press cake	Ultrasound assisted extraction	• Presses cake and tap water (1:2.5) heated up to 60 °C under continuous stirring	• Protein content increased from 19.67% (in coconut cake) to 30.10% (CPP)	Aiello et al. (2022)
		• Ultrasound reactor—conditions: Flow rate (140 L/h), probe dia (41.75 mm), power (4.5 kW), frequency (18 kHz), oscillation amplitude (45–60 μm), residence time (2 min), energy input per sample (117 kJ/L)	• Extraction yields of coconut pressed cake: 24.4 g dry extract/100 g	
		• Processed samples separated via a sieving press (150 μm) and obtained liquid fraction freeze-dried		
Coconut protein powder (enriched with lipid)	Spray drying	• Maltodextrin added to coconut skim milk for obtaining final concentration of 24–25°Brix	• Protein and fat content reported to be 42.22% and 14.55% (wet basis) in CPP	Kaewmungkun and Limpisophon (2023)
		• Spray drying conditions: Inlet air temperature - 190 °C and Outlet air temperature - 80 °C		
Mature coconut kernel	Isoelectric precipitation	• Mature coconut pressed for coconut milk and centrifugation (4000 g for 40 min) for skim milk and cream	• Coconut milk protein powder reported to have protein and fat content as 62.1% and 26.9%	Lad and Murthy (2012)
		• Coconut skim milk is refrigerated (6 ± 2 °C) overnight for supernatant and insoluble precipitate phases		
		• Supernatant phase adjusted to pH 3.9 using 0.1 M HCl, and centrifuged twice (5400 g for 25 min) for precipitates		
		• These protein precipitates dispersed in Millipore water and adjusted to pH 7.0 using 0.1 M NaOH followed by drying at room temperature		

(continued)

Table 6.2 (continued)

Coconut source	Methodology	Conditions	Salient findings	References
Mature coconut	Isoelectric precipitation and Freeze-thaw treatment	• Coconut milk obtained by pressing using hydraulic press (coconut kernel and water—1:1)	• Total protein content in freeze dried coconut cream fractions obtained through isoelectric precipitation method is higher (88.94%) than in freeze-thaw treatment (75.27%)	Onsaard et al. (2006)
		• pH of coconut milk adjusted to 3.9 with 0.1 or 1.0 M CH_3COOH and chilled for 8 h at 4 °C	• While fat content in coconut cream fractions obtained through isoelectric precipitation method (1.90%) than in freeze-thaw treatment (2.45%)	
		• Later, centrifuged at ambient temperature for cream and skim milk phases		
		• Isoelectric precipitation: The obtained cream phase thawed at 35–40 °C in water-bath		
		• Freeze-thaw treatment: The obtained cream phase subjected to freezing at −20 °C for 12 h, thawed in water bath at 40 °C		
		• After thawing in both methods, cream phase centrifuged (5500 g for 30) min to separate oil and protein fractions		
		• The protein fractions rinsed with hexane to remove any residual oil, and freeze-dried for coconut cream protein fractions		

Coconut protein powder from skimmed coconut milk	Ultrafiltration (dead-end filtration) followed by spray drying	• UF conditions: Polysulfone membranes (10 KDa) and polyamide membranes (NF)	• Albumin and globulin fractions in skimmed coconut milk are retained and concentrated in UF process	Ng et al. (2015)
			• Kinetin, and zeatin proteins of UF permeate are concentrated and retained in NF process	
		• Spray drying conditions: Flow rate (1.75 mL/min), nozzle dia (2 mm) feed temperature (25 ± 1 °C), inlet air (170 ± 1 °C), outlet air (85 ± 1 °C), air pressure (7 bar)	• Obtained coconut protein concentrate added with maltodextrin (5%) to maintain 20° Brix and spray dried for concentrated CPs powder	

denaturation and darkened coloration (Chandran et al. 2023). Thus, this method is not suitable for large scale production and there is a need for greener, safe and sustainable methods for producing coconut proteins.

6.5.2 Membrane Processing

Membrane processing is a non-thermal method enabling selective separation and subsequent recovery of target biomolecules from liquid foods. This method utilizes a microporous membrane and facilitates separation by applying external pressure (Yiengveerachon et al. 2020; Li et al. 2018). One such membrane separation method called ultrafiltration (UF) is used to concentrate and purify macromolecular (10^3–10^6 Daltons) solutions, particularly protein solutions. UF method isolates and concentrates proteins from skim milk (Svanborg et al. 2015), soybean whey (Cheng et al. 2017)], and cheese whey (Carter et al. 2021; Ostertag et al. 2023). Molecular weight cut off (MWCO) of membrane, pH of feed, and transmembrane pressure (TMP) affect the recovery of CPs from coconut whey (CW). The yield and retention (%) of CPs from CW are mentioned in Table 6.2.

Vijayasanthi et al. (2020) employed polyether sulfone UF membrane (300 kDa) to concentrate CPs from CW. This study reported protein retention of 83 wt.% and high sugar removal of 84% from coconut whey (pH 4) at a TMP of 4 bar. CW concentrated through UF process followed by spray drying produced concentrated CPs. The total protein content reported an increase of 45.49% (w/w) in concentrated CP powder as compared with CW (2.52% (w/w)). The fat content was also reported to be enriched from 9.49% (w/w) in concentrated CP powder as compared with CW (0.49% (w/w)). The concentrated CPs showed good flow properties, stability and sensory quality (Vijayasanthi et al. 2020).

Ng et al. (2015) concentrated CPs from coconut skim milk by employing UF and spray drying processes. The spray dried CPP was reported to have a total protein content of 32.85 g/100 g and fat content of 0.30 g/100 g. The complex mixture of coconut whey or skim milk causes fouling on the membrane surface, which reduces the effectiveness of the UF process. Unfortunately, the lack of anti-fouling characteristics in traditional membranes causes the UF process to have low flux and separation efficiency (Yiengveerachon et al. 2020). Polymeric UF membranes have been changed recently by adding charged functional groups to the membrane surface to improve the electrostatic repulsion between the charged membrane surface and proteins thereby controlling fouling to a certain extent.

Balaraman et al. (2022) created hybrid PES membranes with functional adjuvants like imidazole, a naturally occurring deep eutectic solvent, and used them to separate the coconut protein (cocosin) from CW. The isolated CPs (53% w/w) were subsequently ultra-purified with a greater purity fold (93-fold) using anion exchange chromatography. Recently, Rastogi et al. (2022) enhanced protein recovery from paneer whey by crosslinking whey proteins with the help of transglutaminase (TG) enzyme followed by UF at 1.5 bar. Cross-linking of proteins before UF reduced fouling by 9% on membrane surface and showed highest protein retention rate of 85%.

6.5.3 Novel Extraction Methods

As an alternative to conventional alkaline/isoelectric precipitation techniques, novel extraction techniques such as ultrasound, microwave, etc., are used to disrupt the cellular structure of plant sources, which in turn leads to a release of proteins from those plant sources. Martínez-Padilla et al. (2022) employed ultrasound and microwave as pre-treatment to coconut milk or coconut gratings-water mixtures and the process conditions are mentioned in Table 6.2. Ultrasound treatment was reported to be more efficient in protein recovery of 29.8–34.83% than microwave treated (21.89–24.71%) and untreated coconut milk (13.84–19.9%) (Martínez-Padilla et al. 2022). CPs are obtained from defatted coconut cake through ultrasound assisted extraction and found that *in-vitro* protein digestibility increased 62.6% in concentrated CPs from 40.8% in raw coconut (Aiello et al. 2022).

6.5.4 Drying Methods

Coconut skim milk and insoluble solid protein (together called coconut whey) obtained as by-products after protease enzyme treatment for VCO were thoroughly mixed and homogenized to obtain a TSS of 20° Brix (Naik et al. 2013). Obtained CW dehydrated through drying methods, i.e., drum drying (110 °C), freeze drying (33–330 mbar), and spray drying to produce CW powder. Spray-dried and freeze-dried CW powders have been found to have a high protein level (177 g/kg), whereas drum-dried powder has a low protein value (~159 g/kg) (Naik et al. 2013, 2014). Naik et al. (2012) developed high protein content (33.1% w/w) and low-fat content (3% w/w) spray-dried CW powder. In comparison to spray-dried (about 65%) and drum-dried (approximately 62%) powders, freeze-dried CW powder had the maximum solubility (nearly 80%) (Naik et al. 2014). Thus, CW powder obtained by freeze–drying ensures better quality and can be directly utilized for different food formulations (Naik et al. 2013).

Drying of aqueous CW at high temperatures could cause the denaturation of proteins and modify their structures as well. At the lab scale and in pharma industries, freeze-drying method is commonly employed to produce protein concentrates. Spray drying is a vital process for producing various concentrated protein powders in the food industries (Zhao et al. 2013). Simple, inexpensive, repeatable, and readily scaled up, spray-drying is especially helpful for encapsulating heat-sensitive biomolecules (Di Giorgio et al. 2019). Spray dried CP powders had characteristic milky, coconut and nutty aroma (Naik et al. 2012), and had a shelf life of 6 months approximately, under ambient conditions (27 °C & 65% RH) (Naik et al. 2013).

Thus, spray drying was found as the most feasible method to produce CPC with better quality.

6.6 Biopeptides from Coconut Protein

In the quest for developing functional foods and dietary supplements promoting human health, bioactive peptides derived from vegetable proteins are gradually increasing. These biopeptides can have immunomodulatory, antimicrobial, antioxidant, antithrombotic, hypocholesterolaemia, and antihypertensive effects depending on the kind, sequence, and molecular weight of amino acids (Montesano et al. 2020). Biopeptides are produced from the plant protein source by enzymatic hydrolysis, fermentation, gastrointestinal digestion (digestive enzymes) or *in vitro* hydrolysis by proteolytic enzymes (Gorguç et al. 2020; Rizzello et al. 2016). Coconut cake albumin undergoes high pressure pretreatment and is sequentially digested with a mixture of enzymes (such as alcalase, favourzyme, pepsin, and trypsin), later freeze dried for CP hydrolysates or biopeptides (Li et al. 2016). Zheng et al. (2019) identified three new antioxidant and ACE-inhibitory peptides made of 6–7 amino acids that were derived from coconut cake albumin. These biopeptides have the potential to be utilized as functional food ingredients due to their strong ACE-inhibitory activity and excellent radical scavenging capacity (Zheng et al. 2019). Furthermore, these biopeptides have the ability to decrease intracellular ET-1 levels and shield vascular endothelial cells from damage caused by reactive oxygen species, suggesting that they may have antihypertensive properties (Li et al. 2016; Zheng et al. 2019).

The globulins and bioactive peptides with good antioxidant activity obtained from fresh coconut kernel (by protease enzyme hydrolysis) could be used as emulsifiers and antioxidants for nutraceutical applications (Ma et al. 2022a). Coconut protein hydrolysates obtained (by alcalase enzyme hydrolysis) from coconut skim milk were reported to stabilize virgin olive and sunflower O/W emulsions (Thaiphanit et al. 2016).

6.7 Functional Properties of Coconut Proteins

Amino acids are the building blocks of proteins, which are important food additives and components. Understanding the functional qualities of CPs, such as their solubility, gelation, emulsifying, and foaming capacities, is crucial for incorporating them into food formulations and novel processed goods with high nutritional value. The functional qualities will also be significantly impacted by the production processes employed for isolating CPs and the processing parameters involved in those processes.

6.7.1 Solubility

The capacity of protein to dissolve in an aqueous solvent is known as its solubility. The isoelectric point of most plant proteins ranges from pH 4 to 5. The majority of CPs' solubility occurs in very acidic and alkaline solutions, with pH 4 exhibiting the least amount of solubility (Rodsamran and Sothornvit 2018a,b). The pH range between 4 and 5 is the minimum solubility of CPs isolated from coconut kernel and coconut whey. The solubility of CP was studied at low concentrations (0.1–0.7%) (Naik et al. 2012, 2014; Thaiphanit and Anprung 2016). The low solubility of CPs limits their food applications.

Increasing the ionic strength of solvents increases the solubility of proteins Kaewmungkun and Limpisophon reported maximum solubility of CPs (2% w/v) when dispersed in 0.1 M citrate buffer at pH 6.2. The salting-in effect caused a considerable increase in protein solubility from 6.20% to 18.58%, when the ionic strength of solvents such as NaCl (0.2–0.5 M) was increased. Although the solubility of CPs was enhanced by raising the pH and NaCl concentrations, the CP suspension eventually precipitated (Kaewmungkun and Limpisophon 2023).

Enzymatic hydrolysis of proteins into smaller fractions of biopeptides is another way to change the solubility (Tan et al. 2023). Coconut proteins are usually denatured at 80 °C or higher temperatures (Patil and Benjakul 2018). Denatured proteins become unfolded and may lose their solubility (Tan et al. 2023). Thus, temperature also has a strong influence on the solubility of CPs. CPs should have high solubility or dispersibility to enhance their food applications.

6.7.2 Gelation

Because of protein unfolding dissociation, association, and aggregation, gelation of proteins results in a three-dimensional cross-linked protein network. A substantial portion of plant proteins are made up of globulins, which have the ability to gel under various process conditions (Tan et al. 2023). The globulin fraction of CPs improves their gelation potential, thus enhancing the use of CPs as a new gelling and thickening agent in food products such as gels, jams, jellies, desserts, cheese like and yoghurt-like products (Yalegama et al. 2024).

6.7.3 Emulsifying Ability

Patil and Benjakul (2018) reported that globulin fractions (accounting for 60–75%) of CPs showed better emulsifying properties than albumin fractions isolated from defatted coconut meat. Recently, coconut protein as an emulsifier gained much attention. CPs function as organic emulsifiers, stabilizing the oil droplets in coconut milk. A significant factor in the stability of coconut milk is the globulin fraction of the coconut (Chen et al. 2023a,b). CPs can be adsorbed rapidly to the oil-water interface; however, they have poor emulsifying ability. Onsaard et al. (2006) isolated CPs from coconut skim milk and reported to stabilize viscous emulsions. In contrast to emulsions made with whey protein isolate, those made with CPs are not as stable. For this reason, thick emulsions used in desserts, yogurts, sauces, and dressings need to be stabilized as much as possible by CPs.

Naik et al. (2012) revealed that compared to defatted soybean powder and skimmed milk, spray-dried CW powder had superior emulsifying qualities. The albumin fraction of CPs showed low emulsifying ability than the globulin fractions in VCO-in-water emulsion. It has been reported that the globulin fraction of CPs stabilized the emulsion more steadily than the albumin fraction (Patil and Benjakul 2017). The emulsifying ability of CPs is improved by various modification methods such as heat treatment (Thaiphanit and Anprung 2016; Ma et al. 2022a,b), ultrasound combined with heating (Sun et al. 2022) ultrasound (Lad and Murthy, 2012), enzymatic hydrolysis (Thaiphanit et al. 2016), and atmospheric cold plasma (Chen et al. 2023a,b) are being studied to enhance CPs applications in food industry.

6.7.4 *Foaming Ability*

The foaming ability of native plant proteins is affected by protein properties such as solubility, molecular weight, conformation, and air-water interface tension (Meenmanee et al. 2022). The compact structure of proteins makes them difficult to unfold and causes them to be slowly adsorbed at the interface (Tan et al. 2023). Compared to defatted coconut cake, CPs isolated from coconut milk cake have a decreased foaming capacity. Additionally, the pH affects the foaming ability of CPs (Mat et al. 2022). Recently enzymatic and non-enzymatic deamidation methods have been employed to improve the foaming stability and capacity of CPs for food applications such as foams, emulsions, whipped cream and toppings, mousses, ice-creams, baked goods and beverages (Meenmanee et al. 2022; Rodsamran and Sothornvit 2018a,b).

6.8 Health Benefits of Coconut Protein

The beneficial effects of CPs in preventing various disease conditions such as cardiovascular diseases, diabetes, neurodegenerative diseases, etc., or having novel therapeutic effects are discussed in this section (Fig. 6.2).

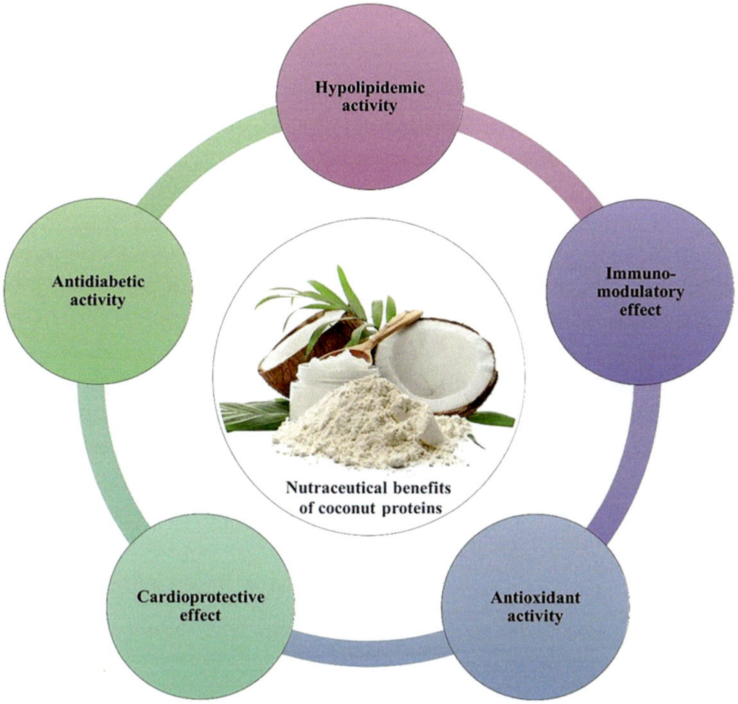

Fig. 6.2 Health benefits of coconut proteins

6.8.1 Anti-diabetic Properties

In recent decades, diabetes mellitus has emerged a prevalent issue, primarily attributed to changes in dietary habits, increasing rates of obesity, and reduced physical activity. Given the global epidemic of diabetes, significant research efforts are underway to formulate novel anti-diabetic drugs (Dahlen et al. 2022). The demand for plant-based products with anti-diabetic activity has been increasing due to their minimal side effects and ease of availability. Thus, plant-based proteins (especially coconut proteins) are gaining interest in the current market. Salil and coworkers conducted research on the impact of coconut proteins (CPs) from the kernel on alloxan induced diabetic rats for 45 days. Diet rats treated with CPs showed a significant decrease in serum glucose and an increase in insulin and hepatic glycogen levels. These results imply that CP supplementation improved pancreatic functions by preserving beta cells, which allowed diabetic rats' carbohydrate metabolism to return to normal (Salil et al. 2011). The same research group further reported that arginine rich CPs modulated the nitric oxide pathway, reduced hyperglycemia, hyperlipidemia and increased the hypolipidemic and antioxidant enzyme level (SOD, CAT) significantly in alloxan induced diabetic rats (Salil et al. 2011, 2012).

6.8.2 Hypolipidemic Activity

Hyperlipidemia also called as "hyperlipoproteinemia", is a disorder characterized by abnormal lipid metabolism, resulting in increased levels lipids in the serum such as triglycerides, cholesterol and low-density lipoprotein cholesterol (LDL-C) (Kang et al. 2019). The hyperlipidemic condition can increase the risk of obesity, diabetes, heart stroke and cardiovascular disease. Salil and Rajamohan group examined the hypolipidemic and antiperoxidative activity of CPs on hypercholesterolemic albino rats induced by high fat diet. Animals supplemented with CPs showed low levels of cholesterol, triglycerides, phospholipids and LDL-C. The HMG CoA reductase (the main rate limiting step in cholesterol biosynthesis pathway) activity showed less in high fat diet rats while CPs treated rats resulted showing high level of HMG CoA. Also, the CPs fed animals resulted in reduced malondialdehyde (lipid peroxide level) and increasing the SOD and catalase in the heart (Salil and Rajamohan 2001). Similar research was performed by Mini and coworker on ethanol fed albino rats. Therefore, the authors concluded that the high content of L-arginine in CPs may be the primary reason for their hypolipidemic activity (Mini and Rajamohan 2004).

6.8.3 Immunomodulatory Activity

Immunomodulatory agents are used to regulating the immune system of the human body and control various life-threatening diseases such as multiple sclerosis, microbial infections and ageing, cancer, etc. Vigila and Baskaran (2008) found that the CPs act as a potent immunomodulatory agent in cyclophosphamide induced albino mice. Animals treated with orally administered CPs exhibited an increased count of blood cells (WBC, RBC, and platelets level in blood).

6.8.4 Cardioprotective Activity

Nowadays plant-based products are gaining significant research attention in managing or preventing cardiovascular diseases (Langyan et al. 2022). Mini and Rajamohan (2002) investigated the cardiovascular effect of CPs on myocardial infarction induced rats. The significant reduction of creatinine phosphokinase, glutamate pyruvate transaminase and glutamate oxaloacetate enzyme levels were observed on CPs administrated animals. However, the nitric acid synthase (NOS) activity level increased in the myocardial infarction-induced rats. The authors compared the enzyme activity level with arginine supplemented rats and concluded that the regular consumption of CPs may help in the prevention of cardiovascular disease. Additionally, CPs with high content of L-arginine are the major factor contributing to cardioprotective effect (Mini and Rajamohan 2002). Similar research was examined by Remya and coworkers on myocardial infarction induced albino rats. The CPs treatment (orally 50 mg/100 g body weight) upregulated the NOS pathway and downregulated the nuclear factor-kappa B and tumor necrosis factor-alpha expression on myocardial infarction induced rats (Remya et al. 2013).

6.8.5 *Antioxidant Activity*

Reactive oxygen species and reactive nitrogen species are two examples of extremely reactive free radicals that develop in excess and lead to oxidative stress. Numerous chronic illnesses, including diabetes, Alzheimer's disease, rheumatoid arthritis, cardiovascular disorders, cancer, and others, can be brought on by these free radicals (Wen et al. 2020). Due to growing consumer demand for highly nutritional and functional proteins, scientists are mainly focusing on plant-based proteins (Dewage et al. 2022).

Zheng and Li (2018) extracted the coconut milk and subjected it to enzyme hydrolysis using protease, alcalase, papain etc. to bioactive peptides. Five different CPs hydrolysate fractionations (Fraction—A to E) were obtained using G-25 gel chromatography. CPs hydrolysate. Fraction-E showed the highest antioxidant activities against hydroxyl free radicals. CPs hydrolysate Fraction-D exhibited the highest protective activities against damage of DNA (Li et al. 2016). Li and co-researchers fractionated the different CPs, i.e., glutelin-1 and glutelin-2, prolamine, albumin and globulin from coconut cake using electrophoretic separations. Prolamine exhibited the highest radical scavenging activity against ABTS, hydroxyl radicals followed by glutelin-2, glutelin-1. Globulin demonstrated significant chelating ability which was much greater than that of standard Butylated hydroxytoluene (Li et al. 2018). Ma et al. (2022b) identified 17 proteins and 9 globulins of coconut through the functional and bioinformatic analysis. These globulins and proteins of coconut, and their corresponding bioactive peptides can be used for emulsifiers and antioxidant applications in future (Ma et al. 2022b).

6.9 Food Applications

Coconut kernel has become a common protein source in the diet of ruminant animals. Despite the high protein content (21.2–21.4%), the essential AAs especially lysine (0.59%) and methionine (0.34%) in coconut kernel are lower in comparison with soybean (2.69% and 0.62%), sunflower (1.00% and 0.5%), and groundnut (1.54% and 0.54%) respectively (Moorthy and Viswanathan 2009). Thus, the use of coconut cake and coconut kernel in human diets has been restricted due to their high fiber content, lack of essential AAs (like lysine and methionine), and low concentrations of essential AAs (especially tryptophan, lysine, methionine, and histidine)

(Mat et al. 2022; Ravindran and Blair 1992; Singh et al. 2022). Therefore, further supplementation of coconut kernel and cake is required for dietary food and nutraceutical applications.

Currently, defatted coconut flour obtained during VCO production is being utilized as functional ingredient in food products. Thomas et al. (2022) incorporated defatted coconut cake (10 g) in ready-to-eat pasta formulations for protein enrichment and found that protein content increased from 6.7 g (in the control sample) to defatted coconut-based pasta (7.04 g). Adeloye et al. (2020) mixed defatted coconut flour (10%) to enrich the protein content in nixtamalized maize flour, and also to improve the antioxidant properties. Adsare and Annapure (2023) developed muffins with good acceptability by replacing refined wheat flour with defatted coconut flour (50%) and protein content increased to 6.87 g in wheat flour-based muffins as compared to coconut flour-based muffins (7.57 g). Thus, defatted coconut cake obtained as by-products from coconut oil and milk processing industries serves as a good source of CPs and can be used for nutraceutical formulations.

Rodsamran and Sothornvit (2018a,b) obtained CPs from coconut cake which later defatted for CP powder, and mixed with concentrated coconut water (CCW) to develop biodegradable CP films. The high total phenolic content in CCW reported to be responsible for highest antioxidant capacity of developed CP films. The dark brown colour of developed CP films might act as UV barrier packaging and extend the shelf-life of food products (Rodsamran and Sothornvit 2018a,b). In recent times, CP-enriched lipid powder can be used as a functional ingredient in food formulations such as emulsion-based products, coffee whiteners, and plant protein drinks (Kaewmungkun and Limpisophon 2023).

6.10 Conclusions and Future Perspectives

Coconut protein isolated from white coconut kernel with a balanced AA profile can be used a protein source in the human diet. CPs reported to have high amino acid compositions, particularly, arginine, glutamic acid, and aspartic acid, but deficient in sulphur containing amino acid (i.e., methionine). Thus, CPs require amino acid supplementation to meet the standard composition as suggested by WHO/FAO.

Arginine of CPs is mainly responsible for anti-diabetic, antioxidant, hypolipidemic, and cardiovascular effect. Thus, coconut protein concentrates with high purity and significant health benefits can serve as excellent dietary supplements and functional ingredients. The digestibility of CPs is affected by their chemical structure, processing/isolation methods, and the presence of other unfavourable compounds. Therefore, the digestibility and nutraceutical properties of CPs are required to be evaluated when replacing animal proteins in the human diet. Additionally, the prospects of consumption of CPs in human health and nutrition need to be elaboratively studied.

There is huge scope for developing more sustainable, low cost and safe methods for isolating high quality CPs. As an alternative to the conventional isoelectric precipitation method, novel processing methods such as deep eutectic solvent, ultrasound and microwave assisted extraction, etc., can be employed to produce CPs. Existing UF membrane processes can be combined with other techniques such as electro-dialysis, ultrasound, cross-linking with enzymes, or membrane surface modification in order to achieve higher recovery of CPs from aqueous coconut whey at large-scale.

References

Adeloye JB, Osho H, Idris LO (2020) Defatted coconut flour improved the bioactive components, dietary fibre, antioxidant and sensory properties of nixtamalized maize flour. J Agric Food Res 2:100042. https://doi.org/10.1016/j.jafr.2020.100042

Adsare SR, Annapure US (2023) Partially defatted coconut flour as a functional ingredient in replacement of refined wheat flour for development of fiber rich muffins. J Food Sci Technol 61:491–502. https://doi.org/10.1007/s13197-023-05857-2

Aiello G, Xu R, Pugliese R, Bartolomei M, Li J, Bollati C, Rueller L, Robert J, Arnoldi A, Lammi C (2022) Quality assessment of the protein ingredients recovered by ultrasound-assisted extraction from the press cakes of coconut and almond beverage preparation. Foods 11:3693. https://doi.org/10.3390/foods11223693

Anoop M, Sirohi S, Singh HP (2023) Effect of risk on irrigation adoption by coconut farmers in Kerala. Indian J Ecol 50(3):870–874

Balaraman HB, Rangarajan V, Rathnasamy SK (2022) Empirical flux modelling for cocosin enrichment from Cocos nucifera whey using natural deep eutectic solvent based affinity membrane. Ind Crop Prod 190:115893. https://doi.org/10.1016/j.indcrop.2022.115893

Briceño-Islas G, Estarrón-Espinosa M, Urías-Silvas JE (2023) Revalorization of coconut from Guerrero, Mexico: isolation and characterization of oils and proteins. ACS Food Sci Technol 3(4):648–657

Carter B, DiMarzo L, Pranata J, Barbano DM, Drake MA (2021) Efficiency of removal of whey protein from sweet whey using polymeric microfiltration membranes. J Dairy Sci 104:8630–8643. https://doi.org/10.3168/jds.2020-18771

Chambal B, Bergenståhl B, Dejmek P (2012) Edible proteins from coconut milk press cake; one step alkaline extraction and characterization by electrophoresis and mass spectrometry. Food Res Int 47:146–151. https://doi.org/10.1016/j.foodres.2011.04.036

Chambal B, Bergenståhl B, Dejmek P (2013) Coconut press cake alkaline extract—protein solubility and emulsification properties. Food Nutr Sci 4:29–37. https://doi.org/10.4236/fns.2013.49a2005

Chandran AS, Suri S, Choudhary P (2023) Sustainable plant protein: an up-to-date overview of sources, extraction techniques and utilization. Sustain Food Technol 1:466–483. https://doi.org/10.1039/d3fb00003f

Chen GQ, Qu Y, Gras SL, Kentish SE (2023a) Separation technologies for whey protein fractionation. Food Eng Rev 15:438–465. https://doi.org/10.1007/s12393-022-09330-2

Chen Y, Yao M, Yang T, Fang Y, Xiang D, Zhang W (2023b) Changes in structure and emulsifying properties of coconut globulin after the atmospheric pressure cold plasma treatment. Food Hydrocoll 136:108289

Cheng J, Xie S, Wang S, Xue Y, Jiang L, Liu L (2017) Optimization of protein removal from soybean whey wastewater using chitosan ultrafiltration. J Food Process Eng 40:1–9. https://doi.org/10.1111/jfpe.12370

Cruz-Solis I, Ibarra-Herrera CC, Rocha-Pizaña MR, Luna-Vital D (2023) Alkaline extraction–isoelectric precipitation of plant proteins. In: Hernández-Álvarez AJ, Mondor M, Nosworthy

MG (eds) Green protein processing technologies from plants: novel extraction and purification methods for product development. Springer International Publishing, Cham, pp 1–29. https://doi.org/10.1007/9783-031-16968-7_1
Dahlen AD, Dashi G, Maslov I, Attwood MM, Jonsson J, Trukhan V, Schiöth HB (2022) Trends in antidiabetic drug discovery: FDA approved drugs, new drugs in clinical trials and global sales. Front Pharmacol 12:1–16. https://doi.org/10.3389/fphar.2021.807548
Dewage E, Sandun N, Nam K, Huang X, Ahn DU (2022) Mechanisms, and applications: a review. Antioxidants 11(1025):1–18
Di Giorgio L, Salgado PR, Mauri AN (2019) Encapsulation of fish oil in soybean protein particles by emulsification and spray drying. Food Hydrocoll 87:891–901. https://doi.org/10.1016/j.foodhyd.2018.09.024
Divya PM, Roopa BS, Manusha C, Balannara P (2023) A concise review on oil extraction methods, nutritional and therapeutic role of coconut products. J Food Sci Technol 60:441–452. https://doi.org/10.1007/s13197-022-05352-0
Gorguç A, Gençdag E, Yılmaz FM (2020) Bioactive peptides derived from plant origin byproducts: Biological activities and techno-functional utilizations in food developments—a review. Food Res Int 136:109504. https://doi.org/10.1016/j.foodres.2020.109504
Gunetileke KG, Laurentius SF (1974) Conditions and protein for the separation from coconut milk of oil emulsion. Food Technol Sec 39:230–233. https://doi.org/10.1111/j.1365-2621.1974.tb02863.x
International Coconut Community (ICC) Statistical Year Book (2021) https://coconutcommunity.org/page-publication/7/4
Kaewmungkun K, Limpisophon K (2023) Characteristics of coconut protein-enriched lipid and the effects of pH, NaCl, and xanthan gum on its dispersibility. J Saudi Soc Agric Sci 22:351–360. https://doi.org/10.1016/j.jssas.2023.03.001
Kang HK, Lee HH, Seo CH, Park Y (2019) Antimicrobial and immunomodulatory properties and applications of marine-derived proteins and peptides. Mar Drugs 17:350. https://doi.org/10.3390/md17060350
Krajcovicova-Kudlackova M, Babinska K, Valachovicova M (2005) Health benefits and risks of plant proteins. Bratisl Lek Listy 106:231–234
Kumar M, Tomar M, Potkule J, Verma R, Punia S, Mahapatra A, Belwal T, Dahuja A, Joshi S, Berwal MK, Satankar V, Bhoite AG, Amarowicz R, Kaur C, Kennedy JF (2021) Advances in the plant protein extraction: mechanism and recommendations. Food Hydrocoll 115:106595. https://doi.org/10.1016/j.foodhyd.2021.106595
Kwon K, Park KH, Rhee KC (1996) Fractionation and characterization of proteins from coconut (Cocos nucifera L.). J Agric Food Chem 44:1741–1745. https://doi.org/10.1021/jf9504273
Lachance PA, Molina MR (1974) Nutritive value of a fiber-free coconut protein extract obtained by an enzymic-chemical method introduction. J Food Sci 39:581–584
Lad VN, Murthy ZVP (2012) Enhancing the stability of oil-in-water emulsions emulsified by coconut milk protein with the application of acoustic cavitation. Ind Eng Chem Res 51:4222–4229. https://doi.org/10.1021/ie202764f
Langyan S, Yadava P, Khan FN, Dar ZA, Singh R, Kumar A (2022) Sustaining protein nutrition through plant-based foods. Front Nutr 8:772573. https://doi.org/10.3389/fnut.2021.772573
Lestari D, Ridho Rahmani A, Ariono D (2021) Production of coconut oil and protein for food and cosmetic ingredients. IOP Conf Ser Mater Sci Eng 1143:012039. https://doi.org/10.1088/1757-899x/1143/1/012039
Li Y, Zheng Y, Zhang Y, Liu L, Zhao S (2016) Purification, characterization, synthesis: In vivo and in vitro antihypertensive activity of bioactive peptides derived from coconut (Cocos nucifera L.) cake globulin hydrolysates. RSC Adv 6:92688–92698. https://doi.org/10.1039/c6ra19971b
Li Y, Zheng Y, Zhang Y, Xu J, Gao G (2018) Antioxidant activity of coconut (Cocos nucifera L.) protein fractions. Molecules 23:1–11. https://doi.org/10.3390/molecules23030707

Ma J, Chen H, Chen W, Wu J, Li Z, Zhang M et al (2022a) Effects of heat treatment and pH on the physicochemical and emulsifying properties of coconut (Cocos nucifera L.) globulins. Food Chem 388:133031

Ma J, Pan C, Chen H, Chen W, Chen W, Zhang M, Zhong Q (2022b) Insight of the functional and biological activities of coconut (Cocos nucifera L.) protein by proteomics analysis and protein-based bioinformatics. Molecules 27:2987. https://doi.org/10.3390/molecules27092987

Mangalasseri A, Singh HP (2023) Effect of risk on irrigation adoption by coconut farmers in Kerala. Indian J Ecol 50(3):870–874. https://doi.org/10.55362/ije/2023/3984

Martínez-Padilla LP, Hernández-Rojas FS, Sosa-Herrera MG, Juliano P (2022) Novel application of ultrasound and microwave-assisted methods for aqueous extraction of coconut oil and proteins. J Food Sci Technol 59:3857–3866. https://doi.org/10.1007/s13197-022-05409-0

Mat K, Abdul Kari Z, Rusli ND, Che Harun H, Wei LS, Rahman MM, Mohd Khalid HN, Mohd Ali Hanafiah MH, Mohamad Sukri SA, Raja Khalif RIA (2022) Coconut palm: food, feed, and nutraceutical properties. Animals 12:2107

Meenmanee S, Rattananukrom A, Thaiphanit S, Suppavorasatit I (2022) Improvement of solubility, foaming, and emulsification properties of coconut (Cocos nucifera L.) protein by non-enzymatic deamidation. LWT 153:112493. https://doi.org/10.1016/j.lwt.2021.112493

Mepba HD, Achinewhu SC (2003) Effects of processing on protein nutritive quality of coconut Cocos nucifera products. Plant Foods Hum Nutr 58:15–25. https://doi.org/10.1023/A:1024006620501

Mini S, Rajamohan T (2002) Cardioprotective effect of coconut kernel protein in isoproterenol administered rats. Indian J Biochem Biophys 39:197–200

Mini S, Rajamohan T (2004) Influence of coconut kernel protein on lipid metabolism in alcohol fed rats. Indian J Exp Biol 42:53–57

Mohd-Razali A, Morni MM, Taib M, Ahmad A (2020) Phytic acid content and digestibility of coconut residues derived-proteins after solid-state fermentation by Aspergillus awamori. Malaysian Appl Biol 49:121–126. https://doi.org/10.55230/mabjournal.v49i4.1601

Montesano D, Gallo M, Blasi F, Cossignani L (2020) Biopeptides from vegetable proteins: new scientific evidences. Curr Opin Food Sci 31:31–37. https://doi.org/10.1016/j.cofs.2019.10.008

Moorthy M, Viswanathan K (2009) Nutritive value of extracted coconut (Cocos Nucifera) meal. Res J Agric Biol Sci 5:515–517

Morris SM (2006) Arginine: beyond protein. Am J Clin Nutr 83:508–512. https://doi.org/10.1093/ajcn/83.2.508s

Naik A, Raghavendra SN, Raghavarao KSMS (2012) Production of coconut protein powder from coconut wet processing waste and its characterization. Appl Biochem Biotechnol 167:1290–1302. https://doi.org/10.1007/s12010-012-9632-9

Naik A, Prakash M, Ravi R, Raghavarao KSMS (2013) Storage study and quality evaluation of coconut protein powder. J Food Sci 78:1784–1792. https://doi.org/10.1111/1750-3841.12267

Naik A, Venu GV, Prakash M, Raghavarao KSMS (2014) Dehydration of coconut skim milk and evaluation of functional properties. CYTA J Food 12:227–234. https://doi.org/10.1080/19476337.2013.833296

Neela S, Prasad NBL (2017) Asian Journal of Food and Agro-Industry Induced fermentative production of virgin coconut oil, As. J. Food Ag-Ind. 2012 (2017) 355–363. www.ajofai.info.

Ng CY, Mohammad AW, Ng LY, Jahim JM (2015) Sequential fractionation of value added coconut products using membrane processes. J Ind Eng Chem 25:162–167. https://doi.org/10.1016/j.jiec.2014.10.028

Onsaard E, Vittayanont M, Srigam S, McClements DJ (2006) Comparison of properties of oil-in-water emulsions stabilized by coconut cream proteins with those stabilized by whey protein isolate. Food Res Int 39:78–86. https://doi.org/10.1016/j.foodres.2005.06.003

Ostertag F, Krolitzki E, Berensmeier S, Hinrichs J (2023) Protein valorisation from acid whey—screening of various micro- and ultrafiltration membranes concerning the filtration performance. Int Dairy J 146:105745. https://doi.org/10.1016/J.IDAIRYJ.2023.105745

Patil U, Benjakul S (2017) Characteristics of albumin and globulin from coconut meat and their role in emulsion stability without and with proteolysis. Food Hydrocoll 69:220–228. https://doi.org/10.1016/j.foodhyd.2017.02.006

Patil U, Benjakul S (2018) Coconut milk and coconut oil: their manufacture associated with protein functionality. J Food Sci 83:2019–2027. https://doi.org/10.1111/1750-3841.14223

Raghavendra SN, Raghavarao KSMS (2011) Aqueous extraction and enzymatic destabilization of coconut milk emulsions. J Am Oil Chem Soc 88:481–487

Rastogi Y, Priya, Gogate PR (2022) Intensified recovery of whey proteins using combination of enzyme in free or immobilized form with ultrafiltration. Chem Eng Process 179:109076. https://doi.org/10.1016/j.cep.2022.109076

Rasyid F, Manullang M, Hansen PMT (1992) Isolation and characterization of coconut protein. Food Hydrocoll 6:301–314. https://doi.org/10.1016/S0268005X(09)80097-0

Ravindran V, Blair R (1992) Feed resources for poultry production in Asia and the Pacific. II. Plant protein sources. Worlds Poult Sci J 48:205–231. https://doi.org/10.1079/WPS19920017

Remya S, Chikku AM, Renjith RS, Arunima S, Rajamohan T (2013) Coconut kernel protein in diet protects the heart by beneficially modulating endothelial Nitric oxide synthase, tumor necrosis factor-alpha, and nuclear factor-kappaB expressions in experimental myocardial infarction. J Food Drug Anal 21:325–331. https://doi.org/10.1016/j.jfda.2013.07.012

Rizzello CG, Tagliazucchi D, Babini E, Sefora Rutella G, Taneyo Saa DL, Gianotti A (2016) Bioactive peptides from vegetable food matrices: research trends and novel biotechnologies for synthesis and recovery. J Funct Foods 27:549–569. https://doi.org/10.1016/j.jff.2016.09.023

Rodsamran P, Sothornvit R (2018a) Physicochemical and functional properties of protein concentrate from by-product of coconut processing. Food Chem 241:364–371. https://doi.org/10.1016/J.FOODCHEM.2017.08.116

Rodsamran P, Sothornvit R (2018b) Bioactive coconut protein concentrate films incorporated with antioxidant extract of mature coconut water. Food Hydrocoll 79:243–252

Salil G, Rajamohan T (2001) Hypolipidemic and antiperoxidative effect of coconut protein in hypercholesterolemic rats. Indian J Exp Biol 39:1028–1034

Salil G, Nevin KG, Rajamohan T (2011) Arginine rich coconut kernel protein modulates diabetes in alloxan treated rats. Chem Biol Interact 189:107–111. https://doi.org/10.1016/j.cbi.2010.10.015

Salil G, Nevin KG, Rajamohan T (2012) Arginine-rich coconut kernel diet influences nitric oxide synthase activity in alloxandiabetic rats. J Sci Food Agric 92:1903–1908. https://doi.org/10.1002/jsfa.5558

Santhi JV, Tavanandi HA, Sharma R, Prabhakar G, Raghavarao KSMS (2020) Differential partitioning of coconut whey proteins and fat using aqueous two phase extraction. Fluid Phase Equilib 503:112314. https://doi.org/10.1016/j.fluid.2019.112314

Singh R, Langyan S, Sangwan S, Rohtagi B, Khandelwal A, Shrivastava M (2022) Protein for human consumption from oilseed cakes: a review. Front Sustain Food Syst 6:1–12. https://doi.org/10.3389/fsufs.2022.856401

Sorde KL, Ananthanarayan L (2019) Effect of transglutaminase treatment on properties of coconut protein-guar gum composite film. LWT 115:108422. https://doi.org/10.1016/J.LWT.2019.108422

Sujatha A, Deepa Balakrishnan S (2023) Properties of high strength lightweight concrete incorporating crushed coconut shells as coarse aggregate. Mater Today Proc. https://doi.org/10.1016/j.matpr.2023.03.201

Sun Y, Chen H, Chen W, Zhong Q, Shen Y, Zhang M (2022) Effect of ultrasound on pH shift to improve thermal stability of coconut milk by modifying physicochemical properties of coconut milk protein. LWT 167:113861. https://doi.org/10.1016/j.lwt.2022.113861

Svanborg S, Johansen AG, Abrahamsen RK, Skeie SB (2015) The composition and functional properties of whey protein concentrates produced from buttermilk are comparable with those of whey protein concentrates produced from skimmed milk. J Dairy Sci 98:5829–5840. https://doi.org/10.3168/jds.2014-9039

Tan M, Nawaz MA, Buckow R (2023) Functional and food application of plant proteins—a review. Food Rev Intl 39:2428–2456. https://doi.org/10.1080/87559129.2021.1955918

Thaiphanit S, Anprung P (2016) Physicochemical and emulsion properties of edible protein concentrate from coconut (Cocos nucifera L.) processing by-products and the influence of heat treatment. Food Hydrocoll 52:756–765. https://doi.org/10.1016/j.foodhyd.2015.08.017

Thaiphanit S, Schleining G, Anprung P (2016) Effects of coconut (Cocos nucifera L.) protein hydrolysates obtained from enzymatic hydrolysis on the stability and rheological properties of oil-in-water emulsions. Food Hydrocoll 60:252–264. https://doi.org/10.1016/j.foodhyd.2016.03.035

Thomas B, Sudheer KP, Saranya S, Kothakota A, Pandiselvam R, Joseph M (2022) Development of protein enriched cold extruded pasta products using hybrid dried processed mushroom powder and defatted flours: a study on nutraceutical, textural, colour and sensory attributes. LWT 170:113991. https://doi.org/10.1016/j.lwt.2022.113991

Vigila AG, Baskaran X (2008) Immunomodulatory effect of coconut protein on cyclophosphamide induced immune suppressed Swiss albino mice. Ethnobotanical Leaflets 12:1206–1218

Vijayasanthi J, Adsare SR, Lamdande AG, Naik A, Raghavarao KSMS, Prabhakar G (2020) Recovery of proteins from coconut milk whey employing ultrafiltration and spray drying. J Food Sci Technol 57:22–31. https://doi.org/10.1007/s13197-01904025-9

Wang L, Zhang Y, Li R, Xiang D (2023) L-lysine moderates thermal aggregation of coconut proteins induced by thermal treatment. Sci Rep 13:1–10. https://doi.org/10.1038/s41598-023-38758-7

Wen C, Zhang J, Zhang H, Duan Y, Ma H (2020) Plant protein-derived antioxidant peptides: Isolation, identification, mechanism of action and application in food systems: a review. Trends Food Sci Technol 105:308–322. https://doi.org/10.1016/j.tifs.2020.09.019

Yalegama LC, Warnakulasuriya SN, Idirisinghe IMSK, Pathirana HH, Wanasundara JP (2024) Coconut: a sustainable source providing plant protein and several coproducts. In: Sustainable protein sources. Academic Press, London, pp 257–283

Yiengveerachon C, Yoshikawa S, Matsumoto H, Ookawara S (2020) Characteristics of coconut protein separation process by means of membrane ultrafiltration. J Food Process Eng 43:1–15. https://doi.org/10.1111/jfpe.13363

Zhao Q, Xiong H, Selomulya C, Chen XD, Huang S, Ruan X, Zhou Q, Sun W (2013) Effects of spray drying and freeze drying on the properties of protein isolate from rice dreg protein. Food Bioproc Tech 6:1759–1769. https://doi.org/10.1007/s11947-012-0844-3

Zheng Y, Li Y (2018) Physicochemical and functional properties of coconut (Cocos nucifera L) cake dietary fibres: effects of cellulase hydrolysis, acid treatment and particle size distribution. Food Chem 257:135–142

Zheng Y, Li Y, Li G (2019) ACE-inhibitory and antioxidant peptides from coconut cake albumin hydrolysates: purification, identification and synthesis. RSC Adv 9:5925–5936. https://doi.org/10.1039/c8ra10269d

Chapter 7
Virgin Coconut Oil: Extraction, Quality Control and Biological Functions

Abdul Rohman and Gunawan Indrayanto

Abstract Virgin coconut oil (VCO) is a premium product of coconut, considered as functional food oil due to its various pharmacological and beneficial effects on humans. The oil industry has developed numerous extraction processes for obtaining VCO from the coconut fruit. These methods include cold and hot extractions, extraction with low pressure, chilling, freezing and thawing, natural fermentation, centrifugation, enzyme extraction, supercritical CO_2 extraction, and expeller pressing. Different extraction methods yield VCO with varying physicochemical characteristics, leading to different products with a wide range of applications. Certain bioactive components in VCO, particularly lauric acid, are reported to exhibit biological effects believed to be beneficial to human health, such as antibacterial and anti-inflammatory properties. Given the high market value of VCO, quality control and analysis to detect potential adulteration are crucial to ensure authenticity and compliance with claimed labels. To address this, various analytical techniques have been optimized, validated, and successfully applied for the quality control and authentication analysis of VCO. Additionally, this chapter discusses various biological functions of VCO.

Keywords VCO · Extraction · Biochemical features · Pharmacological activities · Lauric acid · Functional food

A. Rohman (✉)
Center of Excellence, Institute for Halal Industry & Systems, Universitas Gadjah Mada, Yogyakarta, Indonesia

Department of Pharmaceutical Chemistry, Faculty of Pharmacy, University of Gadjah Mada, Yogyakarta, Indonesia

G. Indrayanto
School of Medicine, Ciputra University, Surabaya, Indonesia

S. V. Ramesh, S. Praveen (eds.), *Coconut-Based Nutrition and Nutraceutical Perspectives*, https://doi.org/10.1007/978-981-97-3976-9_7

7.1 Introduction

The coconut, scientifically known as *Cocos nucifera* L., belongs to the family '*Arecaceae*' and is famously known as "the tree of life." Widely cultivated in tropical regions, particularly in Indonesia, Malaysia, India, and the Philippines, the coconut palm is a vital crop with diverse applications globally. Coconut is grown in extensive plantations and has a presence in more than 80 countries. The composition of the coconut fruit includes a husk comprising approximately 35%, a shell of 28%, meat of 28%, and water with a composition of 15%. It serves as a rich source for manufacturing juice or nut water, milk, and oil, as highlighted by Srivastava et al. (2018). The annual coconut production is estimated at around 55 million tons, with Indonesia contributing approximately 3.1 million hectares, while the Philippines and India contribute approximately 2.7 and 1.5 million hectares, respectively. Therefore, Indonesia, the Philippines, and India stand as the top three coconut producers globally, contributing three-quarters of the total world's coconut production (Srivastava et al. 2018).

The wet processing of fresh coconut kernel results in the production of virgin coconut oil (VCO), one of the most valuable products derived from the coconut. Recognized as a functional food oil due to its pharmacological activities, VCO provides numerous health benefits. It holds economic significance as a value-added product derived from fresh coconuts and is a prominent high-value item in coconut-producing countries. This is primarily attributed to its extensive uses in various products, including food, pharmaceuticals, cosmetics, and hair care (Suryani et al. 2020).

Given its high level of medium-chain saturated fatty acids, particularly lauric acid (C12:0), VCO is resistant to oxidative modifications, making it suitable for cooking (Rajamohan and Archana 2019). The introduction of VCO into the oil industry occurred towards the end of the twentieth century. Some South Asian countries such as The Philippines, Indonesia, Malaysia, Thailand, Sri Lanka, and Vietnam, along with others such as Fiji, India, and Western Samoa, are known as leading exporters of VCO in the global market (Muralidharan and Jayashree 2011), while the USA, European countries, the Middle East, the Pacific, Australia, and South Africa are primary importing countries of VCO.

VCO is derived from the milk extracted from fresh mature coconut kernels through natural means, without undergoing any chemical treatments like refining, bleaching, and deodorizing, which are typical processes for conventional coconut oil or refined-bleached-deodorized (RBD) oil. VCO is characterized by its nearly colorless appearance, a slightly detectable acidic aroma, a sweet and salty taste, as well as a noticeable nutty aroma and flavor (Rohman and Man 2012). Historically, the term 'Virgin oils' referred to vegetable oils fit for human consumption in their natural state, as they are only subjected to purification with natural processes such as washing with water, settling, filtering, and centrifuging. However, Codex Alimentarius standards for coconut oil, primarily commercial RBD coconut oil, allow edible vegetable oils to undergo refining processes using chemicals such as alkali for washing, bleaching, and deodorizing to eliminate unwanted components and extend shelf life (Bawalan 2011). In contrast, the Philippine National Standard defines VCO as vegetable oils obtained by extracting the fresh or mature kernel (meat) of coconut using natural or mechanical tools, with or without the employment of heat, without subjecting to the chemical RBD process, and without changing the oil's nature. Additionally, VCO is suitable for consumption without the need for further processing actions (Bureau of Agriculture and Fisheries Standards 2007).

Chemically, vegetable oils, including virgin coconut oil (VCO), are composed of triacylglycerols, which are glycerol esterified with three fatty acids. VCO, specifically, contains approximately 50% lauric acid (C12:0), categorizing it as medium-chain triglycerides (MCTs). In the human gastrointestinal tract, MCTs are known to be more readily hydrolyzed and absorbed than long-chain triglycerides (LCTs) by certain lipases. Due to its richness in MCTs, the consumption of VCO is correlated with an increase in serum triglyceride (TG) levels. However, the lipid profile may show improvement because of the incorporation of structured lipids (McCarty and DiNicolantonio 2016). VCO is believed to offer more valuable effects than regular coconut oil (CO) since most of the unsaponifiable components are retained in VCO. Additionally, VCO demonstrates various important pharmacological effects in humans, including antioxidant and antimicrobial activities (anti-bacterial, anti-fungal, antiviral, and antiparasitic), along with cardioprotective, hepatoprotective, antidiabetic, and hypolipidemic effects, all of which contribute to its potential health benefits (Salian and Shetty 2018).

In the fats and oils industry, VCO commands a premium price in the market. Therefore, ensuring its quality and analyzing for potential adulteration is crucial to guarantee that VCO is authentic and meets the label claims. To address this task, various analytical techniques have been optimized, developed, and utilized for the quality control and authentication analysis of VCO, particularly in detecting potential adulterants. Spectroscopic and chromatographic-based techniques have been widely employed for the authentication analysis of VCO. These techniques provide detailed information about the characteristics and chemical components responsible for VCO's pharmacological activities. However, the responses generated during spectroscopic and chromatographic measurements often involve large datasets. To extract useful information from this substantial amount of data, chemometrics analysis is employed. Chemometrics involves the application of statistical and mathematical methods to analyze and interpret chemical data, helping to guarantee the accuracy and precision of the analytical results for VCO.

7.2 Extraction (Preparation) of VCO

In 2006, the FAO Regional Office for Asia and the Pacific released a publication entitled "Virgin Coconut Oil: The Production Manual for micro- and village-scale production of VCO," authored by Bawalan and Chapman (2006). This manual extensively covers various preparation and extraction methods for Virgin Coconut

Oil (VCO), including optimized and modified natural fermentation methods, extraction methods applying low-pressure oil, and extraction methods applying high-pressure expellers.

In 2011, the Secretariat of the Pacific Community (SPC) Suva Office in Fiji published a comprehensive book authored by Bawalan (2011), delving into VCO production technologies, GMP (good manufacturing practices), SOP (standard operating procedures) for sanitation, by-product processing, and downstream products derived from VCO. It also provides information on VCO production equipment, standards for VCO, fatty acid profiles, and other chemical components present in coconut oil, formulations, and some procedures for downstream products from VCO, along with other related coconut products presented as annexures. For those seeking more details on extraction methods and preparations of VCO, can refer to the mentioned FAO and SPC Suva publications.

The Indian Council of Agricultural Research (ICAR) has innovated and established a VCO cooker designed for the extraction of VCO using the hot process. However, variations in physicochemical properties can arise during VCO production processes employed in India and other regions, potentially impacting the pharmacological and nutritional qualities of VCO. A study investigating the physicochemical and biological properties of VCO from different processes, including fermentation and enzymatic processes, hot process oil excluded from dried gratings, centrifugation, and conservatively prepared copra coconut oil, was conducted, taking into account the design of the VCO cooker. Multivariate analysis was employed to differentiate VCO samples based on their quality profiles. VCO from the hot process formed a distinct cluster from the other VCOs, characterized by a robust antioxidant potential attributed to its high total phenol content. In contrast, VCO prepared using centrifugal and fermentation methods exhibited relatively weaker antioxidant capacities along with lower phenolic and flavonoid contents (Ramesh et al. 2020).

General methods of extraction and preparation of VCO have been extensively reviewed and discussed in several articles. Srivastava et al. (2018), Rohman et al. (2021), and Ng et al. (2021a, b) have summarized various extraction or preparation techniques, including cold and hot extractions, extraction with low pressure, chilling, freezing and thawing, natural fermentation, centrifugation, enzyme extraction, supercritical CO_2 extraction, and expeller pressing. Ferrer et al. (2018) discussed the preparation of VCO using the extraction combination method of low-pressure oil and a modified kitchen, which can be applied in small and medium-scale coconut communities or farms in the Philippines. Aytaç (2022) compared various extraction techniques for VCO, namely cold pressing, Soxhlet, and supercritical fluid extraction (SFE), with different conditions on the fatty acid contents. SFE extraction was found to be the best method for obtaining VCO with desired qualities in terms of yield, fatty acid compositions, and effects on human health.

The effects on physicochemical properties and antioxidant activity of VCO obtained using different extraction techniques have been investigated by Mohammed et al. (2021). Additionally, Nivya et al. (2023) compared the sensory attributes and some physicochemical properties of VCO prepared by hot extraction, cold centrifugation, and enzymatic methods.

From the results of fatty acid composition, lauric acid (C12:0, a medium-chain fatty acid) is the main fatty acid present in VCOs, accounting for 45.05% to 47.05%. Furthermore, VCO extracted using cold centrifugation contained more lauric acid (approximately 47.05%), tocopherol (approximately 27.68 μg/g), total phenolic content (9.97 μg/g expressed as gallic acid equivalent), and total antioxidant capacity (μg/mg) than that extracted using hot extraction and enzymatic methods.

Negi et al. (2024) reported the effect of selected thermal and non-thermal pretreatments (microwave heating, Ohmic heating, ultrasonication, and pulsed electric field) on the yield and quality parameters of subsequently wet-extracted VCO. The highest VCO yields (>93%) were observed using ultrasonicated and pulsed electric field-treated samples, and all quality parameters complied with international standards. Sundrasegaran and Mah (2020) compared various extraction methods on the yields of phytonutrient profiles of VCO, showing that supercritical fluid extraction was the best extraction technique for VCO preparation. The optimization of process parameters to produce VCO using aerobic fermented *neera* (coconut inflorescence sap) at different levels (5–25%) has been reported (Pandiselvam et al. 2023). These research reports indicate that different methods of VCO preparation could yield different metabolite contents in VCO. Hence, researchers should optimize the method of VCO preparation to produce VCO with desired physicochemical and biological properties, which could potentially affect the nutritional aspects and pharmacological activities.

7.3 Quality Features of VCO

Edible animal fats and vegetable oils play vital roles as ingredients in various food products, including salad and cooking oils, margarine, shortenings, salad dressings, and confectionery coatings. Analysis of these edible fats and oils, including VCO, aims to characterize them based on several parameters such as iodine value used for the measurement of degree of unsaturation, saponification value used for describing the molecular weight (MW) of fatty acids composed fats and oils, peroxide value for the evaluation of peroxides and hydroperoxides levels, and acid value to evaluate the formation of free fatty acids due to hydrolytic and oxidation degradations. Additionally, other parameters related to the oxidation of fats and oils, such as anisidine value and TBARS (Thiobarbituric Acid Reactive Substances), are also measured (Negash et al. 2019). These analyses are crucial for ensuring the quality, stability, and safety of edible fats and oils, including VCO, in various food applications (Negash et al. 2019).

VCO can be prepared from coconut in a straightforward manner under room temperature. As a consequence, the loss of minor components responsible for biological activities, such as unsaponifiable components (phenolics and vitamins), can be avoided (Nevin and Rajamohan 2008). Table 7.1 presents compiled physico-chemical parameters and fatty acid profiles of VCO.

Table 7.1 The physical properties and chemical constants along with fatty acid profiles of virgin coconut oil

Physico-chemical properties	Range or maximum values			
Iodine value	(4.47–8.55)[a]; (5.24–5.32)[b] (g I_2/100 g)			
Saponification value	(252.45–260.67)[a]; (345.70–348.0)[b] (mg KOH/g oil)			
Acid value	(0.13–0.27)[a]; (1.01–1.03)[a] (mg KOH/g)			
Peroxide value	(0.21–0.63)[a] (mEq/kg)			
Anisidine value	(0.16–0.49)[a]			
Total phenolic content	(7.78–29.18)[a] (mg gallic acid equivalent/100 g oil)			
Free fatty acids	(0.13–0.25)[a]; (0.25–0.26)%[b]			
pH	(6.40–6.50)[b]			
Moisture	0.1%[c]			
Volatile matter, 120 °C	0.2%[c]			
Density	(0.915–0.920)g/mL[c]			
Refractive index, 40 °C	(1.4480–1.4492)[c]			
Insoluble impurities	0.05%[c]			
Unsaponifiable matter	(0.2–0.5)%[c]			
Total plate count	0.5[c]			
Color	Colorless			
Fatty acid composition (%)	*CODEX*	Seneviratne and Jayathilaka (2016)	Marina et al. (2009c)	Dia et al. (2005)
Caproic acidor C6:0	nd–0.70	0.40–0.60	0.52–0.69	nd–0.60
Caprylic acidor C8:0	4.60–10.00	5.00–10.00	7.19–8.81	5.98–10.44
Capric acid or C10:0	5.0–8.0	4.50–8.00	5.65–6.59	5.37–6.60
Lauric acid C12:0	45.10–53.20	43.00–50.00	46.89–48.03	47.63–52.55
Myristic acidor C14:0	16.80–21.00	16.00–21.00	16.23–18.90	16.79–20.08
Palmitic acidor C16:0	7.50–10.20	7.50–10.00	7.41–9.55	6.38–10.17
Stearic acidor C18:0	2.00–4.00	2.00–4.00	2.81–3.57	7.45–10.73
Oleic acidor C18:1	5.00–10.00	5.00–10.00	5.72–6.72	5.15–6.03
Linoleic acidor C18:2	1.00–2.50	1.00–2.50	0.90–1.60	nd–0.12
Linolenic acid C18:3	nd–0.20	<0.5	nd	nd

[a]Adapted from Marina et al. (2009b)
[b]From Suryani et al. (2020)
[c]Adapted from Seneviratne and Jayathilaka (2016)

7.4 Authentication Analysis of VCO

In the fats and oils industry, where VCO is highly valued for its perceived health benefits and quality, adulteration poses significant concerns. Adulteration of food products, including edible fats and oils, not only compromises their quality but also poses potential risks to consumer health. Substituting genuine VCO with lower-quality oils or fats may lead to allergenic reactions or adverse health effects for consumers. To combat this issue, various analytical methods have been developed and employed for the authentication of VCO. These methods aim to identify and quantify potential adulterants, ensuring the integrity of the product.

The ban on 166 brands of coconut oil-based products by FSSAI India in 2018 underscores the seriousness of adulteration issues within the coconut oil industry. Adulteration compromises the quality and authenticity of the product, and in the case of edible oils like coconut oil, it can have significant implications for consumer health and safety. Scientists have developed and validated several analytical methods to detect adulteration practices in VCO. These methods include Fourier Transform Infrared (FTIR) spectroscopy (Neves and Poppi 2020), differential scanning calorimetry (Mansor et al. 2012), electronic nose (Marina et al. 2010), and chromatographic-based methods (Xu et al. 2015). These techniques are often coupled with chemometrics, as depicted in Fig. 7.1, to enhance the accuracy and reliability of the analysis.

The combination of FTIR-ATR accessory coupled with multivariate data analysis, such as linear discriminant analysis (LDA), has been successfully employed for the authentication of VCO from the adulterant of palm oil (PO), which has a lower price than VCO. In this study, the levels of PO as an adulterant in VCO ranged from 0.5% to 30% v/v. LDA applied the absorbance values at the whole FTIR spectra as

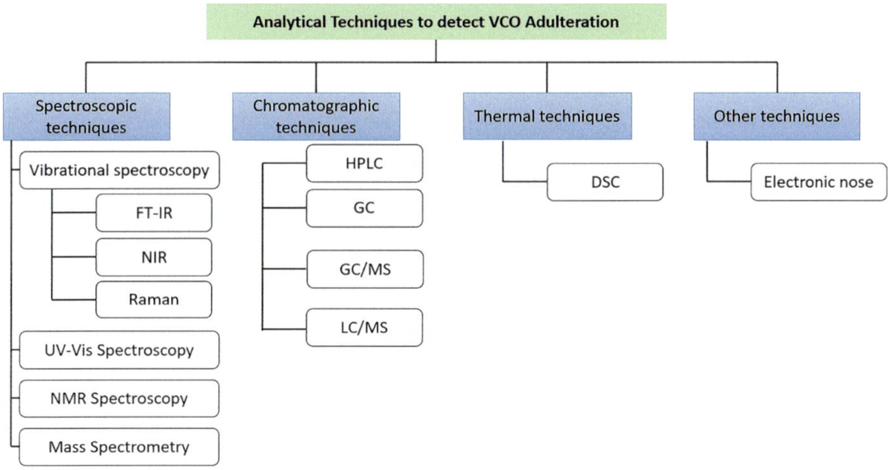

Fig. 7.1 Analytical methods for authentication of virgin coconut oil from potential adulterants (Priya et al. 2022)

variables during chemometrics modeling, showing 100% accurate classification in both calibration and cross-validation groups for all PO blends.

Two multivariate calibrations, namely PCR and PLS-R, were optimized to achieve the best prediction modeling for FTIR normal spectra and FTIR spectral derivatives (1st and 2nd derivatives) at combined wave numbers of 3010–2800 and 1800–700 cm^{-1}. These results indicated that 2nd derivative spectra at wave numbers of 1800–700 cm^{-1} provided acceptable accuracy and precision. Using PLS-R, the highest R^2 and the lowest RMSEP were 0.998 and 0.375% v/v, respectively. Additionally, an R^2 value of 0.998 and an RMSEP value of 0.441% v/v were obtained using PCR. The lowest levels of PO detected in VCO were estimated to be as low as 0.5% v/v (Amit et al. 2023).

Previously, an authentication study of VCO was performed using principal component analysis (PCA) and LDA to create a classification model between VCO and VCO adulterated with paraffin oil and mustard oil (Amit et al. 2020a, b).

The chemometrics of data-driven SIMCA employing absorbance values at wave number regions of 1080–1210 cm^{-1} as variables during chemometrics modeling, previously pre-treated with the first derivative using the Savitzky-Golay method, has been effectively employed for the authentication of VCO with selected vegetable oils such as corn (CO), canola (CaO), sunflower (SFO), and soybean (SO). The developed method was capable of confirming authentic VCO and detecting VCO adulterated with these oil adulterants (CO, CaO, SFO, and SO) in a concentration range of 10–40%. The combination of ATR-FTIR spectroscopic technique combined with data-driven SIMCA was also able to identify these four oils (CO, CaO, SFO, and SO) with a sensitivity of 88–100% and a specificity of 96–100%. ATR-FTIR spectroscopy combined with a one-class strategy based on DD-SIMCA is a fast and reliable method to be routinely used during the quality control of VCO (Neves and Poppi 2020). Additionally, another vibrational spectroscopy technique, namely Raman spectroscopy, has also been successful for the authentication analysis of coconut oil (De Géa Neves and Poppi 2018).

^{13}C-NMR spectroscopy coupled with chemometrics has been effectively employed for the authentication of VCO by classifying VCO samples and those adulterated with other oils (VCO, RBD-CO, VCO mixed with RBD-CO, and old VCO with a shelf life >2 years). Sample extraction was conducted using deuterated chloroform (CDCl3) containing 0.5% v/v trimethylsilyl (TMS). PCA employing two principal components (PC1 and PC2) could clearly separate VCO from RBD-CO. However, some overlapping objects were observed during the classification of VCO and old VCO. The results also indicated that PCA could provide the classification of VCO and its adulterants, but not all adulterated samples could be distinctly separated from pure VCO, particularly VCO with a low level of RBD-CO as an adulterant, which overlapped with pure VCO. Furthermore, PLS-DA using four discriminant components showed a good separation model for VCO and VCO adulterated with RBD-CO, fresh VCO, and old VCO, with an optimum value of Q2 of about 1. A permutation test employing 1000 permutations was applied to validate the OPLS-DA, and the results indicated that all models were valid with a p-value <0.001 (Lagurin et al. 2020).

The molecular spectroscopy of phosphorus-31 (31P) NMR in combination with PCA has been successfully employed for the differentiation of VCO from RBD-coconut oil. The target compounds used for differentiation include mono- and diglycerides, free fatty acids (FFAs), and sterols. Before analysis using 31P-NMR, the target compounds were subjected to derivatization as dioxaphospholane. Different levels of these target compounds were observed, with monoglycerides found to be higher in VCO compared to RBD-CO, while the total diglycerides were lower in VCO than in RBD-CO. Additionally, FFAs and sterols were significantly higher in VCO compared to RBD-CO. Based on the PCA score plot, VCO and RBD-CO could be clearly differentiated, with the variables of 1,2-diglycerides, 1,3-diglycerides, and FFAs being the most important variables contributing to this differentiation (Dayrit et al. 2008).

High-performance liquid chromatography (HPLC) has been widely employed for the authentication of VCO by analyzing potential adulterants. Different types and concentrations of triacylglycerols (TAGs) composing authentic VCO and VCO adulterated with low-priced oils such as palm olein and palm kernel oil (PKO) were explored for this authentication task. Komaram et al. (2021) applied HPLC to detect PKO as an adulterant in VCO through the analysis of three major TAGs: dilaurin-monocaprin/myristin-caprylin-laurin (C34), trilaurin (C36), and dilaurin-monomyristin (C38). Furthermore, investigation of VCO adulterated with palm olein was conducted by quantifying the levels of dipalmitoyl-monoolein (POP) and trilaurin (LaLaLa). Both TAGs were used as detection indices for the quantification of palm olein. Linear correlations were found between the levels of % C36 (x-axis) and the levels of PKO as an adulterant, with an R^2 of 0.9917. Similarly, the R^2 for the correlation between % palm olein in VCO and the ratio of POP: LaLaLa was 0.99694. Additionally, HPLC using an evaporative light scattering detector has been reported as a powerful method for the quality control of VCO through the analysis of lauric acid, monolaurin, dilaurin, and trilaurin (Ponphaiboon et al. 2018).

Liquid chromatography tandem mass spectrometry (LC-MS/MS) using direct infusion electrospray ionization mass spectrometry (ESI-MS) offers a powerful analytical method for detecting soybean oil (SO) as an adulterant in VCO at levels of 2–70%. In the authentication study, certain triacylglycerols (TAGs) were analyzed as TAG markers in VCO, namely LaLaLa, CLaLa, CCLa, LaLaM, and LaMM (where C stands for capric acid, M stands for myristic acid, and La stands for lauric acid). For SO, the TAG marker is LLnP in its ammonium adduct [LLnP + NH4] + (m/z 870.9) (where L stands for linoleic acid, Ln stands for linolenic acid, and P stands for palmitic acid). A linear correlation was found between the levels of LLnP (x-axis) and SO levels (y-axis) with an R^2 value of 0.994. Therefore, it can be concluded that the levels of LLnP could be used as a detection index for the quantification of SO as an adulterant in VCO, with a minimum detection level of 2% for SO (Pizzo et al. 2019).

Gas chromatography coupled with flame ionization detector (GC-FID) is commonly used for authenticating VCO through the analysis of fatty acid (FA) compositions. The FAs present in authentic VCO and VCO adulterants are compared.

Marikkar (2018) developed GC-FID combined with PCA for authenticating VCO from palm oil adulterants, where FAs are converted to volatile fatty acid methyl esters (FAME). The FA compositions were used as variables during PCA modeling for the classification of VCO and VCO adulterated with palm olein. Based on loading plots of PCA, lauric acid (C12:0), palmitic acid (C18:0), and oleic acid (C18:0) were identified as the FAs contributing the most to the discrimination between VCO and VCO adulterated with palm olein. Additionally, Mansor et al. (2011) employed fast-GC, known as electronic nose (e-nose), for authenticating VCO from lard adulteration. Binary mixtures of samples consisting of lard and VCO with a concentration range of lard from 1% to 50% v/v were analyzed using a surface acoustic wave (SAW) detector in fast-GC. Results identified ten different chromatograms as adulterant peaks, with one showing a good relationship with the levels of lard (R^2 value of 0.9344). Gas chromatography coupled with mass spectrometer detector (GC-MS) offers a powerful method for authenticating VCO, either using one column (one-dimensional) or two columns with different polarities (two-dimensional GC). GC x GC-TOF-MS (time of flight) has been successfully used for authenticating VCO from different types of animal fats. Cholesterol and cholestanol as trimethylsilyl ethers (TME) derivatives were applied as chemical markers for differentiating VCO from animal fats (lard, chicken fat, mutton fat, and beef fat). This study confirmed the suitability of GC x GC-TOF-MS for detecting VCO adulteration with animal fats through quantitative analyses of cholesterols in VCO (Xu et al. 2015).

In addition to chromatographic and spectroscopic-based methods, conventional methods along with certain chemical parameters can be exploited as rapid tools for authenticating VCO. Cariappa et al. (2023) utilized total phenolic and flavonoid contents, iodine value, saponification value, and selected fatty acids like lauric acid, myristic acid, palmitic acid, and oleic acid for authenticating VCO from potential adulterants, with a minimum detection limit of adulterant as low as 10%.

7.5 The Nutritional and Health Potential of VCO

Coconut oil is composed of more than 85% saturated fats. Most saturated fats are medium-chain triglycerides (MCTs), of which lauric acid is the dominant fatty acid (Marina et al. 2009a).VCO is indeed well-known for its numerous beneficial effects to human health and is often considered a superfood. Some key nutritional functions of VCO include:

- **100% Natural, Unbleached, and Cold-Pressed:** VCO is typically processed in a way that retains its natural properties. It is unbleached, meaning it has not undergone a bleaching process, and it is often cold-pressed to preserve its nutritional content.
- **Powerful Antioxidants:** VCO contains potent antioxidants that can help combat oxidative stress in the body.

- **Healthy Fatty Acids:** VCO is a rich source of various healthy fatty acids, including lauric acid. Lauric acid is known for its antimicrobial and anti-inflammatory properties.
- **Essential Vitamins:** VCO contains essential vitamins, including vitamin E, which is known for its antioxidant properties and its role in skin health.
- **Medium-Chain Triglycerides (MCTs):** VCO is particularly high in MCTs, which are a type of fatty acid. MCTs are believed to have various health benefits, including being easier for the body to convert into energy compared to long-chain triglycerides (LCTs). They are also thought to be less likely to be stored as fat (Ng et al. 2021a).
- **Promotes Heart Health**: Despite being high in saturated fats, VCO contains medium-chain triglycerides (MCTs) that may improve heart health by raising levels of HDL (good) cholesterol and reducing levels of LDL (bad) cholesterol, thereby potentially lowering the risk of heart disease.
- **Boosts Immunity**: Lauric acid, the predominant fatty acid in VCO, possesses antimicrobial and antiviral properties that can help strengthen the immune system and defend against infections caused by bacteria, viruses, and fungi.
- **Aids Digestion**: MCTs in VCO are easily digested and absorbed by the body, providing a quick source of energy. They also support gut health by promoting the growth of beneficial gut bacteria and reducing inflammation in the digestive tract.
- **Supports Weight Management**: The MCTs in VCO have been shown to increase feelings of fullness and boost metabolism, potentially aiding in weight management efforts by promoting satiety and calorie burning.
- **Enhances Skin and Hair Health**: VCO can be applied topically to moisturize and nourish the skin and hair. Its antibacterial and anti-inflammatory properties may help treat various skin conditions, such as acne and eczema, while also promoting hair growth and scalp health.
- **Provides Antioxidant Protection**: VCO contains antioxidants, such as phenolic compounds and tocopherols, which help neutralize free radicals and protect cells from oxidative damage, thereby reducing the risk of chronic diseases and premature aging.
- **Balances Blood Sugar Levels**: Some studies suggest that MCTs in VCO may improve insulin sensitivity and regulate blood sugar levels, making it a potentially beneficial dietary addition for individuals with diabetes or those at risk of developing the condition.
- **Supports Brain Function**: The MCTs in VCO can cross the blood-brain barrier and serve as a readily available source of energy for the brain. This may enhance cognitive function, improve focus, and protect against age-related cognitive decline.

The complete nutritional features of coconut oil have been discussed (Mikołajczak 2017; Beegum et al. 2024). It's well-established that the qualitative and quantitative compositions of metabolites in plants, including coconut oil, can be influenced by various external factors such as the location of cultivation, age of plants, and methods of harvesting. As a result, the biochemical compositions of coconut oils, and consequently their nutritional values, may differ depending on the geographical origin and cultivation practices. The impact of coconut oils on human health, encompassing their general pharmacological activities, has been the subject of discussion and summarization (Mikołajczak 2017; Rajamohan and Archana 2019; Rohman et al. 2021). Furthermore, research by Rajamohan and Archana (2019), Rohman et al. (2021), and others delve into the pharmacological activities of coconut oil, exploring its potential health benefits and medicinal properties. These studies likely provide valuable insights into how coconut oil consumption may impact human health and well-being. Specifically, investigations by Chatterjee et al. (2020) and Ramesh et al. (2021) offer insights into the dietary effects of coconut oil, particularly in the context of Alzheimer's disease prevention and management. Additionally, the potential cardioprotective effects of virgin coconut oil have been discussed by researchers like Babu et al. (2014) and Beegum et al. (2024), further highlighting the diverse range of health benefits associated with coconut oil consumption.

Virgin coconut oil (VCO) indeed possesses a variety of pharmacological effects that can benefit human health, as indicated by studies such as Villarino et al. (2007) and Nevin and Rajamohan (2004). These effects are likely attributed to its content of short and medium-chain fatty acids like caproic, caprylic, capric, and lauric acids.

Law et al. (2014) observed that VCO consumption during chemotherapy improved the functional status and overall quality of life in breast cancer patients, while also alleviating chemotherapy-related symptoms. Similarly, Famurewa et al. (2018) found that VCO supplementation protected against oxidative toxicity and inflammation induced by methotrexate chemotherapy in rats.

Robinson et al. (2019) reported that short-term supplementation with VCO did not alter blood flow responses during aerobic exercise in young adults. Đurašević et al. (2020) highlighted the differential effects of VCO on glucose and lipid homeostasis in non-diabetic and diabetic rats, while Nikooei et al. (2021) observed improvements in lipid profiles with VCO consumption, including increased HDL cholesterol and decreased triglycerides and fasting blood sugar levels. Contrary to expectations, Jeyakumar et al. (2023) found that VCO consumption in a balanced diet did not increase plasma HDL cholesterol levels in male volunteers. Adeyemi et al. (2020) investigated the anti-obesitogenic effects of VCO in obese male rats, noting significant benefits in biochemical and histological markers. Furthermore, Arunima and Rajamohan (2013, 2014) demonstrated the antioxidant properties of VCO and its positive effects on lipid parameters, suggesting its potential role in preventing oxidative damage and improving lipid metabolism. These findings collectively underscore the diverse health benefits associated with VCO consumption across various physiological contexts. Assunção et al. (2009) found that dietary supplementation with coconut oil did not lead to dyslipidemia but contributed to a reduction in abdominal obesity in women presenting with this condition. Fernando et al. (2023) reported that virgin coconut oil (VCO) did not enhance cognition in individuals with mild-to-moderate Alzheimer's Disease compared to canola oil, but it did improve Mini-Mental State Examination (MMSE) scores in carriers of the apolipoprotein E ε4 allele. Additionally, VCO did not adversely affect lipid profiles or glycated hemoglobin levels, making it safe for consumption (Illam et al. 2017).

Polyphenols present in VCO, as reported by Illam et al. (2017), may protect cells from pro-oxidant insults by modulating cellular antioxidant status, reducing oxidative damage by interacting with free radicals, delaying oxidation reactions, or regulating cellular antioxidant defense systems. Furthermore, Machado et al. (2023) investigated the effects of organic VCO on immune response and obesity-related metabolism, finding that despite its high content of medium-chain saturated fatty acids like lauric acid, VCO had numerous beneficial effects on human health in the context of obesity. It helped reduce lipid accumulation in hepatocytes and adipocytes and regulated immune responses in gut cells. Moreover, Rahim et al. (2017) suggested that VCO could serve as a memory enhancer through mechanisms involving enhanced cholinergic activity, increased antioxidant levels, and reduced oxidative stress. These studies collectively highlight the multifaceted health benefits of VCO, ranging from metabolic improvements to cognitive enhancement and antioxidant protection.

Absolutely, the nutritional and medicinal properties of virgin coconut oil (VCO) can indeed vary depending on several factors such as geographical origin, cultivation practices, and production methods. These variations can result in differences in the metabolite content of VCO, ultimately influencing its health benefits. Metabolomics studies, particularly using liquid chromatography-high resolution mass spectrometry (LC-HR-MS/MS), offer a powerful approach to analyze and characterize the metabolite profile of VCO. By employing this technique, researchers can identify and quantify a wide range of metabolites present in VCO, including fatty acids, phenolic compounds, vitamins, and other bioactive molecules. Through metabolomics analysis, researchers can gain insights into the specific metabolites present in VCO that contribute to its pharmacological effects. This information can help elucidate the mechanisms underlying the health benefits of VCO and provide valuable insights for optimizing its production and consumption.

7.6 Perspectives

VCO stands out from other coconut oil variants due to its antioxidant, anti-inflammatory, lipid-lowering, and cytoprotective properties, which are attributed to its relatively high polyphenol content. Polyphenols in VCO inhibit lipid peroxidation, promote antithrombotic effects, and provide anti-inflammatory benefits, thereby conferring cardiovascular benefits. Moreover, the fatty acid composition of coconut oil, with MCFAs predominating, contributes to its unique health effects. MCFAs are absorbed differently in the intestine, bypassing pancreatic lipase activity and directly transporting to the liver through the hepatic portal vein. This mechanism prevents the accumulation of body fat and weight gain, contributing to anti-obesity effects. Additionally, MCFAs in VCO regulate lipoprotein lipase in adipose tissue, improve insulin sensitivity, and enhance glucose tolerance.

Furthermore, phenolic acids present in VCO, such as rutin, quercetin, and caffeic acid, play a role in regulating insulin resistance and glycemic index, providing additional health benefits. Ingestion of VCO and extra virgin coconut oil influences hepatic lipid metabolism, leading to the mobilization of fat, cholesterol, and triglycerides from the liver to the blood. This results in greater excretion of fecal cholesterol, enhanced energy expenditure, and increased mobility of body fat for bile acid biosynthesis in the liver. The combined action of polyphenols and fatty acids in coconut oil contributes to its antioxidant, anti-inflammatory, and cardiovascular benefits. These findings underscore the potential health advantages of consuming coconut oil, particularly VCO, in promoting overall well-being (Beegum et al. 2024).

The discussion on the health benefits of coconut oil often focuses on its fatty acid composition, overlooking other important phytonutrients such as phytosterols, which also play a significant role in promoting health. Therefore, it is essential to explore the nutraceutical effects of coconut oil-derived phytosterols in addition to its fatty acids. While many clinical studies support the consumption of coconut oil, further research is needed with larger sample sizes, diverse populations, and specific clinical markers to provide more conclusive evidence. Additionally, limitations such as small sample sizes and short study durations should be addressed in future research to ensure the reliability of findings.

7.7 Conclusion

Indeed, as the popularity of virgin coconut oil (VCO) continues to rise, optimizing extraction methods to ensure desired physicochemical characteristics becomes crucial. Given that VCO is rich in medium-chain triglycerides, particularly lauric acid, which imparts various biological activities such as antibacterial and antioxidant properties, understanding its metabolite content is essential for elucidating its health benefits.

Metabolomics studies using liquid chromatography-high resolution mass spectrometry (LC-HR-MS/MS) offer a promising approach to identify and quantify metabolites responsible for these activities accurately. By analyzing the metabolite profile of VCO, researchers can uncover specific compounds contributing to its antibacterial and antioxidant effects, among others.

Additionally, due to the risk of adulteration practices targeting VCO, robust analytical methods are essential for detecting adulterants in VCO. Techniques such as Fourier Transform Infrared (FTIR) spectroscopy, gas chromatography coupled with mass spectrometry (GC-MS), and high-performance liquid chromatography (HPLC) have proven effective in identifying adulterants in VCO, safeguarding its integrity and authenticity.

In summary, leveraging metabolomics studies alongside analytical techniques for detecting adulteration can enhance our understanding of VCO's health benefits and ensure its quality and authenticity in the market.

References

Adeyemi WJ, Olayaki LA, Abdussalam TA, Ige SF, Okesina BK, Abolarin PO, Usman H, Tiamiyu AO, Seidu MO, Opabode AO (2020) Comparative evaluation of the pharmacological value of virgin coconut oil, omega 3 fatty acids, and orlistat in experimental study on obesity with normo/hyper-lipidaemic diet. Pharma Nutr 13:100192. https://doi.org/10.1016/j.phanu.2020.100192

Amit, Jamwal R, Kumari S, Dhaulaniya AS, Balan B, Kelly S, Cannavan A, Singh DK (2020a) Utilizing ATR-FTIR spectroscopy combined with multivariate chemometric modelling for the swift detection of mustard oil adulteration in virgin coconut oil. Vib Spectrosc 109:103066. https://doi.org/10.1016/j.vibspec.2020.103066

Amit, Jamwal R, Kumari S, Dhaulaniya AS, Balan B, Singh DK (2020b) Application of ATR-FTIR spectroscopy along with regression modelling for the detection of adulteration of virgin coconut oil with paraffin oil. LWT 118:108754. https://doi.org/10.1016/j.lwt.2019.108754

Amit, Kumari S, Jamwal R, Suman P, Singh DK (2023) Expeditious and accurate detection of palm oil adulteration in virgin coconut oil by utilizing ATR-FTIR spectroscopy along with chemometrics and regression models. Food Chem Adv 3:100377. https://doi.org/10.1016/j.focha.2023.100377

Arunima S, Rajamohan T (2013) Effect of virgin coconut oil enriched diet on the antioxidant status and paraoxonase 1 activity in ameliorating the oxidative stress in rats-a comparative study. Food Funct 4(9):1402–1409. https://doi.org/10.1039/c3fo60085h

Arunima S, Rajamohan T (2014) Influence of virgin coconut oil-enriched diet on the transcriptional regulation of fatty acid synthesis and oxidation in rats-a comparative study. Br J Nutr 111(10):1782–1790. https://doi.org/10.1017/S0007114514000004X

Assunção ML, Ferreira HS, Dos Santos AF, Cabral CR, Florêncio TMMT (2009) Effects of dietary coconut oil on the biochemical and anthropometric profiles of women presenting abdominal obesity. Lipids 44(7):593–601. https://doi.org/10.1007/s11745-009-3306-6

Aytaç E (2022) Comparison of extraction methods of virgin coconut oil: cold press, soxhlet and supercritical fluid extraction. Sep Sci Technol 57(3):426–432. https://doi.org/10.1080/01496395.2021.1902353

Babu AS, Veluswamy SK, Arena R, Guazzi M, Lavie CJ (2014) Virgin coconut oil and its potential cardioprotective effects. Postgrad Med 126(7):76–83. https://doi.org/10.3810/pgm.2014.11.2835

Bawalan DD (2011) Processing manual for virgin coconut oil, its products and by-products for Pacific Island Countries and Territories. Secretariat of the Pacific Community, Noumea

Bawalan DD, Chapman K (2006) Virgin coconut oil: production manual for micro-and-village-scale processing. In: FAO, 1st edn. FAO Regional Office for Asia and the Pacific, Rome. http://www.fao.org/publications/card/en/c/bfbb8a43-fd11-4ff8-8d55-56a81f2ecb23/

Beegum PS, Ramesh SV, Pandiselvam R, Neema M, Manikantan MR, Hebbar KB (2024) Perspectives on the cardioprotective, neuroprotective and anti-obesity functions of coconut (Cocos nucifera L.), vol 58. Food Biosci, p 103756. https://doi.org/10.1016/j.fbio.2024.103756

Bureau of Agriculture and Fisheries Standards (2007) Philippine VCO standard. Philippine National Standards, pp 1–8

Cariappa MB, Ramesh SV, Chikkanna GS, Venkatesh J, Vishnuvardhana, Hebbar KB, Singh AK (2023) Detection of oil adulteration in virgin coconut oil (VCO) utilizing chemometrics and principal component analysis. Food Anal Methods 16(7):1291–1301. https://doi.org/10.1007/s12161-023-02506-4

Chatterjee P, Fernando M, Fernando B, Dias CB, Shah T, Silva R, Williams S, Pedrini S, Hillebrandt H, Goozee K, Barin E, Sohrabi HR, Garg M, Cunnane S, Martins RN (2020) Potential of coconut oil and medium chain triglycerides in the prevention and treatment of Alzheimer's disease. Mech Ageing Dev 186:111209. https://doi.org/10.1016/j.mad.2020.111209

Dayrit FM, Buenafe OEM, Chainani ET, De Vera IMS (2008) Analysis of monoglycerides, diglycerides, sterols, and free fatty acids in coconut (Cocos nucifera L) oil by 31P NMR spectroscopy. J Agric Food Chem 56(14):5765–5769. https://doi.org/10.1021/jf8005432

De Géa Neves M, Poppi RJ (2018) Monitoring of adulteration and purity in coconut oil using raman spectroscopy and multivariate curve resolution. Food Anal Methods 11(7):1897–1905. https://doi.org/10.1007/s12161-017-1093-x

Dia VP, Garcia VV, Mabesa RC, Tecson-Mendoza EM (2005) Comparative physicochemical characteristics of virgin coconut oil produced by different methods. Philippine Agric Sci 88(4):462–475

Đurašević S, Nikolić G, Zaletel I, Grigorov I, Memon L, Mitić-Ćulafić D, Vujović P, Đorđević J, Todorović Z (2020) Distinct effects of virgin coconut oil supplementation on the glucose and lipid homeostasis in non-diabetic and alloxan-induced diabetic rats. J Funct Foods 64:103601. https://doi.org/10.1016/j.jff.2019.103601

Famurewa AC, Folawiyo AM, Enohnyaket EB, Azubuike-Osu SO, Abi I, Obaje SG, Famurewa OA (2018) Beneficial role of virgin coconut oil supplementation against acute methotrexate chemotherapy-induced oxidative toxicity and inflammation in rats. Integr Med Res 7(3):257–263. https://doi.org/10.1016/j.imr.2018.05.001

Fernando M, Silva R, Fernando B, de Silva A, Wickremasinghe R, Dissanayake A, Martins RN, Williams S (2023) Effect of virgin coconut oil on cognition of mild-to-moderate Alzheimer's disease patients with APOE ε4 Allele. Alzheimers Dement 19(S21):230670. https://doi.org/10.1002/alz.075934

Ferrer PJ, Quilinguen VF, Rosario J, Pestaño LD (2018) Process design of virgin coconut oil (VCO) production using low-pressure oil extraction. MATEC Web Conf 156:1–9. https://doi.org/10.1051/matecconf/201815602003

Illam SP, Narayanankutty A, Raghavamenon AC (2017) Polyphenols of virgin coconut oil prevent pro-oxidant mediated cell death. Toxicol Mech Methods 27(6):442–450. https://doi.org/10.1080/15376516.2017.1320458

Jeyakumar SM, Damayanti K, Rajkumar Ponday L, Acharya V, Koppala SR, Putcha UK, Nagalla B, Vajreswari A (2023) Assessment of virgin coconut oil in a balanced diet on indicators of cardiovascular health in non-obese volunteers: a human metabolic study. Diabetes Metab Syndr 17(9):102844. https://doi.org/10.1016/j.dsx.2023.102844

Komaram AC, Anjaneyulu E, Goswami K, Nayak RR, Kanjilal S (2021) Detection and quantification of palmolein and palm kernel oil added as adulterant in coconut oil based on triacylglycerol profile. J Food Sci Technol 58(11):4420–4428. https://doi.org/10.1007/s13197-020-04927-z

Lagurin LG, Garrovillas MJM, Dayrit FM (2020) The application of 13C NMR and untargeted multivariate analysis for classifying virgin coconut oil. PRO 70(1):54. https://doi.org/10.3390/foods_2020-07718

Law KS, Azman N, Omar EA, Musa MY, Yusoff NM, Sulaiman SA, Hussain NHN (2014) The effects of virgin coconut oil (VCO) as supplementation on quality of life (QOL) among breast cancer patients. Lipids Health Dis 13(1):1–7. https://doi.org/10.1186/1476-511X-13-139

Machado M, Rodriguez-Alcalá LM, Pintado M, Maria Gomes AM (2023) Insights into coconut oil's anti-obesity potential: in vitro modulation of lipidic accumulation, adipolysis, and immune response. Eur J Lipid Sci Technol 125(10):2300037. https://doi.org/10.1002/ejlt.202300037

Mansor TST, Man YBC, Rohman A (2011) Application of fast gas chromatography and fourier transform infrared spectroscopy for analysis of lard adulteration in virgin coconut oil. Food Anal Methods 4(3):365–372. https://doi.org/10.1007/s12161-010-9176-y

Mansor TST, Man YBC, Shuhaimi M (2012) Employment of differential scanning calorimetry in detecting lard adulteration in virgin coconut oil. J Am Oil Chem Soc 89(3):485–496. https://doi.org/10.1007/s11746-011-1936-3

Marikkar JMN (2018) Principal component analysis of fatty acid data to detect virgin coconut oil adulteration by palm olein. Cord 34(1):9. https://doi.org/10.37833/cord.v34i1.24

Marina AM, Che Man YB, Amin I (2009a) Virgin coconut oil: emerging functional food oil. Trends Food Sci Technol 20(10):481–487. https://doi.org/10.1016/j.tifs.2009.06.003

Marina AM, Che Man YB, Nazimah SAH, Amin I (2009b) Chemical properties of virgin coconut oil. J Am Oil Chem Soc 86(4):301–307. https://doi.org/10.1007/s11746-009-1351-1

Marina AM, Che Man YB, Nazimah SAH, Amin I (2009c) Monitoring the adulteration of virgin coconut oil by selected vegetable oils using differential scanning calorimetry. J Food Lipids 16(1):50–61. https://doi.org/10.1111/j.1745-4522.2009.01131.x

Marina AM, Man YBC, Amin I (2010) Use of the SAW sensor electronic nose for detecting the adulteration of virgin coconut oil with RBD palm kernel olein. J Am Oil Chem Soc 87(3):263–270. https://doi.org/10.1007/s11746-009-1492-2

McCarty MF, DiNicolantonio JJ (2016) Lauric acid-rich medium-chain triglycerides can substitute for other oils in cooking applications and may have limited pathogenicity. Open Heart 3(2):e000467. https://doi.org/10.1136/openhrt-2016-000467

Mikołajczak N (2017) Coconut oil in human diet—nutrition value and potential health benefits. J Educ Health Sport 7(9):307–319

Mohammed NK, Samir ZT, Jassim MA, Saeed SK (2021) Effect of different extraction methods on physicochemical properties, antioxidant activity, of virgin coconut oil. Mater Today Proceed 42:2000–2005. https://doi.org/10.1016/j.matpr.2020.12.248

Muralidharan K, Jayashree A (2011) Value addition, product diversification and by-product utilization in coconut. Coconut Dev Board 7(4):1–25

Negash YA, Amare DE, Bitew BD, Dagne H (2019) Assessment of quality of edible vegetable oils accessed in Gondar City, Northwest Ethiopia. BMC Res Notes 12(1):1–5. https://doi.org/10.1186/s13104-019-4831-x

Negi A, Nimbkar S, Thirukumaran R, Moses JA, Sinija VR (2024) Impact of thermal and nonthermal process intensification techniques on yield and quality of virgin coconut oil. Food Chem 434:137415. https://doi.org/10.1016/j.foodchem.2023.137415

Neves MDG, Poppi RJ (2020) Authentication and identification of adulterants in virgin coconut oil using ATR/FTIR in tandem with DD-SIMCA one class modeling. Talanta 219:121338. https://doi.org/10.1016/j.talanta.2020.121338

Nevin KG, Rajamohan T (2004) Beneficial effects of virgin coconut oil on lipid parameters and in vitro LDL oxidation. Clin Biochem 37(9):830–835. https://doi.org/10.1016/j.clinbiochem.2004.04.010

Nevin KG, Rajamohan T (2008) Influence of virgin coconut oil on blood coagulation factors, lipid levels and LDL oxidation in cholesterol fed Sprague-Dawley rats. E-SPEN 3(1):1–8. https://doi.org/10.1016/j.eclnm.2007.09.003

Ng SP, Khor YP, Lim HK, Lai OM, Wang Y, Wang Y, Nehdi IA, Tan CP (2021a) In-depth characterization of palm-based diacylglycerol-virgin coconut oil blends with enhanced techno-functional properties. LWT 145:111327. https://doi.org/10.1016/j.lwt.2021.111327

Ng YJ, Tham PE, Khoo KS, Cheng CK, Chew KW, Show PL (2021b) A comprehensive review on the techniques for coconut oil extraction and its application. Bioprocess Biosyst Eng 44(9):1807–1818. https://doi.org/10.1007/s00449-021-02577-9

Nikooei P, Hosseinzadeh-Attar MJ, Asghari S, Norouzy A, Yaseri M, Vasheghani-Farahani A (2021) Effects of virgin coconut oil consumption on metabolic syndrome components and asymmetric dimethylarginine: a randomized controlled clinical trial. Nutr Metab Cardiovasc Dis 31(3):939–949. https://doi.org/10.1016/j.numecd.2020.11.020

Nivya EM, Panjikkaran ST, Aneena ER, Sharon CL, Gopal KS, Pathrose B, Suman KT, Lakshmy PS, Rajeesha CR, Rammya Molu K (2023) Quality evaluation of virgin coconut oil extracted from different processing methods. Pharma Innov 12(1):44–48. https://doi.org/10.22271/tpi.2023.v12.i1a.18106

Pandiselvam R, Akshay AT, Manikantan MR, Ramesh SV, Patil H, Gopal M (2023) Synergetic effect of fermented coconut inflorescence sap for the production of virgin coconut oil. J Food Biochem 2023:1–12. https://doi.org/10.1155/2023/7125810

Pizzo JS, Galuch MB, Santos PDS, Manin LP, Zappielo CD, Silva Filho OJ, Santos OO, Visentainer JV (2019) Determination of coconut oil adulteration with soybean oil by direct infusion electrospray ionization mass spectrometry. J Braz Chem Soc 30(7):1468–1474. https://doi.org/10.21577/0103-5053.20190042

Ponphaiboon J, Limmatvapirat S, Chaidedgumjorn A, Limmatvapirat C (2018) Optimization and comparison of GC-FID and HPLC-ELSD methods for determination of lauric acid, mono-, di-, and trilaurins in modified coconut oil. J Chromatogr B Anal Technol Biomed Life Sci 1099:110–116. https://doi.org/10.1016/j.jchromb.2018.09.023

Priya RB, Rashmitha R, Preetham GS, Chandrasekar V, Mohan RJ, Sinija VR, Pandiselvam R (2022) Detection of adulteration in coconut oil and virgin coconut oil using advanced analytical techniques: a review. Food Anal Methods 15(11):2917–2930. https://doi.org/10.1007/s12161-022-02342-y

Rahim NS, Lim SM, Mani V, Majeed ABA, Ramasamy K (2017) Enhanced memory in Wistar rats by virgin coconut oil is associated with increased antioxidative, cholinergic activities and reduced oxidative stress. Pharm Biol 55(1):825–832. https://doi.org/10.1080/13880209.2017.1280688

Rajamohan T, Archana U (2019) Nutrition and health aspects of coconut. In: The coconut palm (Cocos nucifera L.)—research and development perspectives. Springer, Singapore, pp 757–777. https://doi.org/10.1007/978-981-13-2754-4_15

Ramesh SV, Pandiselvam R, Thushara R, Manikantan MR, Hebbar KB, Beegum S, Mathew AC, Neenu S, Shil S (2020) Engineering intervention for production of virgin coconut oil by hot process and multivariate analysis of quality attributes of virgin coconut oil extracted by various methods. J Food Process Eng 43(6):1–10. https://doi.org/10.1111/jfpe.13395

Ramesh SV, Krishnan V, Praveen S, Hebbar KB (2021) Dietary prospects of coconut oil for the prevention and treatment of Alzheimer's disease (AD): a review of recent evidences. Trends Food Sci Technol 112(April):201–211. https://doi.org/10.1016/j.tifs.2021.03.046

Robinson SA, O'Brien MW, Grandy SA, Heinze-Milne S, Kimmerly DS (2019) Short-term supplement of virgin coconut oil improves endothelial-dependent dilation but not exercise-mediated hyperemia in young adults. Nutr Res 67:17–26. https://doi.org/10.1016/j.nutres.2019.03.016

Rohman A, Man YBC (2012) Application of fourier transform infrared spectroscopy for authentication of functional food oils. Appl Spectrosc Rev 47(1):1–13. https://doi.org/10.1080/05704928.2011.619020

Rohman A, Irnawati I, Erwanto Y, Lukitaningsih E, Rafi M, Fadzilah NA, Windarsih A, Sulaiman A, Zakaria Z (2021) Virgin coconut oil: extraction, physicochemical properties, biological activities and its authentication analysis. Food Rev Intl 37(1):46–66. https://doi.org/10.1080/87559129.2019.1687515

Salian V, Shetty P (2018) Coconut oil and virgin coconut oil: an insight into its oral and overall health benefits. J Clin Diagn Res 12(1):ZE01–ZE03. https://doi.org/10.7860/JCDR/2018/31409.11051

Seneviratne K, Jayathilaka N (2016) Coconut oil: chemistry and nutrition. Lakva Publisher, Battaramulla. https://www.researchgate.net/publication/322818556

Srivastava Y, Semwal AD, Sharma GK (2018) Virgin coconut oil as functional oil. In: Therapeutic, probiotic, and unconventional foods. Academic Press, London, pp 291–301. https://doi.org/10.1016/B978-0-12-814625-5.00015-7

Sundrasegaran S, Mah SH (2020) Review: Extraction Methods of Virgin Coconut Oil and Palm-pressed Mesocarp Oil and their Phytonutrients. eFood 1(6):381–391. https://doi.org/10.2991/efood.k.201106.001

Suryani S, Sariani S, Earnestly F, Marganof M, Rahmawati R, Sevindrajuta S, Indra Mahlia TM, Fudholi A (2020) A comparative study of virgin coconut oil, coconut oil and palm oil in terms of their active ingredients. PRO 8(4):1–11. https://doi.org/10.3390/PR8040402

Villarino BJ, Dy LM, Lizada MCC (2007) Descriptive sensory evaluation of virgin coconut oil and refined, bleached and deodorized coconut oil. LWT 40(2):193–199. https://doi.org/10.1016/j.lwt.2005.11.007

Xu B, Li P, Ma F, Wang X, Matthäus B, Chen R, Yang Q, Zhang W, Zhang Q (2015) Detection of virgin coconut oil adulteration with animal fats using quantitative cholesterol by GC × GC-TOF/MS analysis. Food Chem 178:128–135. https://doi.org/10.1016/j.foodchem.2015.01.035

Chapter 8
Coconut Inflorescence Sap (Neera): Nutritive Potential and Health Conferring Products

S. V. Ramesh, R. Pandiselvam, P. P. Shameena Beegum, M. R. Manikantan, Murali Gopal, and K. B. Hebbar

Abstract Coconut inflorescence sap, commonly known as *neera*, is a phloem sap obtained from adult coconut palms. Traditional methods of tapping coconut spadix result in a fermented, oyster-white colored sap with a significant amount of ethanol. However, the introduction of the Coco-sap chiller allows the extraction of unfermented inflorescence sap suitable for processing into various value-added products such as sugar and other nutritive items. The unfermented sap, referred to as *Kalparasa*®, can be consumed directly as a refreshing drink when served chilled. Biochemical characterization of *Kalparasa*® has highlighted its nutritive potential due to the presence of phenolics, sugars, minerals, inulin, and essential vitamins. This chapter explores the physical and biochemical features of coconut inflorescence sap, discusses varietal and seasonal influences on neera production, delves into fermentation chemistry and microbiome aspects, explores differences in primary and secondary value-added products, and outlines the health benefits associated with coconut inflorescence sap. In conclusion, future perspectives on the utilization of coconut inflorescence sap are presented.

Keywords Coconut neera · Phloem sap · Bioactives · Nutritive products

8.1 Introduction

Palms are considered among the oldest angiosperms globally, and the economically important palms are coconut (*Cocos nucifera*), African oil palm (*Elaeis guineensis*), date palm (*Phoenix dactylifera*), and arecanut palm (*Areca catechu*). Since time immemorial, various palms have been tapped to yield beverages such as fresh sweet

S. V. Ramesh (✉) · R. Pandiselvam · P. P. Shameena Beegum · M. R. Manikantan · M. Gopal · K. B. Hebbar (✉)
ICAR-Central Plantation Crops Research Institute, Kasaragod, Kerala, India
e-mail: ramesh.sv@icar.gov.in; hebbar.kb@icar.gov.in

S. V. Ramesh, S. Praveen (eds.), *Coconut-Based Nutrition and Nutraceutical Perspectives*, https://doi.org/10.1007/978-981-97-3976-9_8

toddy, fermented toddy, honey (concentrated sap), jaggery and sugar. *Arenga pinnata* is likely one of the earliest sources of sugar for humanity. Historical records in the fourth century BC have documented the custom of producing and consuming *Borassus flabellifer* sugar in India. The process of tapping palms and production of sugar in India dates back over 4000 years. Also there are reports detailing the production of jaggery and treacle using the sap of palm *Caryota urens* in Sri Lanka. In Africa, palm sap primarily serves the traditional purpose of wine production. This usage has historical documentation in Egypt, where date palm sap was utilized since time immemorial, and along the Guinea coast, as reported by early navigators in the fifteenth century (Rangaswami 1997).

In certain palm species such as coconut, palmyra, and kithul, the primary tapping is done on the inflorescence. Nevertheless, tapping of stem for sap is common in date palms in contrast tapping in oil palm involves both the stem and inflorescence. Among these tapping methods, stem tapping of palms causes severe damage and necessitates an extended recovery period whereas least or no damage occurs when palm inflorescences are tapped for the sap and sugar production. Improper tapping techniques may lead to palm fatalities if not executed correctly (Francisco-Ortega and Zona 2013). *Neera* or coconut sap holds significant importance as a traditional beverage obtained by tapping the coconut spadix, predominantly consumed by rural communities. This phloem sap, containing sugars, proteins, elemental minerals, vitamins, phenolics, flavonoids etc., helps in the normal growth and development of coconuts. Coconut trees yield approximately 12–14 inflorescences (spadices) annually, averaging one per month. Each spadix has the capacity to support around 25 mature or tender coconuts. While maturity of a coconut takes a complete year, the tender nuts are harvested during the period of 6–8 months maturity. If a spadix is allowed to produce tender coconuts and considering water content of 500 mL/nut a total water content of 12–13 L is obtained in a spadix. Nevertheless, if the spadix is appropriately tapped, 60–70 L of sap could be attained in a span of 40–45 days. Additionally, phytochemical composition of the sap is richer in nutrients than tender nut water. Tapping coconut palms for inflorescence sap has been found to be energy efficient from plant physiological standpoint than growing palms for tender nut purpose (Hebbar et al. 2015).

Harvesting unfermented sap proves to be a challenging endeavor due to its slow flow and high susceptibility to fermentation. The inner lining of sap collection vessels is coated with lime to arrest the process of fermentation, but despite this addition, the sap can turn white with an unpleasant odor, rendering it unsuitable as a healthy beverage. The fermented sap is referred to as 'toddy,' characterized by a strong odor making it unappealing despite its nutritional content. However, instead of utilizing open earthen pots for sap collection, a specially designed collection device called the Coco-sap chiller has been designed (Hebbar and Augustine 2021) (Fig. 8.1). The sap collection process takes place at low temperatures, resulting in sap that differs significantly from *neera* collected through other traditional methods. This distinctive product is appropriately rechristened as "*Kalparasa*," (Trade Mark No. 2813919 dated: 22-09-2014). As already stated, the conventional approach to collecting *neera* involves the addition of preservatives or lime, resulting in a pH of

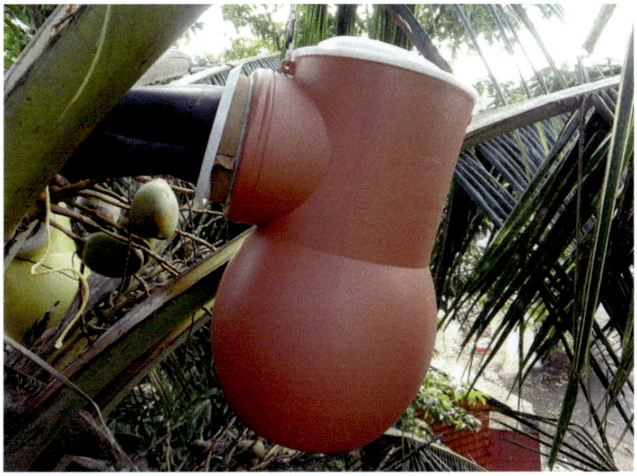

Fig. 8.1 Coco-sap chiller: A devise developed to tap coconut inflorescence sap (*neera*) in an unfermented form. (Source: Hebbar et al. 2022; https://link.springer.com/article/10.1007/s12355-021-01101-3. Reprinted with permission from Springer Nature)

approximately 5.5. In contrast, the sap obtained through from 'Coco-sap chiller' has a pH of approximately 7 and higher. The distinctive characteristics of sap collected using Coco-sap chiller and other traditional practices are outlined (Table 8.1). Delicious golden brown colour, free from extraneous materials such as insects, pollen and dust are some of the unique features of the sap collected using Coco-sap chiller. In addition, various health conferring biomolecules such as phenolics, vitamins, minerals and free amino acids are found in the sap (Hebbar et al. 2020). Beyond serving as healthy beverage, it serves as a perfect substrate for producing premium natural value-added products such as coconut sugar, jaggery, neera honey, etc. (Hebbar et al. 2013). Additionally, it can be used as a substrate for generating silver nanoparticles (Rajesh et al. 2020) and is rich in probiotic microbes (Gopal et al. 2021).

8.2 Varietal and Seasonal Influence of Neera Production

Understanding the influence of variety and season on coconut inflorescence sap production is crucial for farmers. This knowledge allows for the regulation of tapping times, identification of suitable varieties, and the implementation of irrigation practices to enhance sap production. Tall coconut varieties prove to be more effective than dwarf varieties when it comes to coconut inflorescence sap production. Among the varieties tested, WCT and DxT hybrids demonstrated the highest sap production, with averages of 960 mL and 880 mL, respectively. In contrast, COD exhibited very low sap production and was deemed unsuitable for tapping. In terms of sugar content, WCT displayed the highest total sugar content at 11.44 g/100 mL,

Table 8.1 Comparative nutritional constituents of coconut inflorescence sap collected through traditional and Coco-sap chiller methods

Nutritional components	Traditional sap	Coco-sap chiller method
Biochemical constituents/features		
Brix° (soluble solids)	13–15	15–18
pH	6 or low	7–8
Total sugars (g)	16.20 ± 0.33	9.20 ± 0.97
Reducing sugars (g)	0.68 ± 0.01	1.24 ± 0.87
Free amino acids (g)	1.03 ± 0.10	0.413 ± 0.09
Total phenolic content (mg GAE)	21.7 ± 0.48	14.8 ± 1.03
Total flavonoids (mg CE)	0.817 ± 0.19	0.177 ± 0.02
Vitamins		
Vitamin C (mg)	16.3 ± 0.76	19.6 ± 0.95
Niacin (μg)	14.9 ± 2.80	11.4 ± 0.7
Pyridoxine (μg)	1.32 ± 0.12	2.35 ± 0.01
Pantothenic acid (μg)	1.64 ± 0.11	3.99 ± 0.08
Biotin (μg)	0.07 ± 0.01	0.09 ± 0.01
Thiamine (μg)	0.02 ± 0.00	0.07 ± 0.02
Cholecalciferol (μg)	0.062 ± 0.00	0.056 ± 0.00
Ergocalciferol (μg)	0.028 ± 0.00	0.074 ± 0.01
Tocopherol (μg)	2.94 ± 0.46	7.20 ± 0.93
Vitamin K1(μg)	0.601 ± 0.09	1.73 ± 0.19
Vitamin K2(μg)	0.428 ± 0.12	0.771 ± 0.12
Mineral nutrition		
Sodium (mg)	–	90.6
Potassium (mg)	–	168.4
Phosphorus (mg)	–	3.9
Iron (mg)	–	0.053
Copper (mg)	–	0.031
Zinc (mg)	–	0.020

Adapted from Hebbar et al. (2015, 2020)

while DxT had a notable high reducing sugar content of 0.37 g/100 mL. It has been identified that tapping from the mid-monsoon to the start of ensuing winter season is ideal. Tapping during the summer, especially under rainfed conditions, should be avoided (Samsudeen et al. 2013). A study conducted in the Philippines, focusing on the Sequential Coconut Toddy and Nut Production (SCTNP) scheme in six coconut hybrids and cultivars across two experimental sites in Zamboanga City, revealed significant variations in sap and nut yields. The dwarf x tall hybrids and a local tall cultivar, Laguna, exhibited notably higher yields compared to the Catigan dwarf, Catigan dwarf hybrid (CAT x CAT), and a dwarf cultivar (Tacunan). Aside from differences in coconut varieties, the study highlighted the substantial influence of climatic conditions and the nutritional status of the palms on sap and nut yields (Secretaria et al. 1998). Sap flow in coconut is influenced by the variety (leaf area of palm) and soil conditions (such as soil depth, water holding capacity) in which the palm is cultivated.

8.3 Physical and Biochemical Features of *Kalparasa*®

Table 8.1 delineates the differential physico-chemical features of neera obtained through Coco-sap chiller (*Kalparasa*®) and that obtained through traditional extraction methodologies. *Kalparasa*® exhibits a slightly alkaline nature with a pH range of 7–8, a golden-brown color, and is characterized by a sweet and delicious taste. In contrast, neera is white in colour, possesses a pH of 6 or less, and emits a harsh odour. *Kalparasa*®, apart from its high sugar content, contains elevated levels of amino acids, and antioxidants (polyphenols, flavonoids), with respective increases of 2.5, 1.8, 1.5, and 4.6, folds compared to neera that was obtained in traditional methods (Hebbar et al. 2020). The vitamins such as Vitamin C and niacin are found enriched in *Kalparasa*®. In addition, similar qualitative biochemical features of amino acids, antioxidants (polyphenols and flavonoids), are found in the derivatives of *Kalparasa*® including sap derived sugar, sap concentrate (honey or syrup) etc., (Hebbar et al. 2020).

The coconut inflorescence sap exhibits distinctive characteristics, featuring a high ash content of 0.27% and a pH of 5.52. While it is relatively low in Total Soluble Solids (TSS) at 12 to 14°Brix, indicating a lower sugar content and acidity compared to sugar palm and sugarcane juices, it is rich in minerals. The coconut sap's lighter color (L value) and low browning index make it advantageous for food handlers in sugar preparation. Additionally, the coconut sap is abundant in antioxidants. In terms of sugar composition, the coconut sap is characterized with relatively high content of fructose and glucose and a low quantity of sucrose when compared to sugar palm and sugarcane juices. In comparison to sugar palm and cane juice, coconut sap is characterized by elevated levels of Vitamin C, Vitamin B1, Vitamin B3, Vitamin B4 and Vitamin B10. Given these attributes, coconut sap emerges as a promising source for the production of healthier sugar (Asghar et al. 2020).

An untargeted metabolomic profiling of fresh coconut inflorescence sap uncovered a diverse array of secondary metabolites, sugars, lipids, and peptides. The mass spectrometry (MS) profile, when analyzed in the positive mode, indicated that the coconut inflorescence sap consists mainly of secondary metabolites (64%), whereas among the primary metabolites sugars (9%)lipids (12%) and protein-derived peptides (9%) predominate. Conversely, in the negative mode, the composition of the sap has secondary metabolites (33%), sugars (20%), 9% lipids (9%), and peptides (11%) (Rajesh et al. 2020). The primary metabolites identified in fresh coconut inflorescence sap included polyphenols belonging to the flavonoid class, such as 3,3′,4′,5,6,8-hexamethoxyflavone (22 mg L^{-1}), as well as xanthones like gentisin (22 mg L^{-1})· Additionally, alkaloids including (R)-boschniakine (20 mg L^{-1}) and atherosperminine (18 mg L^{-1}), along with 4-coumaroyl-2-hydroxyputrescine

(18 mg L^{-1}), were identified. Furthermore, dipeptides such as glutamylmethionine were present (10 mg L^{-1}) (Rajesh et al. 2020).

Twenty-one compounds, accounting for over 98% of the volatile content in fresh neera were identified. Key flavor constituents in the volatile profile of fresh inflorescences sap included ethyl lactate, phenyl ethyl alcohol, 3-hydroxy-2-pentanone, farnesol, 2-methyl tetrahydrofuran, and tetradecanone. Neera when clarified exhibited diminished volatile content, with 13 compounds. Ethyl lactate, phenyl ethyl alcohol, 1-hexanol, 2-methyl tetrahydrofuran, 3-hydroxy-2-pentanone, and 2-hydroxy-3-pentanone are the prominent flavor components. Fermented neera presented a higher volatile content, with 12 compounds representing over 95% of the volatile compounds. Ethyl lactate, phenyl ethyl alcohol, and farnesol were retained from the original seven compounds found in fresh neera (Borse et al. 2007). Thirteen phenolic acids and seven flavonoids were detected in coconut inflorescence sap. The primary phenolic acids identified include vanilic acid, syringic acid, trans-cinnamic acid, and p-hydroxybenzoic acid. Among the flavonoids, catechin, hesperitin, and myricetin were predominant (Hebbar et al. 2020). The vitamin content in the sap obtained through Coco-sap chiller method was markedly higher than that collected by traditional method of tapping. Among the water-soluble vitamins investigated, vitamin C exhibited a higher concentration in the sap obtained from Coco-sap chiller (19.6 mg/100 mL) compared to the sap collected in traditional methods (16.3 mg/100 mL). Additionally, the sap collected from Coco-sap chiller contained significantly elevated levels of niacin, tocopherol, pantothenic acid, and pyridoxine (Hebbar et al. 2020) (Table 8.1).

8.4 Dynamics of Physico-Chemical Features of Coconut Inflorescence Sap Upon Storage

The fresh sap from coconut inflorescence typically exhibits a slightly alkaline pH ranging from 7.5 to 8, with minor variations observed from tree to tree. Upon exposure to ambient temperature, fermentation initiates within 2–3 h, leading to a gradual decrease in pH. The completely fermented sap typically reaches a pH of 3.5. Conversely, when stored in sub-zero conditions the sap remains fresh, without any alterations in pH due to the arrest of the activities of the microbes involved in fermentation. Fresh sap, with an initial pH of 7.5, contains approximately 15% sugars, which decreases to about 6% as the pH drops to 4. Simultaneously, the level of reducing sugars increases up to 5%. The coconut inflorescence undergoes the process of natural fermentation process in three stages: conversion of sugars into lactic acid in an initial lactic acid fermentation, followed by conversion of lactic acid into alcohol in a subsequent alcoholic fermentation during the middle stage, and finally, an acetic fermentation in the last stage. At each of these stages, the microbial activity plays a crucial role in facilitating the metabolite(s) conversions in the succeeding stage (Atputharajah et al. 1986). Hebbar et al. (2015) also delineated that fresh inflorescence sap undergoes lactic acid fermentation followed by alcoholic fermentation in the later stage due to the microbial actions when the sap was left abandoned to atmospheric exposure.

8.5 Coconut Inflorescence Sap Microbiome

The high sugar content of the coconut inflorescence sap serves as a suitable substrate for the growth of variety of microorganisms including aerobic mesophils. Throughout the process of neera tapping, collection in containers, transportation, and storage of sap, a substantial presence of acetic acid bacteria, lactic acid bacteria, and yeasts is observed (Nwachukwu et al. 2006; Ogbulie et al. 2007). Yeast, particularly *Saccharomyces cerevisiae*, dominates the sap immediately after tapping, multiplying rapidly under ambient conditions and leading to a significant accumulation of alcohol content within a few hours, contrary to previous studies indicating such changes occurring after 3 days of the start of fermentation (Amoa-Awua et al. 2007). Further exploration of the natural fermentation process of coconut inflorescence sap identified 166 yeast isolates and 39 bacterial isolates. Seventeen yeast species, belonging to eight genera, were found to be involved in biochemical changes during the process of natural fermentation (Atputharajah et al. 1986). Metagenomic analysis of fresh *Kalparasa*® (pH 7.2) and fermented sap (pH 4.5) revealed that unfermented sap showed high bacterial species diversity and low fungal diversity compared to the sap that underwent fermentation (Gopal et al. 2021). The predominance of probiotic-type bacterial genus *Leuconostoc*, followed by equal proportions of other bacteria such as *Gluconobacter*, *Acetobacter*, and *Fructobacillus* along with yeasts genera namely *Saccharomyces* and *Hanseniaspora* were observed. It suggests that the fermentation process of *Kalparasa*® is likely due to the combined activities of acetic acid bacteria and non-*Saccharomyces* yeasts. Predictions related to the bacteriome function in fresh neera revealed the enrichment of nucleoside metabolism along with glycerophospholipid and ABC transporters. This indicates that the unfermented sap could be promoted as a healthy live probiotic-type beverage (Gopal et al. 2021).

8.6 Primary and Secondary Products of Coconut Inflorescence Sap

The primary product derived from coconut *Kalparasa* is not just an excellent health beverage but also serves as an optimal substrate for manufacturing high-quality natural value-added products. These include neera concentrate, syrup, coconut sugar, coconut jaggery, and various other items, including Bengal sweets (Fig. 8.2).

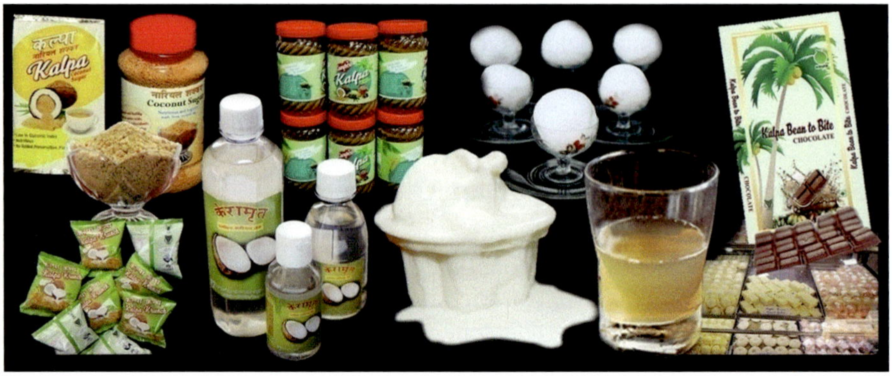

Fig. 8.2 Various products derived from coconut inflorescence sap (The figure depicts various food products such as coconut sugar, frozen coconut delicacy, sweets, bean to bite chocolate, kalpa drinking chocolate etc. obtained from processing coconut inflorescence sap). (Photo Credits: ICAR-CPCRI, Kasaragod)

Coconut sugar is a premier natural sweetener, derived from coconut inflorescence sap, boasting numerous health benefits that contribute to its high market potential despite its premium price. The nutritional profile of coconut sugar includes essential coenzymes such as Vitamin C, Vitamin E, and minerals like potassium, iron, zinc, and phosphorus. Additionally, it contains phytonutrients such as anthocyanidins, flavonoids, and polyphenols (Hebbar et al. 2020). Coconut sap sugar stands out for its significant content of inulin, with approximately 4.7 g/100 g. Inulin plays a crucial role in the production of short-chain fatty acids like propionate, acetate, and butyrate. This conversion of fermentable inulin into short-chain fatty acids contributes to enhancing the functional aspects of coconut sugar and syrup.

Coconut syrup, in particular, contains both dietary fiber and inulin, offering a combination of nutritional benefits. The presence of inulin enriches the syrup with its prebiotic properties, promoting gut health and overall well-being. Additionally, the dietary fiber content further enhances the digestive benefits of coconut syrup (Trinidad 2015). Overall, the inulin in coconut sap sugar and syrup adds to their nutritional value and functional properties, making them attractive options for individuals seeking healthier sweetening alternatives.

Coconut sugar is increasingly used as an alternative sweetener in confectionery, pastries, beverages, and various culinary applications (Okoma et al. 2020) owing to its equivalent sweetening power to sucrose. Its low glycemic index (GI) ranging from 35 to 54 per serving, as reported by Trinidad et al. (2010), positions coconut sugar as a favorable choice for those looking to reduce the risk of chronic diseases, including diabetes, through a low GI diet.

In the food and beverage industry, coconut sugar serves as a versatile ingredient with various applications. It is commonly used in the preparation of a wide range of bakery items, including biscuits, cakes, brownies, and confectionery products such as chocolates. Whether it's adding sweetness to baked goods or enhancing the flavor profile of confections, coconut sugar offers a unique taste and texture that appeals to many consumers. In biscuits, coconut sugar can provide a subtle sweetness and caramel-like flavor, complementing the other ingredients in the recipe. Similarly, in cakes and brownies, it adds depth of flavor and moisture, resulting in rich and indulgent treats. In confectionery products like chocolates, including dark chocolate and drinking chocolate, coconut sugar can be used as a natural sweetener, offering a healthier alternative to refined sugar while imparting a distinct taste. It serves as a sweetener for tea, juice, and other beverages and can also be used as a seasoning agent. In comparison to other sugars, coconut sugar demonstrates nutritional superiority (Sarkar et al. 2023).

Coconut sugar finds diverse applications, extending beyond sweetening, and is employed in the production of chocolate, cakes, ice cream, sweet soy sauce, food coatings, and traditional Bengali sweets, as documented by Hebbar et al. (2017). Additionally, various secondary products made from coconut sugar are as follows:

1. **Kalpa Bar:** This is a chocolate product based on coconut sugar, crafted entirely from plant-origin ingredients, and free from dairy milk. The collaboration between ICAR-CPCRI and CAMPCO has resulted in the development of Kalpa Bar, a unique dark chocolate product that caters to health-conscious consumers. This chocolate bar is formulated with carefully selected ingredients, including cocoa powder, coconut sugar, natural vanilla extract, and GMO-free sunflower lecithin. One of the key features of Kalpa Bar is its low glycemic index, which is beneficial for individuals monitoring their blood sugar levels or following a low-glycemic diet. By using coconut sugar as a sweetener, the chocolate maintains a lower glycemic index compared to traditional sugar-sweetened chocolates. Furthermore, Kalpa Bar is free from added artificial ingredients, making it a healthier choice for those seeking natural and minimally processed foods. The inclusion of natural vanilla extract enhances the flavor profile of the chocolate, providing a satisfying and indulgent experience for consumers. An additional advantage of Kalpa Bar is its ability to be stored at room temperature without melting, thanks to its carefully balanced formulation. This feature makes it convenient for consumers to enjoy the chocolate without the need for refrigeration.
2. **Kalpa Drinking Chocolate:** This product involves blending low glycemic index coconut sugar with fine cocoa powder to craft a delightful drinking chocolate. This carefully curated blend results in a beverage that offers a rich and satisfying chocolate experience without the drawbacks of high-glycemic sweeteners. This drinking chocolate is designed to dissolve instantly in both hot and cold milk, allowing for quick and convenient preparation. Upon preparation, the drinking chocolate releases a tantalizing aroma of rich cocoa, further enhancing the sensory experience for consumers. The aroma invites indulgence and sets the stage for a truly enjoyable beverage moment. In summary, this drinking chocolate offers a convenient and delicious way to enjoy the classic combination of cocoa and sweetness. With its low glycemic index and instant dissolvability, it provides a guilt-free indulgence

3. **Kalparasa-Based Milk Sweets:** The concentrated neera or Kalparasa replaces the traditional sweeteners in the preparation of sweets in West Bengal, India. This alternative method of preparing sweets serves as a means of long-distance transport for neera. These sweets not only provide minerals, vitamins, and valuable fibers absent in cane sugar-based milk sweets but also have a low glycemic index, making them suitable for a healthy lifestyle and sweet indulgence (Ghosh et al. 2016).
4. **Nutribar:** Crafting an energy-rich nutri bar from Kalparasa involves concentrating the coconut sap to a thick consistency measuring 75–80° Brix, which should constitute approximately 80% of the ingredients. This concentrated Kalparasa is then combined with protein-rich elements like roasted peanuts and green gram, along with cocoa powder. This energy-rich nutri bar offers a delicious and wholesome snack option that provides sustained energy and essential nutrients, making it ideal for fueling active lifestyles (Anonymous 2019).
5. **Kalpa Bean to Bite Dark Chocolate:** Recently, there has been a shift towards incorporating palm sugar in chocolate production, presenting a healthier alternative. Addition of natural sugars offers manifold health benefits owing to their relatively low glycemic index properties. A standardized protocol for production of dark chocolate in cottage level set up, referred to as 'Bean to Bite' or 'Bean to Bar,' has been established. This protocol involves the use of well-fermented and dried cocoa beans along with sugar, with or without cocoa butter. This specific composition results in a dark chocolate product that is not only flavorful but also rich in flavonoids, polyphenols, and essential mineral nutrition (Beegum et al. 2022b).
6. **Frozen Coconut Delicacy:** The creation of a coconut-based frozen delicacy exclusively using coconut ingredients, including coconut milk, coconut sugar, tender coconut water, and pulp, results in a premium product that is entirely natural and considered healthy. By exclusively incorporating natural coconut ingredients and sweetening with coconut sugar, this frozen delicacy offers a decadent and indulgent treat that is not only delicious but also healthier compared to traditional desserts (Beegum et al. 2022a). Notably, this frozen delicacy is suitable for individuals with lactose intolerance since it does not contain milk. Moreover, the replacement of refined sugar with coconut sugar contributes to its low glycemic index (GI) and elevated vitamin and mineral content, making it a healthier option.

8.7 Levan from Coconut Inflorescence Sap

Coconut inflorescence sap has been utilized as a substrate, acted upon by *Bacillus subtilis*, for the production of levan demonstrating notable thermal and functional properties, making it a potential replacement for icing sugar. This levan product, a polysaccharide with diverse biological activities, exhibits robust emulsifying, foaming, water, and oil holding capacities. Remarkably, levan also showcases anti-inflammatory and non-hemolytic activities. Its antioxidant potential is demonstrated through assays such as DPPH (2,2-diphenyl-1-picrylhydrazyl) and FRAP (Ferric Reducing Antioxidant Power), indicating its ability to scavenge free radicals and reduce oxidative stress. Moreover, in vitro studies have unveiled levan's antimicrobial activity, particularly at concentrations of 100 and 200 μg/mL. This antimicrobial efficacy underscores levan's potential as a natural agent for combating microbial infections and supporting overall health. The sensory evaluations of levan have revealed its sweetness, surpassing that of icing sugar. A cake cream formulation combining 25% icing sugar with 75% levan garnered the highest overall acceptability, indicating levan's suitability for use in confectionery applications. Furthermore, levan's versatility extends to its production from sucrose-rich substrates such as sugar cane molasses and pineapple extract alone or in combination with coconut inflorescence sap. These alternative sources offer opportunities for sustainable levan production and broaden its potential applications. In addition to its sensory appeal and diverse sources, levan exhibits robust biological activities, including antioxidant, anti-inflammatory, and antimicrobial properties against pathogenic microorganisms. These qualities position levan as a valuable ingredient in pharmaceutical and biomedical industries, where natural bioactive compounds are highly sought after. Moreover, levan's role as a bio-emulsifier underscores its potential as an eco-friendly alternative to synthetic chemical emulsifiers, aligning with the growing demand for sustainable and natural food additives (Mummaleti et al. 2022).

8.8 Inflorescence–Sap Based Starter Culture for VCO Production

The fermentation technique employed for Virgin Coconut Oil (VCO) production incurs significant expenses, primarily due to the initial investment in acquiring pure microbial strains. However, an alternative, potentially more cost-effective approach to enhance VCO fermentation involves using fermented neera. A treatment involving 8-h fermented neera at a 10% concentration produced VCO, meeting FSSAI standards (Pandiselvam et al. 2023).

8.9 Silver Nano Particles from Coconut Inflorescence Sap

The green synthesis of nanoparticles involves utilizing various biological extracts as substrates for nanoparticle synthesis, providing an environmentally friendly alternative to chemical methods. In this context, coconut neera was employed to synthesize silver nanoparticles (AgNPs). The resulting particles were crystalline, predominantly spherical with a smooth (thin) shell, and poly-dispersed, exhibiting diameters varying from 10 to 30 nm. Treatment with aqueous solutions of AgNPs significantly reduced contamination in arecanut in vitro culture media without adversely affecting the normal development of arecanut plantlets. Furthermore, the antimicrobial efficacy of AgNPs synthesized from coconut neera was evaluated against *Escherichia coli, Salmonella typhimurium,* and *Vibrio parahaemolyticus*. The study confirmed the antibacterial activity of AgNPs through various mechanisms, including the production of reactive oxygen species (ROS) and leakage of proteins from bacterial cells. The unfermented inflorescence sap, characterized by an above-neutral pH, demonstrated its efficacy as a potent reducing agent for the synthesis of AgNPs from Ag+ ions. This highlights the potential of coconut neera as a natural source for the production of antimicrobial nanoparticles, offering a sustainable and eco-friendly alternative for combating bacterial pathogens (Rajesh et al. 2020).

8.10 Health Benefits of Coconut Inflorescence Sap and Its Products

The low glycemic index (GI) of coconut sap is associated with slow glucose uptake in the bloodstream, contributing to the fight against diabetes by reducing insulin requirements. The Food and Nutrition Research of India's study revealed that coconut sugar has a glycemic index of 35, which is notably lower than that of many other commercially available sugars. This low glycemic index makes coconut sugar an attractive option for individuals seeking to manage their blood sugar levels more effectively. The presence of phytochemicals including flavonoids, and phenolics, acts as protective agents against hyperglycemia, improving glucose uptake in the body. The phytonutrients present in coconut inflorescence sap have been found to have implications for glycogen metabolism and energy regulation within the body.

Palm sap is notable for containing significant levels of glutamic acid, a pivotal amino acid serving as a precursor for protein production. Enriched with vitamins and electrolytes, the sap acts as a source of coenzymes and cofactors in various metabolic processes, offering protection against diseases and enhancing overall immunity (Jose et al. 2017). The probiotic *Lactobacilli* species found in coconut inflorescence sap have been shown to interact with the gut epithelium, effectively colonizing gut cells. This interaction leads to a boost in both adaptive and innate immunity, as supported by studies conducted by Somashekaraiah et al. (2019) and Gopal et al. (2021).

The fresh sap exhibits a higher content of ascorbic acid, demonstrating its capability to neutralize radicals like hydroxyl, hydrogen peroxide and superoxide anion, in comparison to fermented sap (Chen et al. 2011). Despite lower levels of ascorbic acid in fermented sap, it is observed to safeguard DNA from damage, attributed to the formation of higher concentrations of phenolic components during the fermentation process. Moreover, analogous studies suggest that the sap may potentially prevent cancers by inhibiting the neoplastic transformation of cells in organs such as the colon, lung, and oral cavity. The rich mineral content of coconut inflorescence sap plays a critical role in maintaining the body's electrolyte balance, which is essential for avoiding or reducing dehydration, help regulate fluid balance within cells and tissues and contributes to maintaining normal body temperature. It is recognized as a potent natural beverage for preserving body fluids and is also deemed beneficial as a post-operative drink (Asha et al. 2019). The protective and curative effects of coconut inflorescence sap on alloxan-induced pancreatic cytotoxicity likely involve a combination of mechanisms, including the regulation of carbohydrate metabolism and the repair of pancreatic islet cells. Coconut inflorescence sap may support the repair of islet cells in the pancreas. Islet cells, particularly beta cells, are responsible for producing insulin. Alloxan-induced cytotoxicity can damage these cells, leading to decreased insulin production and glucose intolerance. Coconut inflorescence sap may possess properties that promote the regeneration or repair of damaged islet cells, restoring their function and enhancing insulin secretion (Renjith and Rajamohan 2012).

The unfermented sap derived from the tender, unopened inflorescence of coconut trees is recognized for its significant health benefits. In light of the thermal degradation concerns associated with the traditional evaporation process for producing coconut sugar, a low-temperature method of coconut sugar production was devised [Coconut Sap Powder, registered as COCOZEN™] (Jose et al. 2017; Ratheesh et al. 2017). This method not only ensures the preservation of micronutrients in the coconut sugar but also preserved the sugar-derived bioactive molecules that confer multiple health benefits including normal functioning of kidney, liver and anti-oxidant and anti-inflammatory properties (Jose et al. 2017; Ratheesh et al. 2017). Furthermore, preliminary findings, indicate its substantial ergogenic activity during both aerobic and anaerobic exercises, suggesting its potential as a natural agent to enhance physical performance. Notwithstanding its high carbohydrate nature (80%), the beneficial effect of this CSP could be due to its rich micronutrient profile (Mammen et al. 2020).

In the contemporary era, drug-induced nephrotoxicity stands out as a leading cause of renal damage. A study investigated the nephroprotective and curative effects of a coconut sugar in powder formulation derived from micronutrient-enriched, unfermented coconut flower sap in Wistar rat models (Jose et al. 2017). It suggested the potential of this natural agent in safeguarding and treating kidney-related issues, providing a promising avenue for addressing drug-induced nephrotoxicity and the broader pathogenesis of kidney diseases. The inflammatory response triggered by oxidized low-density lipoprotein (LDL) is recognized as a crucial factor in the development of atherosclerosis. Consequently, a study investigating the anti-inflammatory properties of a new formulation of coconut inflorescence sap has uncovered the ability of coconut inflorescence sap in down regulating and reversing the alterations induced by oxidized LDL (ox-LDL). This suggests a potential anti-inflammatory effect mediated through the Toll-like receptor (TLR)-NF-κB signaling pathway (Ratheesh et al. 2017). In addition, arterial stiffness and blood pressure are crucial indicators of cardiovascular health as individuals age. Plant derived products, offer promise in effectively reducing both BP and arterial stiffness associated with aging, thereby mitigating the risk of cardiovascular diseases. Coconut sap powder (CSP), has been demonstrated to decrease systolic BP and mitigate arterial stiffness in adults (Carlini et al. 2023). The administration of coconut sugar orally to Wistar rats with streptozotocin-induced diabetes has demonstrated several health benefits. The study observed positive outcomes, particularly in terms of bringing back carbohydrate and lipid metabolism to normal levels in diabetic rats. Additionally, the use of coconut sugar yielded favorable results in addressing oxidative stress associated with diabetes (Shetty et al. 2023).

Overall, the ability of coconut inflorescence sap to normalize glucose and lipid levels in diabetic rats highlights its potential as a natural therapeutic agent for diabetes management. These findings suggest that coconut sugar may have potential therapeutic effects in managing diabetes-related complications in humans too. Further research is warranted to elucidate the underlying mechanisms and evaluate its efficacy and safety in human subjects.

8.11 Conclusion and Prospects

The coconut inflorescence sap emerges as a valuable gift from the coconut tree, traditionally revered for its perceived medicinal properties and it is commonly utilized as a refreshing health drink. Remarkably, it is a non-alcoholic bio-beverage with numerous health benefits and devoid of any alcohol content. Globally promoted for its nutritional value and potential for value addition, this beverage contributes to cooling the human body and facilitating digestion. With an impressively low glycemic index, it does not elevate blood sugar levels like conventional fruit juices, making it a safe option even for diabetic individuals. Regular consumption of this sap is believed to prevent diseases such as jaundice, promoting overall health. As a natural detoxifying drink, it is lauded for its absence of side effects. Exploring the creation of novel nutritive products from coconut inflorescence sap constitutes a crucial area of research. The high sugar content in this sap can serve as a valuable substrate for developing products with prebiotic properties, specifically fructo-oligosaccharides. Coconut inflorescence sap holds great potential as a substrate for producing products with prebiotic benefits. Furthermore, there is a need to explore the probiotic properties of neera to formulate nutritive products enriched with probiotic organisms. However, scientific and technological attention is imperative for ensuring the quality and safety of coconut inflorescence sap, given its susceptibility to rapid fermentation. Challenges persist throughout the entire process, spanning from tapping to transportation, processing, and storage. Collecting fresh sap from farmers, transporting it to a cold storage center, processing it into value added products such as sugar, packing, labeling, and marketing require detailed planning and operationalization. This process involves significant manpower, material resources, and a carefully managed workflow from collection to reaching the consumer safely. The substantial investment in coconut sugar production contributes to its high cost. Indeed, integrating automation practices such as the Internet of Things (IoT), wireless communications, machine learning, artificial intelligence (AI), and deep learning into the tapping and processing of coconut inflorescence sap holds significant promise for optimizing production processes and reducing costs. Moreover, automation can enhance product quality and traceability, meeting the increasingly stringent requirements of consumers and regulatory authorities.

References

Amoa-Awua WK, Sampson E, Tano-Debrah K (2007) Growth of yeasts, lactic and acetic acid bacteria in palm wine during tapping and fermentation from felled oil palm (Elaeis guineensis) in Ghana. J Applied Microbiol 102(2):599–606

Anonymous (2019) Annual report 2018–19. ICAR-CPCRI, Kasaragod

Asghar MT, Yusof YA, Mokhtar MN, Ya'acob ME, Mohd Ghazali H, Chang LS, Manaf YN (2020) Coconut (*Cocos nucifera* L.) sap as a potential source of sugar: antioxidant and nutritional properties. Food Sci Nutr 8(4):1777–1787

Asha S, Ratheesh M, Jose SP, Krishnakumar IM, Sandya S (2019) Neera: a nonalcoholic nutritious beverage from unopened inflorescence of coconut palm. In: Natural beverages. Elsevier, pp 339–360. https://doi.org/10.1016/b978-0-12-816689-5.00012-2

Atputharajah JD, Widanapathirana S, Samarajeewa U (1986) Microbiology and biochemistry of natural fermentation of coconut palm sap. Food Microbiol 3:273–280

Beegum PS, Nair JP, Manikantan MR, Pandiselvam R, Shill S, Neenu S, Hebbar KB (2022a) Effect of coconut milk, tender coconut and coconut sugar on the physicochemical and sensory attributes in ice cream. J Food Sci Technol 59:2605–2616. https://doi.org/10.1007/s13197-021-05279-y

Beegum PPS, Pandiselvam R, Ramesh SV, Sugatha P, Nooh A, Neenu S, Gupta A et al (2022b) Sensorial, textural, and nutritional attributes of coconut sugar and cocoa solids based "bean-to-bar" dark chocolate. J Texture Stud 53(6):870–882

Borse BB, Rao LJM, Ramalakshmi K, Raghavan B (2007) Chemical composition of volatiles from coconut sap (*neera*) and effect of processing. Food Chem 101(3):877–880

Carlini NA, Romanowski S, Rabalais EN, Kistler BM, Campbell MS, Krishnakumar IM, Harber MP, Fleenor BS (2023) Coconut sugar derived from coconut inflorescence sap lowers systolic blood pressure and arterial stiffness in middle-aged and older adults: a pilot study. J Appl Physiol 134(3):508–514

Chen W, Zhu Q, Xia Q, Cao W, Zhao S, Liu J (2011) Reactive oxygen species scavenging activity and DNA protecting effect of fresh and naturally fermented coconut sap. J Food Biochem 35(5):1381–1388. https://doi.org/10.1111/j.1745-4514.2010.00506.x

Francisco-Ortega J, Zona S (2013) La savia dulce de las palmeras, una fuente de bebidas, alcohol, vinagre, miel y azu'car. VIERAEA 41:91–113

Ghosh DK, Bandyopadhyay A, Baidyanath D, Kaushik G, Hebbar KB, Chowdappa P (2016) Method of the preparation of fresh coconut inflorescence sap (Kalparasa) based sweets. Patent Application No. 201631013187

Gopal M, Shil S, Gupta A, Hebbar KB, Arivalagan M (2021) Metagenomic investigation uncovers presence of probiotic-type microbiome in *Kalparasa*® (fresh unfermented coconut inflorescence sap). Front Microbiol 12:662783. https://doi.org/10.3389/fmicb.2021.662783

Hebbar KB, Augustine (2021) Cocosap chiller. Patent no 373309

Hebbar KB, Mathew AC, Arivalagan M, Samsudeen K, Thomas GV (2013) Value added products from Neera. Indian Coconut J 56(4):28–33

Hebbar KB, Arivalagan M, Manikantan MR, Mathew AC, Thamban C, Thomas GV, Chowdappa P (2015) Coconut inflorescence sap and its value addition as sugar–collection techniques, yield, properties and market perspective. Curr Sci 109:1411–1417

Hebbar KB, Manikantan MR, Chowdappa P (2017) Kalparasa to boost rural economy. Indian Hortic 62(1):71–74
Hebbar KB, Arivalagan M, Pavithra KC, Roy TK, Gopal M, Shivashankara KS, Chowdappa P (2020) Nutritional profiling of coconut (*Cocos nucifera* L.) inflorescence sap collected using novel coco-sap chiller method and its value added products. J Food Meas Charact 14(5):2703–2712
Hebbar KB, Ramesh SV, Ghosh DK, Beegum PS, Pandiselvam R, Manikantan MR, Mathew AC (2022) Coconut sugar-a potential storehouse of nutritive metabolites, novel bio-products and prospects. Sugar Tech 24(3):841–856
Jose SP, Asha S, Krishnakumar IM, Ratheesh M, Santhosh S, Sandya S, Kumar G, Pramod C (2017) Nephro-protective effect of a novel formulation of unopened coconut inflorescence sap powder on gentamicin induced renal damage by modulating oxidative stress and inflammatory markers. Biomed Pharmacother 85:128–135
Mammen R, John F, Krishnakumar IM, Maliakel B, Mohanan R, Fleenor B (2020) Safety and influence of a novel powder form of coconut inflorescence sap on glycemic index and lipid profile. Bioact Carbohydr Diet Fibre 23:100217
Mummaleti G, Sarma C, Kalakandan SK, Gazula H, Sivanandham V, Anandharaj A (2022) Characterization of levan produced from coconut inflorescence sap using *Bacillus subtilis* and its application as a sweetener. LWT 154:112697. https://doi.org/10.1016/j.lwt.2021.112697
Nwachukwu IN, Ibekwe VI, Nwabueze RN, Anyanwu BN (2006) Characterisation of palm wine yeast isolates for industrial utilisation. African J Biotechnol 5(19):1725–1728
Ogbulie TE, Ogbulie JN, Njoku HO (2007) Comparative study on the microbiology and shelf life stability of palm wine from Elaeis guineensis and Raphia hookeri obtained from Okigwe, Nigeria. African J Biotechnol 6:914–922
Okoma DM, Konan KJ, Assa RR (2020) Vitamin and osidic composition of table sugars from the inflorescences sap of 03 coconut cultivars (*Cocos nucifera* L.) in Ivory Coast. Food Nutr Sci 11(12):1117–1126
Pandiselvam R, Akshay AT, Manikantan MR, Ramesh SV, Patil H, Gopal M (2023) Synergetic effect of fermented coconut inflorescence sap for the production of virgin coconut oil. J Food Biochem 2023:7125810. https://doi.org/10.1155/2023/7125810
Rajesh MK, Muralikrishna KS, Nair SS, Krishna KB, Subrahmanya TM, Sonu KP, Subaharan K, Sweta H, Keshava PT, Neeli C, Karunasagar I (2020) Facile coconut inflorescence sap mediated synthesis of silver nanoparticles and its diverse antimicrobial and cytotoxic properties. Mater Sci Eng C 111:110834
Rangaswami G (1997) Palm tree crops in India. Outlook Agric 9(4):167–173
Ratheesh M, Svenia JP, Asha S, Sandya S, Girishkumar B, Krishnakumar IM (2017) Anti-inflammatory effect of a novel formulation of coconut inflorescence sap against ox-LDL induced inflammatory responses in human peripheral blood mononuclear cells by modulating TLR-NF-κB signaling pathway. Toxicol Mech Methods 27(8):615–621
Renjith R, Rajamohan T (2012) Protective and curative effects of Cocos nucifera inflorescence on alloxan-induced pancreatic cytotoxicity in rats. Indian J Pharmacol 44(5):555–559. https://doi.org/10.4103/0253-7613.100368
Samsudeen K, Niral V, Jerard BA, Kumar M, Sugatha P, Hebbar KB (2013) Influence of variety and season in the inflorescence sap production in *Cocos nucifera* L. J Plant Crop 41(1):57–61
Sarkar T, Mukherjee M, Roy S, Chakraborty R (2023) Palm sap sugar an unconventional source of sugar exploration for bioactive compounds and its role on functional food development. Heliyon 9:e14788. https://doi.org/10.1016/j.heliyon.2023.e14788
Secretaria MI, Ebuna RM, Madrazo RM, Magat SS, Maravilla JN, Santos GA, Baylon GB (1998) Sequential coconut toddy-nut production (SCTNP) scheme in different coconut cultivars and hybrids: production and processing of product. Philippine J Crop Sci 23(Suppl. 1):76
Shetty SS, Ramesh SV, Arivalagan M, Roopashree PG, Manikantan MR, Hebbar KB, Kumari S (2023) Coconut (*Cocos nucifera* L.) inflorescence sap-derived sugar restores the glucose

and lipid homeostasis in streptozotocin-induced diabetic Wistar rat model. Biomedicine 43(3):859–866

Somashekaraiah R, Shruthi B, Deepthi BV, Sreenivasa MY (2019) Probiotic properties of lactic acid bacteria isolated from neera: a naturally fermenting coconut palm nectar. Front Microbiol 10:1–11. https://doi.org/10.3389/fmicb.2019.01382

Trinidad TP (2015) Characterizing coconut sap sugar and syrup as a promising functional food/ingredient. Department of Science and Technology, Food and Nutrition Research Institute, Taguig. https://doi.org/10.1136/bmjopen-2015-forum2015abstracts.79

Trinidad TP, Mallillin AC, Sagum RS, Encabo RR (2010) Glycemic index of commonly consumed carbohydrate foods in the Philippines. J Funct Foods 2:271–274. https://doi.org/10.1016/j.jff.2010.10.002

Chapter 9
Coconut Sugar: Nutritive Potential and Prospects

S. V. Ramesh, S. Sudharshana, Anjitha Jacob, P. P. Shameena Beegum, R. Pandiselvam, M. R. Manikantan, Murali Gopal, and K. B. Hebbar

Abstract Coconut sugar is derived from the concentration of inflorescence sap (also known as *neera* or *Kalparasa®*) collected by tapping the unopened coconut spadix. The original sap contains around 15% sucrose, which is concentrated by heating it to 90–95 °C until it forms crystalline or amorphous sugar. The resulting coconut sugar is brown in color and typically contains 2–3% moisture. In contrast to commercially available sugars that are high in calories, palm-based sugars like coconut sugar are rich in amino acids, vitamins, minerals, polyphenols, and antioxidants. Each of these constituents plays a role in determining the physico-chemical, microbiological, and antioxidant characteristics of coconut sugar. Additionally, coconut sugar has a relatively low glycemic index (GI), making it a suitable and healthy sweetener option for individuals of all ages. The micro- and macro-components isolated from coconut sugar encompass a range of chemical compounds that contribute to its unique characteristics and health benefits. This chapter discusses the method of preparation of coconut sugar, its biochemical features and health benefits; multiple food products produced from it and propose a way forward.

Keywords Sweeteners · Food industry · Biochemical features · Coconut sugar · Glycaemic potential · Mineral nutrition

9.1 Introduction

Coconut sap, a valuable value-added product, plays a crucial role in improving the livelihoods of coconut farmers. Extracted from unopened coconut inflorescences, this nutrient-rich phloem sap is known for its multiple health benefits. However, its high nutrient content and the extended collection time often lead to fermentation

S. V. Ramesh (✉) · S. Sudharshana · A. Jacob · P. P. Shameena Beegum · R. Pandiselvam · M. R. Manikantan · M. Gopal · K. B. Hebbar (✉)
ICAR-Central Plantation Crops Research Institute, Kasaragod, Kerala, India
e-mail: ramesh.sv@icar.gov.in; hebbar.kb@icar.gov.in

S. V. Ramesh, S. Praveen (eds.), *Coconut-Based Nutrition and Nutraceutical Perspectives*, https://doi.org/10.1007/978-981-97-3976-9_9

caused by microbial activity, making it challenging to collect in a hygienic and unfermented state (Hebbar et al. 2018).

Traditionally, sap collection involves using earthen pots or bamboo sacs lined with lime. However, the sap collected through this traditional method typically undergoes partial fermentation, resulting in a semi-transparent, oyster-white liquid known locally as neera. Unfortunately, this method exposes the sap to contaminants like insects and pollen, often resulting in an unpleasant smell, rendering it unsuitable for fresh juice markets. Instead, it is commonly used to produce sugar, toddy, and vinegar, with the addition of chemicals (Nathanael 1959).

To address these challenges and enable the collection of fresh, unfermented sap, the ICAR-Central Plantation Crops Research Institute (ICAR-CPCRI) in Kasaragod, Kerala, developed a patented solution known as the coco-sap chiller (Patent Number: 373309) (Hebbar et al. 2015). This innovative technique involves a portable, double-jacketed device with a PVC pipe and a 2–3 L collection container placed within ice cubes. Just half a kilogram of ice is sufficient to maintain a cool interior temperature for 10–12 h. Unlike the traditional method, the coco sap chiller collects sap in a closed system, protecting it from insects, dust, and ants. The unopened inflorescence is secured with coir or plastic rope to prevent bursting. It is then conditioned twice daily for a week using a mallet and hand massage to loosen the tightly packed spikelet within the inflorescence, facilitating the smooth flow of sap. After conditioning, the tip of the inflorescence is removed, and within a day or two, the sap begins to ooze out from the cut surface of the spadix. The sap harvested using this method can be kept unfermented for extended periods when stored at refrigerated conditions (−1 to −3 °C). Moreover, additional value-added products such as sap concentrate and coconut sugar can be produced (Hebbar et al. 2022) (Fig. 9.1). Palm sap sugar and sweet sap from palmyra palm (*Borassus flabellifer*), nipa palm (*Nypa fruticans* Wurmb), sugar palm (*Arenga pinnata*), and coconut palm (*Cocos nucifera*) serve as alternative sweeteners. These sweeteners have the potential to substitute sucrose in food products. The sweet sap can be consumed in its fresh state, processed into sugar or syrup, or fermented to produce vinegar or alcoholic beverages. Widely utilized in traditional foods across Southeast and Southern Asia, this sugar plays a crucial role in shaping the colour and flavour profiles of various culinary creations (Saputro et al. 2020; Francisco Ortega and Zona 2013).

In 2019, exports of products derived from palm sugar or coconut sap amounted to 36.5 thousand tons, valued at US$49.3 million. These exported products are required to adhere to the food regulations of their respective destination countries, including European countries (EFSA) and the United States (FDA). The global palm sugar industry is projected to reach a total value of $1.7 billion by 2027, compared to its current value of $630 million. This significant growth is attributed to the potential of palm sugar to be utilized as a sucrose substitute in various food products (Market Data Forecast 2024).

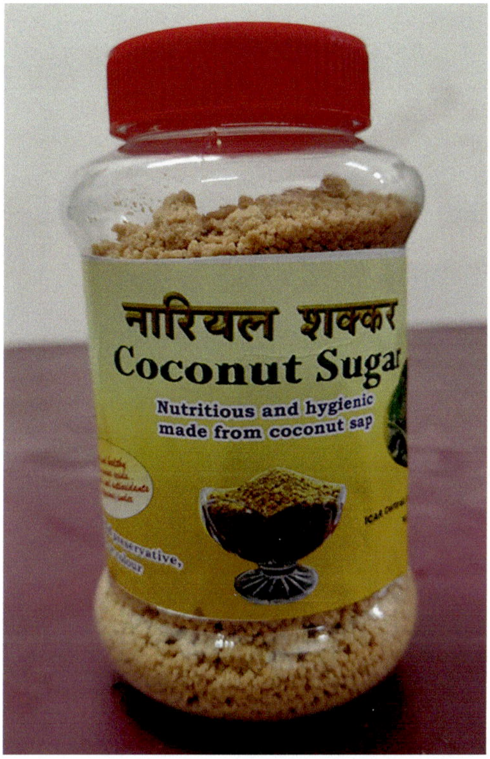

Fig. 9.1 Coconut sugar produced from coconut inflorescence sap. (Photo courtesy: ICAR-CPCRI)

9.2 Preparation of Coconut Sugar

Coconut sugar, renowned for its natural sweetness and distinctive flavor, is a cherished ingredient in numerous traditional dishes and beverages. Its popularity extends to confectionery and baking, where it adds a unique taste and color.

Figure 9.2 depicts the comparative methods of preparation of coconut sugar in a traditional and ICAR-CPCRI methodology. The process of preparing coconut sugar involves heating the sap to 90 °C in a double-jacket cooker, a device developed by ICAR-CPCRI. This batch-type cooker employs thermal fluid to indirectly and uniformly heat the sap and features a mechanical stirring system powered by an electric motor and reduction gearbox (Manikantan et al. 2018). As the sap undergoes controlled heating, its consistency undergoes significant changes. Initially, the fresh sap has a pH of 6.7–7.5 and a Brix of 14–16. As heating progresses, the sap thickens, forming a syrup at 50 Brix. Further heating leads to the formation of a dense syrup with a Brix of 60–70, which eventually boils and thickens to a very high viscosity, crystallizing into clods containing 3–4% moisture. These clods are then processed by rubbing and passing through a 60-mesh sieve to produce sugar with uniformly sized particles (Fig. 9.2).

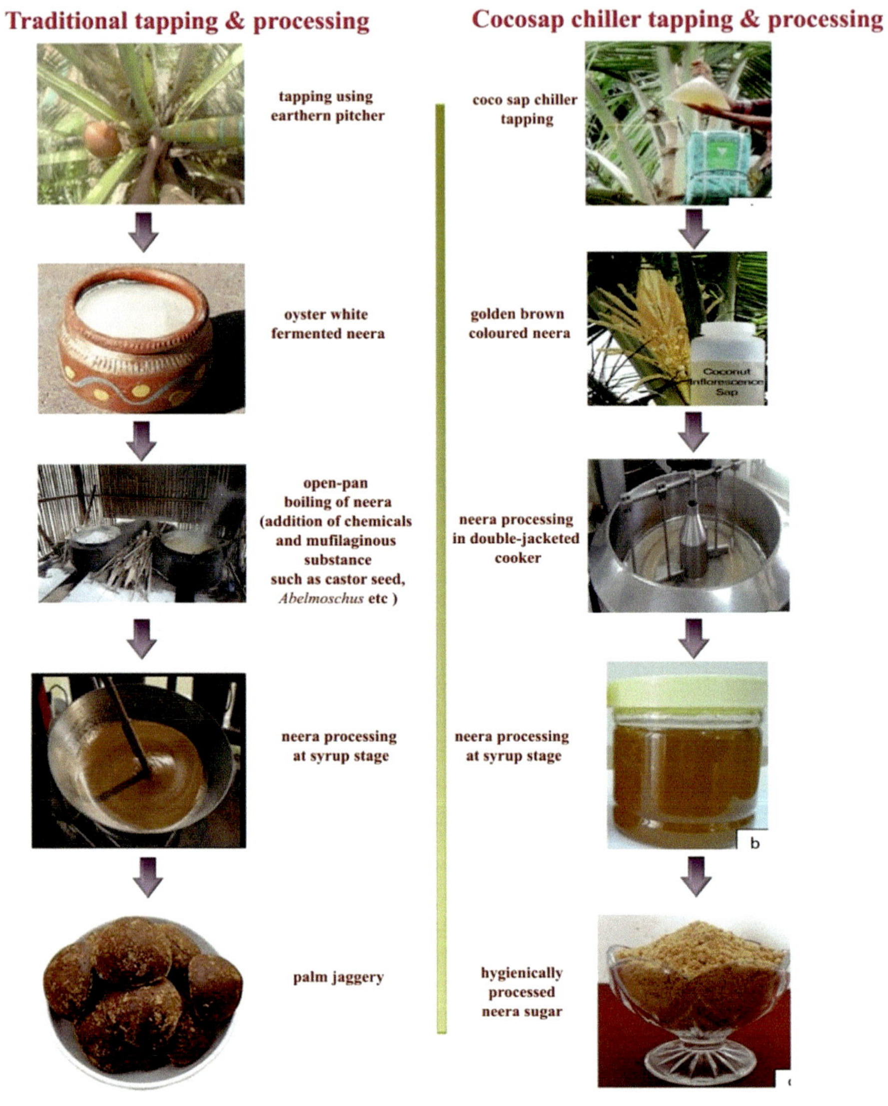
Traditional tapping & processing
Cocosap chiller tapping & processing
tapping using
earthern pitcher
coco sap chiller
tapping
oyster white
fermented neera
golden brown
coloured neera
Coconut
Inflorescence
Sap
open-pan
boiling of neera
(addition of chemicals
and mufilaginous
substance
such as castor seed,
Abelmoschus etc)
neera processing
in double-jacketed
cooker
neera processing
at syrup stage
neera processing
at syrup stage
b
palm jaggery
hygienically
processed
neera sugar

Fig. 9.2 Processing of coconut inflorescence sap for the production of coconut sugar in traditional (left panel) and in coco-sap chiller based extraction and processing in double jacketed cooker (right panel). (Source: Hebbar et al. 2022)

Traditionally, the process of cooking sugar syrup involves several stages, discerned through experiential knowledge:

1. Thread Stage: The syrup forms fine threads or settles into a clump at the bottom of water when cooled and pulled between the thumb and forefinger.

2. Soft Ball Stage: Dropping syrup into cold water results in the formation of a soft ball or clump with some structure, which flattens over time.
3. Firm Ball Stage: The syrup forms a more defined, pliable ball or clump in water.
4. Soft Crack Stage: Pliable threads bend slightly before snapping, accompanied by a distinct cracking sound.
5. Hard Crack Stage: The syrup forms long threads that begin to break as sugar crystallizes.

These stages aid in determining the precise cooking point to achieve the desired consistency for various confections (Hebbar et al. 2022).

9.3 Sugar Preparation Techniques

The production of coconut sugar involves various evaporation methods, each with its own set of advantages and characteristics:

1. Open Heat Evaporation: This process entails continuous heating of the sap with stirring in an open environment. The resulting sugar can range in color from light to dark brown. After collection, the sugar is sieved to achieve a finely textured product (Saraiva et al. 2023). While open-pan evaporation offers high antioxidant activity, it often leads to significant browning, classifying the syrup as low-grade (Naknean and Meenune 2015).
2. Microwave Evaporation: Microwave technology provides rapid heating compared to conventional methods, offering uniform, clean, and environmentally friendly energy transfer processes (Leonelli and Mason 2010). While microwave technology efficiently concentrates sap syrup by rapidly evaporating moisture, it is less suitable for sugar crystallization due to the need for constant stirring during the final vaporization of moisture.
3. Rotary Evaporation: This method, utilized in the sugar processing industry, operates under vacuum conditions at a temperature of 60 °C. It offers enhanced physicochemical characteristics, reduced energy consumption, and shorter processing durations. Rotary evaporation minimizes thermal decomposition, preserving product quality (Asghar et al. 2020). The syrup produced through rotary evaporation at 60 °C exhibits reduced antioxidant activity compared to those produced using open-heat evaporation and microwave techniques, indicating distinct characteristics (Philippe et al. 2014; Swain et al. 2016).

The rotary evaporation process has several notable advantages. It boasts a remarkably short production duration of 12.2 min and operates at a low temperature of 54.8 °C. In comparison, microwave evaporation and open heat evaporation take longer and operate at higher temperatures. The syrup produced through rotary evaporation has a light brownish hue, higher monosaccharide content, and lower disaccharide content. Additionally, the energy consumption for rotary evaporation is minimal compared to open heat evaporation (Asghar et al. 2020).

9.4 Comparative Profile of Coconut Sugar Produced in Traditional Method and Other Modern Drying Methods

Traditionally, coconut sap undergoes heating and continuous stirring in an open environment at temperatures ranging from 90 to 100 °C. The resulting sugar is collected, manually ground, and sieved.

Comparing different drying methods like vacuum drying and spray drying against the traditional method reveals distinct characteristics. Spray-dried coconut sugar powder exhibits reduced moisture content due to its rapid drying process and increased surface area from atomization. Conversely, traditional coconut sugar powder exhibits the lowest water absorption at each water activity (a_w) level compared to coconut sugar powder from other treatments. This difference can be attributed to the predominantly crystalline structure of traditional coconut sugar, whereas drying methods typically produce amorphous or semi-crystalline structures.

The presence of sharp and well-defined peaks in crystalline materials, as observed in traditional coconut sugar, contrasts with the dispersed bands and wide peaks in amorphous materials produced through drying methods. Traditional coconut sugar powder (TCS) primarily consists of a dominant crystalline structure, comprising approximately 90.5% of the powder. This form also possesses the lowest monolayer moisture content and hygroscopic rate, as well as lower L* values and higher a* and b* values compared to products obtained through drying methods.

Moreover, TCS powder tends to dissolve slowly due to its impermeable particles, whereas amorphous powder particles dissolve rapidly. Vacuum-dried coconut sugar powder achieves a higher powder recovery compared to spray drying, likely due to differences in the drying process.

In conclusion, while drying techniques like vacuum and spray drying effectively produce coconut sugar powder with distinctive properties, traditional methods yield crystalline TCS powder with unique characteristics. These findings underscore the importance of understanding and selecting appropriate drying methods to achieve desired product attributes in the production of coconut sugar powder.

9.5 Nutritional Features of Coconut Sugar

The current food market offers a wide array of low-sugar, sugar-free, and synthetic sweetener products, yet many of these options are associated with potential health hazards, including weight gain and increased risks of brain tumors and bladder cancer. Consequently, there is a pressing need for healthier sugar alternatives. Coconut sugar, derived from the evaporation of coconut sap, presents itself as a nutrient-dense crystalline sugar alternative that closely mimics regular sugar in appearance, taste, and properties. However, it stands out for being entirely natural, unprocessed and unrefined crystalline sweetener (Abdullah et al. 2014). Its melting behaviour nearly identical to regular sugar. However, it offers a far superior flavour profile.

The color of coconut sugar is brown, and it contains 2–3% moisture. Due to its plant-based, natural, and minimally processed nature, coconut sugar serves as a healthier alternative that can be readily integrated into numerous vegan diets (Abdullah et al. 2014). The manufacturing processes of coconut sugar exhibit significant diversity, influenced by local, traditional, and indigenous practices. These factors contribute to the wide range of appearances, tastes, and flavors observed among the various types of coconut sugar available in the market.

The quality of coconut sugar, including its color, texture, flavor, and aroma, is influenced by the quality of the sap used and chemical changes occurring during heating, notably non-enzymatic browning through caramelization and Maillard reactions (MR). The rate of browning of coconut sugar has been directly linked to MR products such as acrylamide and 5-hydroxymethylfurfural, and high levels of these products can pose health risks (Asikin et al. 2014; Hebbar et al. 2022). In this context, it's important to highlight the research conducted by (Phaeon et al. 2021) which examined the presence of acrylamide in both coconut sap and coconut syrup. While acrylamide was not detected in coconut sap, reported levels in coconut syrup were found to be 867 μg/kg. In addition to being potent antioxidants, many MR products have beneficial biological effects.

Traditional sap collection practices, such as collecting sap in open earthen pots over extended periods, can lead to sugar degradation into alcohol and acid, resulting in an undesirable odor and rendering the sap unsuitable for consumption or crystallization without the use of chemicals. Therefore, ensuring the collection of high-quality sap becomes crucial in the coconut sugar production process. Due to the higher antioxidant content in coconut sap, coconut sugar would have better antioxidant properties (Asghar et al. 2020). The coconut sap contain high ash content (0.27%) as compared to sugar palm and sugarcane juice (0.25% and 0.17%, respectively). A high ash content suggests that coconut sap has a greater mineral content. Thus, converting coconut sap into sugar could yield a sugar product enriched with minerals (Hebbar et al. 2015) (Table 9.1).

Over 100 different compounds can be found in coconut sugar and syrup, including carbohydrates, free amino acids, proteins, minerals, vitamins, aromatic compounds, and phenolics (Saraiva et al. 2023). Coconut sugar boasts essential nutrients such as vitamin C, vitamin E, and minerals like potassium, iron, zinc, and phosphorus. It could potentially offer greater nutritional benefits due to its high levels of vitamin C, B1, B3, B4, and B10. It also contains phytonutrients such as flavonoids, antioxidants, polyphenols, and anthocyanidins. Additionally, coconut sugar is rich in inulin, a prebiotic fiber known for its role in producing short-chain fatty acids like propionate, acetate, and butyrate. This conversion underscores the potential health benefits of coconut sugar or syrup, making them promising functional foods.

Coconut sap exhibits notably higher levels of sodium, potassium, and iron compared to sugar palm and sugarcane juices. While other minerals in coconut sap are similar to those in sugar palm and sugarcane juices, overall, the total mineral content in coconut sap surpasses that of sugarcane and sugar palm juices. This suggests

Table 9.1 Nutritional composition of coconut sugar obtained from *Kalparasa*® or unfermented coconut inflorescence sap

Biochemical characteristics	Content
Sugars and fibres	
Total sugars (g/100 g)	91.8 ± 1.01
Reducing sugars (g/100 g)	4.69 ± 0.60
Dietary fiber (g/100 g)	3.1
Antioxidants	
Total phenolics (mg GAE/100 g)	47.2 ± 20.7
Total flavonoids (mg CE/100 g)	4.76 ± 1.21
Ferric reducing antioxidant power (mg ascorbic acid equivalent/100 g)	22.9 ± 4.12
Vitamins	
Pyridoxine (μg/100 g)	101 ± 0.3
Niacin (μg/100 g)	34.7 ± 2.1
Thiamine (μg/100 g)	14.3 ± 1.16
Tocopherol (μg/100 g)	19.6 ± 3.5
Vitamin K1 (μg/100 g)	7.35 ± 0.95
Vitamin K2 (μg/100 g)	5.57 ± 0.61
Sodium (mg/100 g)	568
Potassium (mg/100 g)	1002
Iron (mg/100 g)	2.2
Zinc (mg/100 g)	2.1
Protein and amino acids	
Protein (g/100 g)	2.6
Valine (mg/100 g)	40.68
Threonine (mg/100 g)	45.81
Leucine (mg/100 g)	16.01
Lysine (mg/100 g)	136.5
Methionine (mg/100 g)	54.55
Histidine (mg/100 g)	3.48
Phenylalanine (mg/100 g)	57.66
Tyrosine (mg/100 g)	5.68

Source: Hebbar et al. (2022)

that coconut sap-derived sugar could potentially be a rich source of minerals (Asghar et al. 2020). Since coconut sap contains less sucrose and more glucose and fructose, it might be useful for diabetic patients. Therefore, coconut sugar, with elevated levels of fructose and glucose and reduced sucrose content, contributes to its lower glycemic index (GI) value (Saputro et al. 2017).

With a sweetness comparable to saccharose, coconut sugar has become a popular alternative sweetener in various culinary applications, including confectionery, pastries, beverages, and other gastronomic uses. Studies have shown that when blended with different sweeteners like cane sugar, palm sugar, and sorbitol with wheat flour, coconut sugar demonstrates nearly identical levels of starch digestibility. This versatility and nutritional profile contribute to the growing popularity of coconut sugar as a healthier sugar alternative.

9.6 Comparative Features of Coconut Sugar and Cane Sugar

Coconut sugar provides both calories and essential nutrients, unlike cane sugar, which only offers calories. It has a significant level of mineral content, including high levels of potassium, magnesium, zinc, and iron. Moreover, it contains all the essential amino acids necessary for protein synthesis and is packed with vitamins such as B1, B2, B3, and B6. Compared to unrefined cane sugar, coconut sugar contains significantly higher amounts of iron, magnesium, and zinc, with ratios of two, four, and ten times respectively.

The nutritional analysis comparing coconut jaggery to cane sugar revealed that coconut jaggery had significantly higher levels of moisture (8.92%), ash (2.09%), protein (1.91%), fat (0.14%), and fiber (0.05%) while having lower levels of total starch and total sugar (Pathirana et al. 2022; Wrage et al. 2019).

The research by (Maryani et al. 2021) revealed that when analyzing simple sugars in coconut sugar and cane sugar, the composition was as follows: coconut sugar contained 86.86% sucrose, 4.64% glucose, and 3.70% fructose, whereas cane sugar had 94.75% sucrose with no detectable levels of glucose or fructose.

9.7 Glycemic Potential of Coconut Sugar

The glycemic index (GI) is a scale used to measure how quickly foods containing carbohydrates raise blood glucose levels (Vega-López et al. 2018). It ranges from 0 to 100, with lower values indicating slower increases in blood glucose levels after consumption (Russell et al. 2016). Foods with a low GI are generally considered healthier choices.

Coconut sugar has a relatively low glycemic index of 35, making it a suitable sweetening option for individuals concerned about blood sugar levels (Saraiva et al. 2023). In comparison, palm sugar (*Borassus flabellifer*) has a GI of 42, and sugarcane sugar (*Saccharum officinarum* L.) has GI values ranging from 58 to 82. This lower GI of coconut sugar makes it a favorable choice for individuals seeking healthier alternatives to traditional sugars. In summary, due to its low glycemic index, coconut sugar is considered an appropriate and healthy sweetening option for individuals of all ages.

9.8 Health Benefits of Coconut Sugar

Coconut sugar reduces brachial systolic blood pressure and stiffness in the carotid artery among middle-aged and older adults, suggesting that coconut sugar could serve as an innovative nutraceutical for addressing cardiovascular issues associated with aging. Consuming coconut sugar was found to be safe and well-tolerated at a dosage of 15 g/day over a 90-day study period. It exhibits a relatively low glycemic index (GI) of 52.47 and causes a less pronounced increase in post-meal blood glucose compared to pure glucose, showing no adverse effects on hematology or biochemical parameters related to liver, heart, and kidney functions. Notably, there was evidence of lipid-lowering effects and an increase in hemoglobin (Hb) levels by the end of the study, indicating potential health benefits. However, the mechanisms underlying these effects, particularly concerning the presence and interaction of micronutrients within the carbohydrate matrix of coconut sugar, warrant further investigation (Mammen et al. 2020).

A study involving 43 patients with type 2 diabetes, all of whom were overweight, was conducted to compare the postprandial blood glucose responses to glucose, cane sugar, and coconut jaggery. The participants had an average age of 48.19 ± 7.95 years and were assessed with initial health screenings. Despite differences in nutritional composition, there were no significant variations in peak blood glucose concentrations or incremental areas under the curve in blood glucose response between the two types of sweeteners (Pathirana et al. 2022). Coconut sugar exhibited a few health benefits in diabetic rats by reversing the impaired glucose and lipid metabolism to normal state and also offered encouraging outcomes in case of oxidative stress (Shetty et al. 2023).

9.9 Coconut Sugar Derived Food Products

Coconut sugar is considered as a valuable product due to its plethora of health benefits, making it an excellent natural sweetener option despite being expensive (Hebbar et al. 2022). There is a great demand for coconut sugar in the food and beverage industry, especially for baked goods such as biscuits and making chocolate, cake, sweet soy sauce, food coating, ice cream, and typical Bengali sweets. Coconut sugar can be used to make a wide variety of coconut by products, such as Kalpa bar-a chocolate infused with coconut sugar, exclusively formulated with plant-based ingredients and completely free from dairy components. The dark chocolate formulation with coconut sugar was optimized to consist of 45% cocoa liquor, 30% coconut sugar, and 25% cocoa butter. This product is abundant in polyphenols, flavonoids, antioxidants, and minerals (Hebbar et al. 2022); Kalpa drinking chocolate**:** A delicious drinking chocolate made from low GI coconut sugar and fine cocoa powder; Milk sweets**-** the concentrated form of coconut inflorescence sap is used directly in West Bengal sweets in place of other sweeteners (Ghosh et al. 2018).

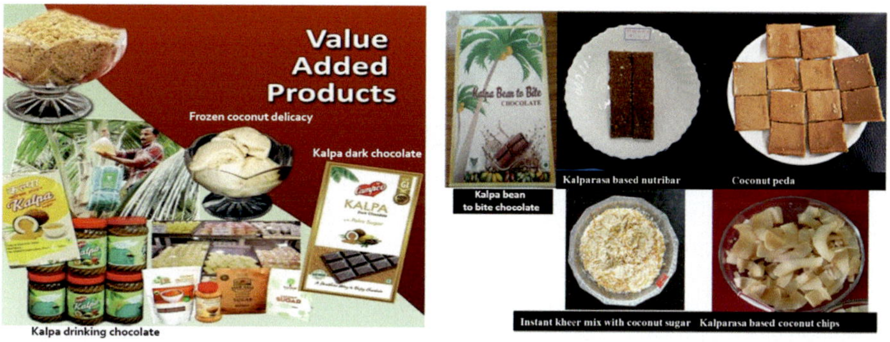

Fig. 9.3 Value added products and second line of food products developed using coconut sugar. (Source: Hebbar et al. 2022)

These sweets offer essential minerals, vitamins, and valuable fibers and it is low in glycemic index, making them suitable for both a healthy and sweet indulgence. Frozen Coconut Delicacy- made of coconut ingredients such as coconut milk, coconut sugar, tender coconut water and pulp. The addition of coconut sugar enhanced the flavour and taste of the delicacy (Beegum et al. 2022). This product is suitable for individuals with lactose intolerance since it does not contain any dairy ingredients. Coconut chips is one of the important coconut-based value added product gaining popularity due to its taste and texture. The dried superior quality coconut chips produced with osmotic dehydration using coconut inflorescence sap contains markedly higher levels of ash, phenolics, and antioxidant activity compared to chips made solely with a cane sugar solution. Besides food products such as coconut peda, instant kheer mix, nutribar are produced using coconut sugar (Hebbar et al. 2022) (Fig.9.3).

9.10 Detection of Adulteration in Coconut Sugar

The price of coconut sugar is relatively high due to its superior quality and cost economics. Consumers are willing to pay 20 to 65 times more for coconut sugar than for conventional refined sugar. It's also common for sugar-rich products to be replaced with cheaper sugar sources without proper labelling (Moore et al. 2012). For instance, starch-derived sugar syrups, high-fructose corn syrup, glucose syrup, and sucrose syrups, sourced from sugar beet or cane sugar, are employed in the adulteration of coconut sugar. Incorporating other sugar sources can alter the proportions of glucose, fructose, and sucrose, as well as modify the $^{13}C/^{12}C$ isotope ratio.

Detecting the presence of cane sugar (C4 plant) and high-fructose corn syrup (C4) through $^{13}C/^{12}C$ isotope analysis is feasible, whereas identifying the addition of beet sugar (C3) is challenging, presenting a significant issue (Tosun 2013). Due to its elevated sucrose content, coconut sugar tends to clump together during storage.

Therefore, it's crucial to include an anti-caking agent such as tricalcium phosphate (TCP) to maintain its stability for use in food applications. TCP coats the surface of coconut sugar powder, reducing its hygroscopicity and enhancing its flowability (Swain et al. 2016).

Additionally, as palm sugar and coconut sugar are similarly produced, differentiation between these two products is often difficult. Coconut sugar can maintain its quality and nutritional benefits when processed from clean, unfermented sap. However, if low-quality *neera* is used, additional chemicals and additives such as gluten, starch, and sugars from C4 plants like coconut or palm oil are required to facilitate crystallization. To prevent overboiling, coconut quarters and oil are added (Levang 1988), while starch absorbs moisture to prevent agglutination. Unfortunately, these additives, including gluten and sugars from C4 plants, may have adverse effects on human health, potentially impacting the coconut sugar market.

Organically sourced coconut sugar, known for its caramel aroma, has unfortunately become a target for adulteration. A study aimed at detecting such adulterations identified minor metabolites serving as chemical markers for coconut blossom sugar (Bachmann et al. 2022). Profiling these metabolites proved instrumental in uncovering potential adulterations in products. Hydroxymethyl furfural (HMF) was absent in all samples examined (Bachmann et al. 2022). However, pyroglutamic acid was detected at a notably higher concentration, surpassing other distinctive metabolites in coconut sugar, such as inositol or shikimic acid. Therefore, HMF emerges as a promising marker metabolite for coconut sugar authentication. To further enhance the identification of coconut sugar's unique metabolic profiles, the combined use of LC-MS/MS and NMR techniques is recommended (Saraiva et al. 2023).

Apart from concerns regarding food adulteration, ensuring food safety is paramount. Coconut sugar offer valuable nutritional and functional advantages to consumers provided it is produced from high-quality inflorescence sap collected, preserved, and processed according to good manufacturing practices (GMP). However, the use of inferior-quality sap and processing under unhygienic conditions pose significant risks, including contamination by insects and microorganisms. Therefore, it is crucial to conduct thorough studies to assess the potential presence of other contaminants. While research on contaminants arising from food processing (e.g., acrylamide), agrochemicals (plant protection chemicals), heavy metals (e.g., mercury, lead, arsenic, cadmium), microbial toxins (e.g., mycotoxins), and cleaning agents (e.g., detergents) or disinfectants (e.g., quaternary ammonium compounds) has been increasingly undertaken for other natural sweeteners and sugar products, it remains largely absent for coconut sugar and syrup.

9.11 Organic Trends

In the context of sustainability and traceability concerns, organic certification emerges as a crucial quality benchmark that enhances the credibility of coconut sugar in the European market. This is particularly relevant given that most coconut sugar exporters hail from developing nations. In addition to organic certification, the growing emphasis on natural and organic trends further underscores the importance of adhering to these standards. Export traders have the opportunity to highlight that coconut sugar is traditionally produced by small farmers, with palm trees cultivated organically alongside other crops. Moreover, they can emphasize that coconut sugar boasts very low fructose content and lower glycemic index values compared to traditional refined beet or cane sugar. These factors collectively contribute to the marketability and appeal of coconut sugar as a sustainable and health-conscious alternative (CBI n.d.).

9.12 Concluding Remarks and Prospects

Sweeteners play a crucial role in crafting palatable food items and are significant for both health and sustainability concerns. Comparing commercially available sugars, coconut sugar emerges as a healthier option, as its fructose and glucose are readily absorbed and converted into energy, unlike sucrose which requires initial breakdown into monosaccharides. Additionally, coconut sugar provides abundant levels of copper, iron, zinc, and manganese in comparison to palm and cane sugar. In response to the preferences of health-conscious consumers, food industries are integrating coconut sugar, sap, and syrup into their products. The process of collecting the sap from the coconut tree, transporting, storing, and then processing it requires significant manpower and resources. Consequently, the production cost of coconut sugar is higher when compared to cane sugar which can be addressed in the future by adopting AI-based technologies. Also, research intervention is imperative for the detection of adulteration in coconut sugar to eradicate the spurious products in the market.

References

Abdullah WG, Rianse U, Iswandi RM, Taridala SAA, Widayati W, Rianse IS, Baka LR, Baka WK (2014) Potency of natural sweetener: brown sugar. Adv Environ Biol 8(21):374–386

Asghar MT, Yusof YA, Mokhtar MN, Ya'acob ME, Mohd. Ghazali H, Chang LS, Manaf YN (2020) Coconut (Cocos nucifera L.) sap as a potential source of sugar: antioxidant and nutritional properties. Food Sci Nutr 8(4):1777–1787

Asikin Y, Kamiya A, Mizu M, Takara K, Tamaki H, Wada K (2014) Changes in the physico-chemical characteristics, including flavour components and maillard reaction products, of non-centrifugal cane brown sugar during storage. Food Chem 149:170–177

Bachmann R, Horns AL, Paasch N, Schrieck R, Weidner M, Fransson I, Schrör JP (2022) Minor metabolites as chemical marker for the differentiation of cane, beet and coconut blossom sugar. From profiling towards identification of adulterations. Food Control, 135, p.108832. https://doi.org/10.1016/j.foodcont.2022.108832

Beegum PPS, Nair JP, Manikantan MR, Pandiselvam R, Shill S, Neenu S, Hebbar KB (2022) Effect of coconut milk, tender coconut and coconut sugar on the physico-chemical and sensory attributes in ice cream. J Food Sci Technol 59:2605–2616

CBI (n.d.) Exporting palm sugar to Europe? Centre for the Promotion of Imports from developing countries (Netherlands). https://www.cbi.eu/sites/default/files/marketinformation/product-factsheet-palm-sugar-germany-honey-sugars-2014.pdf

Francisco Ortega J, Zona S (2013) Sweet sap from palms, a source of beverages, alcohol, vinegar, syrup, and sugar. Vieraea Folia Sci Biol Canar 41:91–113

Ghosh DK, Bandyopadhyay A, Das S, Hebbar KB, Biswas B (2018) Coconut sap (Neera)-untapped opportunity of spinoff gains in West Bengal, India. Int J Curr Microbiol Appl Sci 7(9):1883–1897

Hebbar KB, Arivalagan M, Manikantan MR, Mathew AC, Thamban C, Thomas GV, Chowdappa P (2015) Coconut inflorescence sap and its value addition as sugar–collection techniques, yield, properties and market perspective. Curr Sci 109:1411–1417

Hebbar KB, Pandiselvam R, Manikantan MR, Arivalagan M, Beegum S, Chowdappa P (2018) Palm sap—quality profiles, fermentation chemistry, and preservation methods. Sugar Tech 20(6):621–634

Hebbar KB, Ramesh SV, Ghosh DK, Beegum PPS, Pandiselvam R, Manikantan MR, Mathew AC (2022) Coconut sugar-a potential storehouse of nutritive metabolites, novel bio-products and prospects. Sugar Tech 24(3):841–856

Leonelli C, Mason TJ (2010) Microwave and ultrasonic processing: now a realistic option for industry. Chem Eng Process Process Intensif 49(9):885–900

Levang P (1988) Le cocotier est aussi une plante sucrière. Oléagineux (Paris) 43(4):159–164

Mammen R, John F, Krishnakumar IM, Maliakel B, Mohanan R, Fleenor B (2020) Safety and influence of a novel powder form of coconut inflorescence sap on glycemic index and lipid profile. Bioact Carbohydr Diet Fibre 23:100217

Manikantan MR, Pandiselvam R, Beegum S, Mathew AC (2018) Harvest and postharvest technology. In: Krishnakumar V, Thampan P, Nair M (eds) The coconut palm (Cocos nucifera L.)—research and development perspectives. Springer, Singapore, pp 635–722

Market Data Forecast (2024) Palm sugar market growth, size, share, trends and forecast to 2027. https://www.marketdataforecast.com/market-reports/palm-sugar-market

Maryani Y, Rochmat A, Khastini RO, Kurniawan T, Saraswati I (2021) Identification of macro elements (sucrose, glucose and fructose) and micro elements (metal minerals) in the products of palm sugar, coconut sugar and sugar cane. In: 2nd and 3rd International Conference on Food Security Innovation (ICFSI 2018–2019). Atlantis Press, pp 271–274

Moore JC, Spink J, Lipp M (2012) Development and application of a database of food ingredient fraud and economically motivated adulteration from 1980 to 2010. J Food Sci 77(4):R118–R126

Naknean P, Meenune M (2015) Impact of clarification of palm sap and processing method on the quality of palm sugar syrup (Borassus flabellifer Linn.). Sugar Tech 17:195–203

Nathanael WRN (1959) Chemical and technological investigations on coconut products. National Science Foundation, Colombo

Pathirana HPDTH, Wijesekara I, Yalegama LLWC, Garusinghe C, Jayasinghe MA, Waidyarathne KP (2022) Comparison of blood glucose responses by cane sugar (Saccharum officinarum) versus coconut jaggery (Cocos nucifera) in type 2 diabetes patients. J Futur Foods 2(3):261–265

Phaeon N, Chapanya P, Mueangmontri R, Pattamasuwan A, Lipan L, Carbonell-Barrachina ÁA, Sriroth K, Nitayapat N (2021) Acrylamide in non-centrifugal sugars and syrups. J Sci Food Agric 101(11):4561–4569

Philippe RN, De Mey M, Anderson J, Ajikumar PK (2014) Biotechnological production of natural zero-calorie sweeteners. Curr Opin Biotechnol 26:155–161

Russell WR, Baka A, Björck I, Delzenne N, Gao D, Griffiths HR, Hadjilucas E, Juvonen K, Lahtinen S, Lansink M (2016) Impact of diet composition on blood glucose regulation. Crit Rev Food Sci Nutr 56(4):541–590

Saputro AD, Van de Walle D, Aidoo RP, Mensah MA, Delbaere C, De Clercq N, Van Durme J, Dewettinck K (2017) Quality attributes of dark chocolates formulated with palm sap-based sugar as nutritious and natural alternative sweetener. Eur Food Res Technol 243(2):177–191. https://doi.org/10.1007/s00217-016-2734-9

Saputro AD, van de Walle D, Dewettinck K (2020) Physicochemical properties of coarse palm sap sugars as natural alternative sweetener. Food Biosci 38:100780

Saraiva A, Carrascosa C, Ramos F, Raheem D, Lopes M, Raposo A (2023) Coconut sugar: chemical analysis and nutritional profile; health impacts; safety and quality control; food industry applications. Int J Environ Res Public Health 20(4):3671

Shetty SS, Ramesh SV, Arivalagan M, Roopashree PG, Manikantan MR, Hebbar KB, Kumari S (2023) Coconut (Cocos nucifera L.) inflorescence sap-derived sugar restores the glucose and lipid homeostasis in streptozotocin-induced diabetic Wistar rat model. Biomedicine 43(3):859–866

Swain S, Din M, Ram C, Gangaiah B (2016) Post harvest processing and value addition in coconut, arecanut and spices in Islands. In: Integrated farming systems for tropical islands of India. CIARI, Port Balir, pp 152–157

Tosun M (2013) Detection of adulteration in honey samples added various sugar syrups with 13C/12C isotope ratio analysis method. Food Chem 138(2–3):1629–1632

Vega-López S, Venn BJ, Slavin JL (2018) Relevance of the glycemic index and glycemic load for body weight, diabetes, and cardiovascular disease. Nutrients 10(10):1361

Wrage J, Burmester S, Kuballa J, Rohn S (2019) Coconut Sugar (Cocos nucifera L.): production process, chemical characterization, and sensory properties. LWT Food Sci Technol 112:108227

Chapter 10
Coconut Based Food Products: Repertoire and Biochemical Features

R. Pandiselvam, Anjitha Jacob, and M. R. Manikantan

Abstract The chapter "Coconut-Based Food Products: Repertoire and Biochemical Features" delves into the diverse world of coconut-derived culinary creations, emphasizing their nutritional value, health benefits, and production methods. While traditionally, coconuts have been processed into staples like copra and coconut oil, the global market demands innovation and diversification. This has led to the emergence of a wide array of value-added products, including coconut vinegar, Nata de coco, virgin coconut oil, coconut chips, coconut milk, snowball tender nuts, neera, coconut sugar, and more. Coconut milk and cream, rich in medium-chain triglycerides (MCTs) and essential nutrients, feature prominently in both sweet and savory dishes, offering a creamy texture and distinct tropical flavor. Virgin coconut oil, produced without chemical refinement, retains its nutritional integrity and is sought after for its purported health benefits. Incorporating coconut-based ingredients like coconut milk residue and virgin coconut oil cake into extruded products enhances their nutritional profile, providing consumers with healthier snack options. Coconut's versatility extends to frozen desserts, where it imparts a delightful tropical twist to ice creams and other treats. From crispy coconut chips to tender snowball nuts, coconut-derived snacks offer both flavor and nutrition. Desiccated coconut powder finds its way into various confectionery and culinary delights, while coconut jam and vinegar provide unique flavors and culinary possibilities. The chapter also explores the functional properties of coconut water, serving as a natural isotonic beverage and electrolyte replacement. Neera, the sap collected from coconut inflorescences, offers sweetness and nutritional benefits, while coconut sugar adds depth to bean-to-bite chocolate, appealing to health-conscious consumers with its low glycemic index and rich antioxidant content. Overall, this chapter showcases the vast potential of coconut-based food products, offering a glimpse into a world of flavor, nutrition, and culinary innovation.

R. Pandiselvam (✉) · A. Jacob · M. R. Manikantan
Physiology, Biochemistry and Post-Harvest Technology Division, ICAR–Central Plantation Crops Research Institute, Kasaragod, Kerala, India
e-mail: r.pandiselvam@icar.gov.in

S. V. Ramesh, S. Praveen (eds.), *Coconut-Based Nutrition and Nutraceutical Perspectives*, https://doi.org/10.1007/978-981-97-3976-9_10

Keywords Value addition · Functional food products · Extrusion · Virgin coconut oil · Chips · Neera

10.1 Introduction

The coconut palm, scientifically referred to as *Cocos nucifera* L., stands as a tropical tree cherished for its multifarious uses and benefits. Often hailed as the "tree of heaven" or "*kalpavriksha*," it bestows a plethora of essential products upon humanity (Hebbar et al. 2020). Satisfying fundamental human needs, it serves as a source of food, drink, shelter, fuel, furniture, medicines, decorations, and more. Furthermore, the by-products derived from coconut processing have found commercial application across a wide spectrum of products and purposes. Nevertheless, it's crucial to note that the structure and characteristics of coconuts and their resulting by-products can vary significantly based on factors such as species, origin, and processing methods. In India, approximately half of the annual coconut yield is allocated for culinary and religious practices, while 35% undergoes copra processing. A small percentage, around 2%, is allocated for the production of value-added products, 11% is utilized as tender nut and in related applications, and another 2% is dedicated to seedling production and associated purposes (Sangamithra et al. 2013).

The primary components of the coconut fruit include the exocarp, comprised of dense fibers, which encases the hard shell known as the endocarp. Within the endocarp lies the inner white, meaty kernel referred to as the endosperm, containing the nutritionally invaluable coconut water (Prithviraj et al. 2021). Coconut remains in high demand due to its versatility and ability to thrive in diverse climates and soils. Setting it apart from other oil seeds or horticultural crops, coconut boasts a multitude of applications. Adding value to coconut is crucial for developing innovative products that can enhance the income of both cultivators and processors. The various products and by-products of coconut hold potential for industrial exploitation across a range of purposes (Sangamithra et al. 2013).

Coconut oil, coconut milk from mature nuts, virgin coconut oil (VCO), and coconut water from tender coconuts stand as widely recognized value-added products derived from coconuts (Madhavan et al. 2010). Moreover, in numerous regions worldwide, coconut is cultivated specifically as a beverage crop. Additionally, innovative value-added products like coconut chips, coconut flakes, and coconut-based extrudates such as Kalpa Krunch, biscuits, and rusks have been introduced to capitalize on the potential of coconut as a snack food. Furthermore, coconut yields a variety of value-added items such as coconut neera honey, syrups, vinegar, jelly, coconut jaggery, coconut sugar, and frozen coconut delicacies. The introduction of value-added products derived from coconut is anticipated to bolster the growth of the coconut industry, enhance coconut product diversity and variation, and globalize the market, thereby augmenting the competitiveness of future industries.

This chapter primarily focuses on various coconut based food products. It also attempts to highlight the nutritional value, health benefits, and various production procedures of coconut value added products.

10.2 Coconut Based Food Products

Traditionally, coconuts have undergone processing into edible copra, coconut oil, coir, and coir-derived products following harvest. However, beyond copra and coconut oil, coconut-based products offer extensive potential for development, value addition, and commercialization. Recognizing the impact of globalization, there has been a growing acknowledgment of the opportunity to diversify coconut into a wide array of new value-added products. These include coconut vinegar, Nata de coco, virgin coconut oil, coconut chips, coconut milk, snowball tender nut, neera, and coconut sugar.

Figure 10.1 illustrates a variety of coconut-based value-added food products currently available in the market.

10.2.1 Coconut Kernel Based Product

10.2.1.1 Flavored Coconut Milk

Commercialization and production of plant-based milks have experienced significant exponential growth worldwide (Sethi et al. 2016). Water-soluble extracts made from oilseeds, cereals, pseudocereals, seeds, and/or legumes constitute plant-based milk alternatives. Other ingredients, such as flavors, sugar, and stabilizers, may be added to enhance the taste and overall quality of the product. Coconut milk serves not only as a beverage but also as a key ingredient in numerous sweet and savory recipes. Coconut milk is abundant in essential vitamins and minerals such as iron, calcium, potassium, magnesium, and zinc. Moreover, it contains considerable quantities of both vitamin C and E (Seow and Gwee 1997).

Flavored coconut milk typically refers to coconut milk that has been infused or enhanced with various flavorings to add depth, richness, or a unique taste profile (Uzodinma et al. 2020). Flavored coconut milk starts with a base of coconut milk, which is extracted from grated coconut flesh and water. This base provides the creamy texture and distinct coconut flavor. Various flavorings can be added to coconut milk such as vanilla, strawberry, chocolate, mango, cinnamon and ginger to create different flavored variations. Depending on the desired flavor profile, sweeteners such as sugar, honey, agave syrup, or alternative sweeteners like stevia may be added to enhance sweetness. Some flavored coconut milk products may contain thickeners or stabilizers to improve texture and shelf stability. Common thickeners include guar gum or xanthan gum. Flavored coconut milk retains the nutritional benefits of coconut milk, including being rich in healthy fats, vitamins, and minerals such as potassium and magnesium. However, the addition of flavorings and sweeteners may alter the overall nutritional profile and increasing the sugar content.

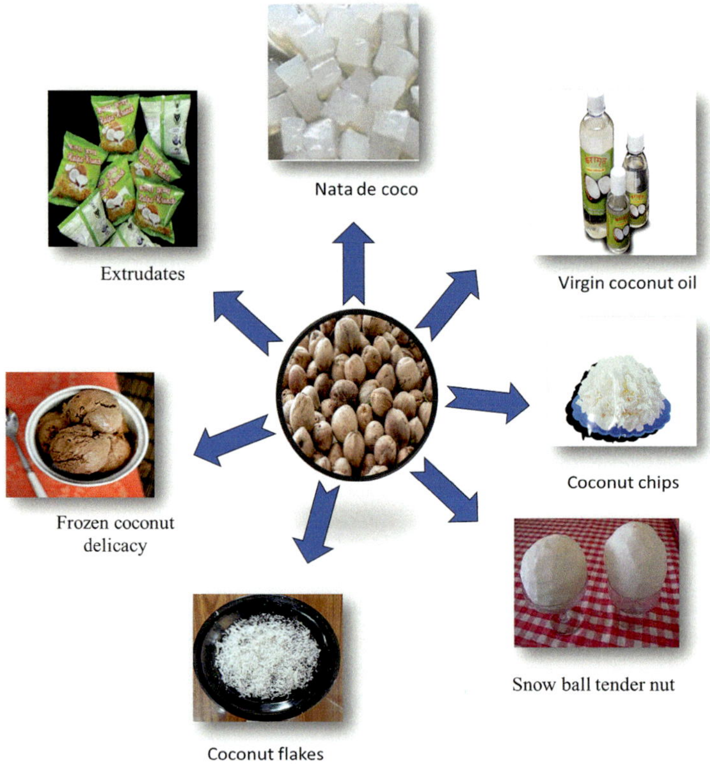

Fig. 10.1 Coconut based value added food products. Various value added products such as coconut chips, snow ball tender nut, coconut flakes, frozen coconut delicacy, extrudates-based food products are presented herein

10.2.1.2 High-Fat Coconut Cream

Coconut-based products are characterized by the presence of medium-chain triglycerides (Nimbkar et al. 2022). Coconut cream is an emulsion produced from mature coconut endosperm with or without addition of water, with a fat content of at least 20% (Codex Allimentarius Commission 2022). The thicker cream fraction obtained from centrifuging coconut milk yields higher fat levels. Nutritionally, coconut cream is high in healthy fats, including medium-chain triglycerides (MCTs), which are believed to offer various health benefits. Additionally, coconut cream contains essential vitamins and minerals like iron, potassium, and manganese.

10.2.1.3 Virgin Coconut Oil

Virgin coconut oil (VCO) is derived from the mature coconut kernel using mechanical or natural methods, with or without the application of heat, and it does not undergo any chemical refining, bleaching, or deodorizing (RBD) processes.

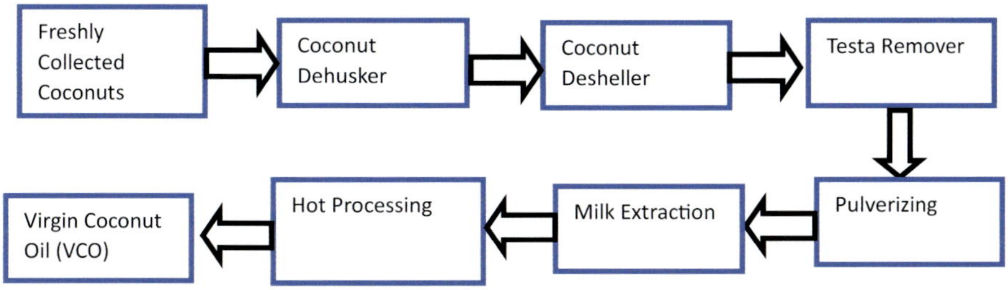

Fig. 10.2 Process Flow chart for the production of virgin coconut oil (VCO)

Figure 10.2 shows process flow chart for the production of virgin coconut oil. It is abundant in vitamin E, medium-chain fatty acids especially lauric acid, as well as vitamins, minerals, and antioxidants and it is known for its high digestibility. The VCO can be obtained directly from fresh coconut meat or coconut milk. Various techniques are used, including hot-processing, natural fermentation, centrifugation, and direct micro-expelling. The selection of the appropriate method is greatly influenced by factors such as the scale of production, the level of mechanization, available investment, and market demand. Several studies have reported the higher levels of phenolic compounds in VCO, and this is associated with increased antioxidant activity when compared to refined coconut oil (Marina et al. 2009). The ideal quality characteristics of VCO are mentioned in Table 10.1.

10.2.1.4 Extrudates Products

Extrusion technology is the most affordable and versatile method for producing innovative cereal-based snacks. Cereals, particularly rice and maize, are widely employed as key ingredients in the production of extruded products because of their functional attributes, cost-effectiveness, and easy accessibility (Deshpande and Poshadri 2011). The practice of food fortification with essential nutrients represents an innovative method for addressing a range of diseases and nutrient-dependent disorders. A variety of extruded products, including noodles, pasta, and snacks, can also be made with coconut flour. Currently, coconut flour is underutilized in the coconut industry and its food use is extremely limited. A commercial processing technique is essential to enhance coconut flour's utilisation. Improvement in the nutritional content of extruded products can be achieved by integrating nutritionally rich coconut-based products and byproducts, such coconut milk residue, virgin coconut oil (VCO) cake, and extrudates infused with neera honey with the commercially available ingredients. This is an efficient approach to enhance the overall nutritional quality of the products especially dietary fibre.

Coconut haustorium develops as a spongy tissue during the germination of coconuts, is abundant in nutrients such as dietary fibre, iron, phenolics, and antioxidants (Manivannan et al. 2018). The inclusion of 20% coconut haustorium in 50% rice and 30% maize led to the production of healthy and nutritious extrudates (Arivalagan et al. 2018).

Table 10.1 Ideal quality characteristics of VCO

Properties	Specification
Colour	Water-clear
Free fatty acid (as lauric acid)	<0.1%
Moisture (matter volatile at 105 °C)	<0.1%
Peroxide Value	<3
Lauric fatty acid content	47–55%
Aroma	Fresh coconut, mild to intense

Source: ICAR-CPCRI Technical Bulletin (2016)

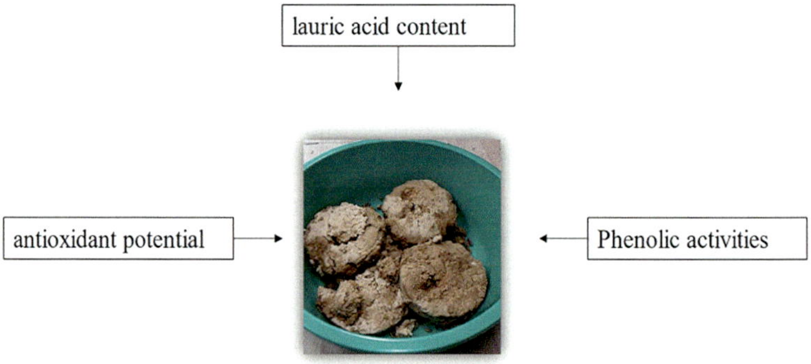

Fig. 10.3 VCO cake

The lauric acid content, phenolic activities and antioxidant potential of VCO cake (Fig. 10.3) will be beneficial in enhancing the immune system. The optimised combination of 28.7% virgin coconut oil cake, 14% feed moisture, and a screw speed of 300 rpm led to noticeable enhancements in the protein content as well as overall acceptability of sensory attributes of extrudate (Shameena Beegum et al. 2019).

Neera honey is abundant in magnesium, potassium, iron, and zinc and it serves as a natural provider of the 12 vital B-complex vitamins and vitamin C. The predominant sugars in coconut neera honey are fructose (38–40%) and glucose (33–35%) (Pandiselvam et al. 2023). The blend of 60% rice flour, 25% corn flour, 15% coconut milk residue samples with the addition of neera honey up to 16% feed moisture was determined to be appropriate for producing nutritious extruded products (Fig. 10.4).

10.2.1.5 Frozen Coconut Delicacy

Incorporation of coconut products in ice cream and other frozen desserts adds a delightful tropical twist, imparting a unique and creamy coconut flavor to these sweet treats. The Frozen Coconut Delicacy is a delectable dessert that encapsulates the tropical essence of coconuts. It is created solely using coconut components, including coconut milk, coconut sugar, tender coconut water and tender coconut

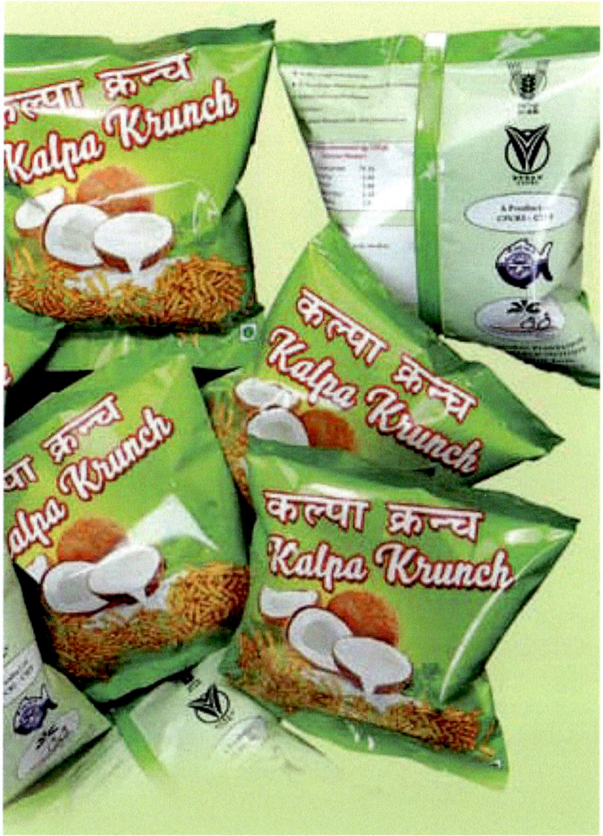

Fig. 10.4 Kalpa Krunch, ready to eat extruded snack prepared from coconut milk residue

pulp. It represents high-quality, completely natural, and wholesome product. It boasts a nutritional profile abundant in vitamins, minerals, and healthy fatty acids. The addition of coconut sugar gives favorable impact on the flavor and taste of the treat (Beegum et al. 2022a). Since it is devoid of dairy milk, it is suitable for individuals with lactose intolerance. Unlike refined sugar, coconut sugar has a low GI and a high vitamin and mineral content.

10.2.1.6 Coconut Chips

Coconut chips, characterized by their natural white colour, delightful crispiness, and healthy non fried snack prepared from fresh kernel subjected to osmotic dehydration. This preparation involves a forced hot air electrical dryer maintained at a temperature of 70–80 °C for 5–6 h, ensuring that the moisture content is reduced to below 3%. The production of sweet coconut chips consist of removal of husk, deshelling, testa removal, slicing of kernel to obtain thin slices, blanching of slices,

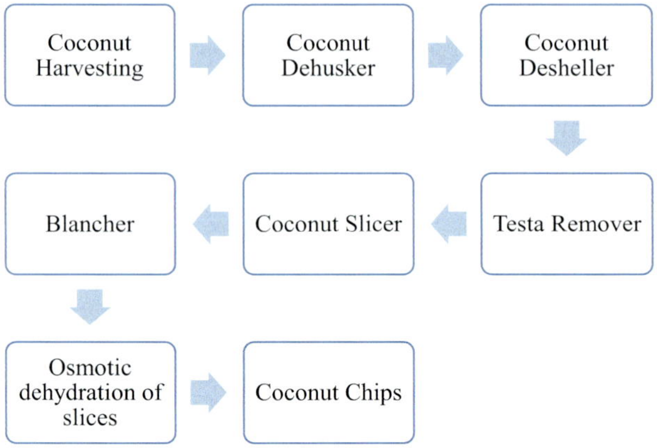

Fig. 10.5 Process flow chart for the production of coconut chips

osmotic dehydration of slices, drying of osmotically dehydrated slices in hot air dryer and then packaging in aluminium foil. It comprises 46% carbohydrates, 1.24% protein, 48% beneficial fats, 6.13% dietary fibre, and 1.36% essential minerals. Utilizing an osmosis-based drying technique, the process involves partially dehydrating sliced fresh coconut kernels by immersing them in a sugar solution, followed by hot air drying (Kumari et al. 2020). This approach yields a product with superior flavour compared to freeze drying and does so at a lower cost. Consequently, the resulting coconut chips contain health-enhancing compounds and present no health risks. Figure 10.5 depicts the process flow chart for the production of coconut chips.

10.2.1.7 Snow Ball Tender Nut

Snowball tender nuts are tender coconuts without the husk, shell, or testa. Its white colour and ball shape makes it visually appealing to consumers. The optimal age for producing a snowball tender nut is around 7–8 months maturity. The white ball consists of tender coconut water and consumers can easily consume it by inserting a straw through the upper part of the soft, white coconut kernel. It is typically presented in an ice cream cup. The procedure for making snow ball tender nut (SBTN) was devised at ICAR-CPCRI, Kasaragod. The snowball is extracted from the shell by using a scooping tool to separate it from the tender kernel and shell. The sterility of the tender coconut water is maintained as it remains unexposed to the surrounding atmosphere (Sangamithra et al. 2013).

10.2.1.8 Desiccated Coconut

Desiccated Coconut Powder is produced by drying and grinding or shredding the coconut kernel after removing its brown outer layer (Sebastian 2017). It is commonly utilized in confectionery, puddings, and various culinary products as a replacement for freshly grated coconut. The desiccated coconut powder processing procedure involves choosing nuts that have reached the appropriate maturity (11–12 months old), removing the husk, shell, and testa, blanching, pulverizing, drying, and then packaging the resulting products. In the drying process, the final moisture content is regulated to be between 2.5% and 3.0% (w.b.) (Pandiselvam et al. 2022).

Desiccated coconut contains healthy saturated fats and serves as a valuable source of dietary fibre. According to FSSAI standards, Grated Desiccated Coconut must contain a minimum of 55% oil content with moisture and ash content not exceeding 3% and 2.5% respectively. Additionally, it typically comprises 18–20% carbohydrates, 6.0–6.6% protein, and 4–6% crude fiber (Manikantan et al. 2018). Lauric acid, derived from coconut fat, possesses antiviral, antibacterial, and antiprotozoal properties. Similarly, capric acid, another fatty acid present in coconut, exhibits antimicrobial characteristics. Multiple research studies have suggested that coconut flour can lower glycemic levels. This is believed to be due to the mix of simple carbohydrates and high fibre found in coconut meat, resulting in a flour that has a minimal effect on blood sugar levels (Sebastian 2017).

10.2.1.9 Coconut Jam

There is a white endosperm in the flesh of the young coconut, which is edible, soft, and jelly-like structure. It tastes sweet and it is an excellent source of minerals like phosphorus, iron, and zinc (Silva 2008). When the water from the kernels is removed, the pulp left over can be transformed into value-added products such as jams. Jam is a type of intermediate moisture food made from the coconut pulp that remains after extracting water from the kernels (Sangamithra et al. 2013). To prepare coconut jam, the pulp is cooked with sugar, pectin, acid, and various additives such as preservatives, colourings, and flavourings until it reaches a thick enough consistency to keep the fruit tissues intact (Lal et al. 1960).

Jams can be made using either a single type of fruit or by combining two or more fruits. In a study (Sindumathi and Amutha 2014), coconut jam was made by mixing different ratios of pineapple pulp and guava pulp with coconut pulp to improve the jam's desirability. It was found that the jam comprising 75% tender coconut pulp and 25% pineapple pulp demonstrated the highest sensory approval among the mixed jam varieties (Estoquia and Teleron 2022), also conducted research on preparing coconut jam by incorporating grated coconut and banana for added flavor. The inherent physical and chemical attributes of coconut pulp render it suitable for consumption in its natural state. Moreover, coconut pulp serves as an outstanding raw material for the jam industry. Coconut, recognized as a functional food, contains fatty acids that provide energy and act as precursors for antimicrobial activity and monoglycerides. The primary fatty acid in coconut, lauric acid, is renowned for its antiviral, antibacterial, and antiprotozoal properties (Sindumathi and Amutha 2014).

10.2.2 Coconut Water-Based Products

10.2.2.1 Coconut Water

Coconut water is located within the cavity of the coconut and varies in its nutrient contents depending on the stage of harvest or development (Prithviraj et al. 2021). In addition the volume of water also varies depending on the maturity stage of coconut (Pandiselvam et al. 2019). It is a clear, colourless liquid extracted directly from coconuts, without expressing their meat. It takes around 11–12 months period for the development of nuts (Beegum et al. 2022b). The coconut water is primarily categorized as either tender coconut water (TCW) or mature coconut water (MCW). TCW is a natural and nourishing beverage that is extracted from the nut at the age of 6–7 months. On the other hand, the principal edible products from coconut fruit that has reached 12 months of maturity are coconut meat (kernel or endosperm) and mature coconut water (MCW). Sugars, minerals, vitamins, enzymes, amino acids, volatile aromatic compounds, and other biological components are present in coconut water (Yong et al. 2009). Despite the high levels of sugar in coconut water, it contains very little oil, proteins, and salts, all of which contribute to its extremely low dietary energy level of 44 calories per liter (Prades et al. 2012a). Since coconut water has excellent nutritional values as well as proven health benefits, it has become one of the most popular refreshing drinks of the Indian and international markets (Pummer et al. 2001). Even though the nutritional benefits of both young and mature coconut water are recognized, the water from the young nuts is commonly consumed as a health drink and can be consumed straight from the tender nuts or can be consumed after processing (Mahayothee et al. 2016).

10.2.2.2 Prebiotic Drinks Based on Coconut Water

Coconut water serves as a superb natural isotonic beverage, with its notable functional properties including the abilities to facilitate rehydration and serve as an electrolyte replacement (Dias et al. 2015). The development of prebiotic drink from coconut water provides not only the refreshing qualities of coconut water but also the added advantage of promoting a healthy gut microbiota through the inclusion of prebiotic components. The term probiotic refers to "live microorganisms that confer health benefits on the host when administered in adequate amounts" (Hill et al. 2014). Food with probiotic bacteria can be used as a nutritional supplement in functional foods. Lactic acid bacteria (LAB) are predominantly employed for such intentions (Plessas et al. 2017). Lactic acid bacteria (LAB) and other starter cultures modify the biochemical and sensory attributes of substances, generate diverse metabolites, and enhance beverages/foods with micronutrients like minerals, vitamins, amino acids, probiotics, prebiotics, and digestive enzymes (Ray et al. 2016). The fermentation of coconut water with probiotic lactic acid bacteria can yield a unique probiotic beverage, offering both hydration and probiotic advantages to consumers.

The utilization of the potential probiotic *Lactobacillus plantarum* DW12 in fermenting mature coconut water (MCW) with the addition of 0.5% monosodium glutamate (MSG) or a combination of 0.5% MSG and 1% sugarcane during a 48-h fermentation period enhances the nutritional value of MCW. This process results in the production of beneficial components such as γ-aminobutyric acid (GABA), vitamin B12, antioxidants, and antimicrobial compounds, contributing significantly to health benefits (Kantachote et al. 2017). The good adaptation of *B. coagulans* in the tender coconut water showed that if a potential probiotic strain is used as a starter culture, then it might produce a fermented product with defined and consistent characteristics and possibly health-promoting properties. Fermented coconut water gives the advantages of plant-based products, and the presence of live bacteria with probiotic qualities enhances the benefits.

10.2.2.3 Novel Electrolyte Beverage

The natural sweetness and refreshing qualities of coconut water make it a popular choice in many tropical regions. It is valued for its high sugar and mineral content and is extracted directly from the inner portion of the coconut fruit (Walter et al. 2014). The rehydrating properties of coconut water also make it a good natural alternative to the carbohydrate-electrolyte sports drinks (Ismail et al. 2007). However, owing to its low pH and high-water activity, along with high sugar content, this product allows rapid microorganism growth, which requires extra care during use (Prades et al. 2012b). The nutritional benefits and convenience of coconut water make it an excellent choice to combine with functional ingredients (Gopalakrishnan 2020) to develop a functional beverage that not only inhibits diarrhea-causing pathogens, modulates intestinal microbiota, and restores electrolyte balance while maintaining hydration. It is possible to integrate the polyphenol-rich bioactive grape pomace extract (GPE) into coconut water through its encapsulation in microparticles, specifically in alginate (GPE-Alg) or chitosan (GPE-CS) (Costa et al. 2021). Coconut beverages, being non-dairy functional options, are suitable for consumption by individuals who are vegetarians or lactose intolerant.

10.2.2.4 Vinegar

Coconut vinegar is the end product of the acetic and alcoholic fermentation of coconut water enriched with sugar, and is a great alternative to synthetic vinegar. Vinegar is usually used as a flavouring agent and food preservatives. It is widely used in pickles, sauces, and salad dressings as a flavouring and preservative. It contains a wealth of vitamins and minerals, including calcium, phosphorus, iron, and sodium, and has been discovered to possess anti-inflammatory and antimicrobial characteristics. The matured coconut water consists of 1–3% sugar which is increased to a concentration of 15% by adding sugar after the filtration process. Once cooled, the pasteurized mixture is inoculated with 1.5 g/L of active dry yeast, *Sacharomyces cerviseae*. Following 5–7 days of alcoholic fermentation, the transparent liquid is siphoned off and inoculated with mother vinegar or starter culture having *Aceteobacter* for effective acetic acid fermentation. After up to 7 days of the acidification process, the coconut vinegar is extracted by siphoning. The vinegar generator assembly is made up of a receiving vat for collecting vinegar, an acidifier, and a feed vat (Sangamithra et al. 2013).

10.2.2.5 Nata-de-Coco

Nata de coco is a clear, jelly-like food product created from the fermentation of mature coconut water using cellulose-producing bacteria, specifically *Acetobacter aceti* subspecies *xylinium*. Figure 10.6 depicted the process flow chart for the production of coconut chips. The microorganism can be cultivated in either coconut water or skimmed coconut milk. It is commonly sweetened and used as a confection or dessert, and it can be served alongside a variety of items such as beverages, ice cream, puddings, and fruit mixes (Cannon and Anderson 1991). It is highly valued for its abundant dietary fiber, zero cholesterol and low fat. Its rich fibre content assists in promoting intestinal health and preventing constipation in humans.

Coconut water is first strained and then combined with specified amounts of sugar and glacial acetic acid. For every liter of coconut water, 100 g of refined sugar and 5 g of monobasic ammonium phosphate are added. This mixture is boiled for 10 min and subsequently allowed to cool. Following that, a solution containing *Acetobacter xylinium* culture (150 mL) and glacial acetic acid (10 mL) is introduced. The resulting mixture is poured into glass trays or wide-mouthed jars, covered with muslin cloth, and left undisturbed for duration of 2–3 weeks. Meanwhile, a jelly-like substance, often white or cream-colored, produced and floats on the

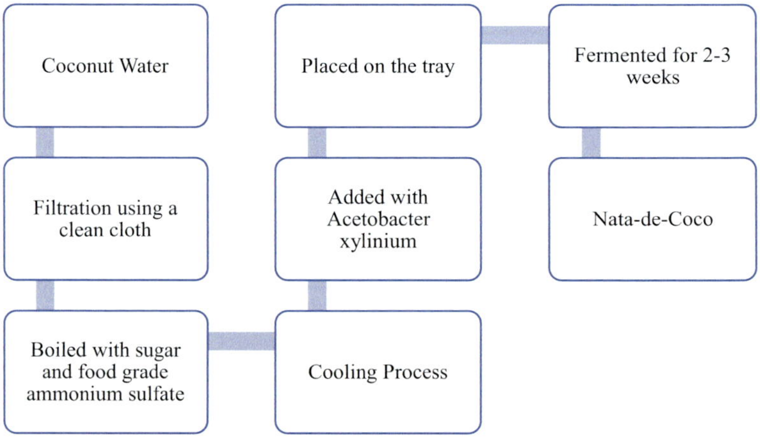

Fig. 10.6 Process Flow chart for the production of coconut chips

surface of the culture medium. The jelly is separated, and to eliminate any acids adhering to its surface, it is washed with water. Subsequently, the washed jelly is sliced into pieces and packaged.

10.2.3 Neera Based Products

10.2.3.1 Coconut Inflorescence Sap (*Neera*)

Coconut inflorescence sap or *neera* is collected from the matured inflorescence of the coconut or palm tree (Hebbar et al. 2018). The sap is tapped from the spadix and is typically used up in rural areas across the world. It ranges from honey to oyster white colours and is translucent and sweet-tasting. "*Neera*," "*Pathaneer*," and "*Kalparasa*" are common vernacular names for the sap, which is discharged by the phloem within a network of sieve tubes (Nguyen et al. 2016). In rural areas, along with coconut trees palmyrah is also traditionally utilized for collecting palm sap, by systematic practice for its local consumers. Basically, the unfermented sweet sap is called *neera* which obtained before fermentation. In order to stimulate sap flow, the tapping technique to release palm sap entails bruising the interior of the developing inflorescences with wooden sticks or bones. A cut is made at the head of the inflorescence to collect the sap. Inflorescence sap is collected twice a day, normally in the morning and evening (Hebbar et al. 2020). A collecting vessel is used to hold the inflorescence in order to collect sap. As the sap oozes drop by drop and is exposed to the environment in the open container for a long time, it spontaneously ferments. The rapid fermenting process converts palm sap into the alcoholic drink known as toddy (Hebbar et al. 2018). In India, lime is applied to the inner surface of earthen pots to prevent the process of fermentation of palm sap.

This nutritious liquid contains a wide range of macro and micronutrients, including sugars, minerals, antioxidants, and vitamins (Table 10.2). The palm sap is subjected to boiling at temperatures exceeding 100 °C for a period of 3–4 h to generate brown sugar characterized by its sweet flavour and aroma (Apriyantono et al. 2002; Ho et al. 2007). The sugars in palm sap undergo the Maillard reaction and caramelization as a result of heating. The palm sugar is characterized by low-glycemic index (GI 35) (Trinidad et al. 2010; Ghosh et al. 2018; Hebbar et al. 2018). The biochemical and mineral composition of Kalparasa is listed in Table 10.2.

10.2.3.2 Coconut Jaggery

Coconut sap contains approximately 15% sugars as well as significant amounts of nutrients that can be processed into various value-added products (Vengaiah et al. 2013). Removal of water through evaporation of unfermented sap at 115 °C yields coconut sugar and jaggery. It can be consumed directly or used in the preparation of sweet confectionary items and ayurvedic medicine. To make coconut honey or

Table 10.2 Biochemical and mineral composition of Kalparasa (per 100 mL)

Biochemical parameters	Quantity
pH	7.18
Total sugar(g)	15.18
Reducing sugar (g)	0.554
Amino acid (g)	0.245
Protein (g)	0.165
Phenolics (mg)	5.10
Antioxidant activity (mm TE)	0.321
Sodium (mg)	90.6
Potassium (mg)	168.4
Phosphorus (mg)	3.9
Manganese (mg)	0.012
Copper (mg)	0.031
Zinc (mg)	0.020
Iron (mg)	0.053

Source: ICAR-CPCRI Technical Bulletin, Kasaragod

syrup, the viscous, hot liquid (Brix 60° to 70°) is cooled. On further heating, sap becomes thicker and more viscous, and is poured into moulds of coconut leaf or steel resulting in jaggery. This jaggery is considered a suitable alternative to sugar in all kinds of food. Its biochemical composition is comparable to that of *neera*. It is therefore equally nutritious as raw palm sap. In contrast to brown sugar and refined cane sugar, it contains more minerals and serves as an excellent source of potassium, magnesium, zinc, and iron. It also has all of the essential amino acids needed for protein synthesis and is a good source of B complex vitamins, which encompass B1, B2, B3, and B6. As a supplementary super food, palm jaggery can also be beneficial in treating diseases including diabetic acidosis and post-operative convalescence. It acts as a diuretic. Additionally, it aids in balancing the body's potassium depletion (Upadhyaya and Sonawane 2023).

10.2.3.3 Coconut *Neera* Honey

The sap from coconut inflorescence is also known as *neera* is an excellent source of nutrients. Coconut Neera Honey is a value-added product made from the sap of coconut inflorescences, which has a pH of 6.0–6.5.The Honey is prepared in the same way as jaggery, however, prolonged heating should be avoided, which can cause charring and alterin colour (Hebbar et al. 2013). Neera honey is a natural source of the 12 essential vitamins B complex and vitamin C, and it is high in potassium, magnesium, zinc, and iron. The two main sugars found in coconut neera honey are fructose (38–40%) and glucose (33–35%). Neera honey is suitable for diabetics due to its low glycaemic index (GI). Neera honey also tends to be more sticky because of its elevated sugar levels and low glass transition temperatures (Pandiselvam et al. 2023).

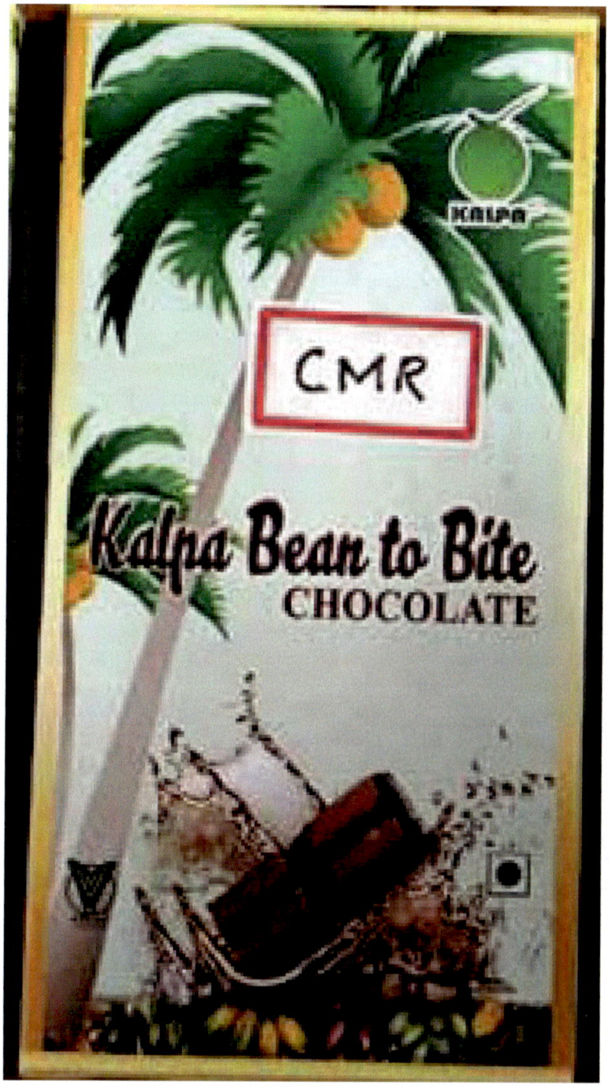

Fig. 10.7 Kalpa Bean to Bite Chocolate

10.2.3.4 Bean to Bite Chocolate

Bean to bite chocolate made from coconut sugar, consisting of sugar and well-fermented cocoa beans, possibly with or without cocoa butter (Fig. 10.7). The chocolate production with palm sugar has become popular as a healthier option, offering several health benefits due to the low glycemic index of natural sugars. Coconut sugar-infused dark chocolate contained 45% cocoa liquor, 30% coconut sugar, and 25% cocoa butter for optimum flavor and texture Polyphenols, flavonoids, antioxidants, and minerals are the major constituents of the chocolate (Hebbar et al. 2022).

10.3 Conclusion

Coconut stands out as a nutritious food source, driving a substantial market demand for the transition towards value-added products like coconut jaggery, coconut chips, coconut vinegar, and coconut neera honey, as mentioned previously. To achieve broad commercial success, these products must be manufactured, packaged, and presented in ways that align with consumer preferences. Given the significant culinary, medicinal, cosmetic, and industrial applications of coconut, it is crucial to exert concerted efforts in promoting value-added coconut products both domestically and internationally. However, the limited advancement of coconut by-products within the agro-industry presents a framework for research challenges. There is a pressing need to emphasize the importance of conducting preliminary research before proceeding with the commercialization of coconut byproducts. Furthermore, developing preservation protocols for coconut products is essential to ensure their quality and shelf life. Additionally, establishing food standards for novel coconut products is imperative to guarantee their safety and adherence to regulatory requirements. These measures are vital for driving the growth and acceptance of value-added coconut products in the market.

References

Apriyantono A, Aristyani A, Lidya Y, Budiyanto S, Soekarto ST (2002) Rate of browning reaction during preparation of coconut and palm sugar. Int Congress Ser 1245:275–278

Arivalagan M, Manikantan MR, Yasmeen AM, Sreejith S, Balasubramanian D, Hebbar KB, Kanade SR (2018) Physiochemical and nutritional characterization of coconut (Cocos nucifera L.) haustorium based extrudates. LWT 89:171–178

Beegum PPS, Nair JP, Manikantan MR, Pandiselvam R, Shill S, Neenu S, Hebbar KB (2022a) Effect of coconut milk, tender coconut and coconut sugar on the physico-chemical and sensory attributes in ice cream. J Food Sci Technol 59:2605–2616

Beegum PPS, Pandiselvam R, Ramesh SV, Thube SH, Pandian TP, Khanashyam AC, Manikantan MR, Hebbar KB (2022b) A critical appraisal on the antimicrobial, oral protective, and anti-diabetic functions of coconut and its derivatives. Qual Assur Saf Crop Foods 14(2):86–100

Cannon RE, Anderson SM (1991) Biogenesis of bacterial cellulose. Crit Rev Microbiol 17(6):435–447

Codex Alimentarius Commission (2022) Standard for aqueous coconut products– Coconut Milk and Coconut Cream. Food and Agricultural Organization of the United Nation, World Health Organization, 2(4), 1–5

Costa JR, Monteiro MJ, Tonon RV, Cabral LMC, Pastrana L, Pintado ME (2021) Fortification of coconut water with microencapsulated grape pomace extract towards a novel electrolyte beverage: Biological, sensorial and quality aspects. Futur Foods 4:100079

Deshpande HW, Poshadri A (2011) Physical and sensory characteristics of extruded snacks prepared from Foxtail millet based composite flours. Int Food Res J 18(2):751–756

Dias FM, Figueiredo RM, Souza JR, Santana CMP (2015) Qualidade microbiológica da água de coco comercializada em carrinhos ambulantes, na região central do município de Vitória da Conquista, BA. Rev Bras Prod Agroindustriais 17(1):97–103

Estoquia LQ, Teleron JI (2022) Operations research on product development, sensory evaluation, consumer's acceptability of coco sweet jam. Int J Adv Eng Res Sci 7:289–292

Ghosh DK, Bandyopadhyay A, Das S, Hebbar KB, Biswas B (2018) Coconut sap (Neera)-untapped opportunity of spinoff gains in West Bengal, India. Int J Curr Microbiol Appl Sci 7(9):1883–1897

Gopalakrishnan RG (2020) Yummy Coconut Products Growing Demand in US Markets. Indian Coconut J 1–5

Hebbar KB, Mathew AC, Arivalagan M, Samsudeen K, Thomas GV (2013) Value added products from Neera. Indian Coconut J LVI(4):28–33

Hebbar KB, Pandiselvam R, Manikantan MR, Arivalagan M, Beegum S, Chowdappa P (2018) Palm sap—quality profiles, fermentation chemistry, and preservation methods. Sugar Tech 20(6):621–634

Hebbar KB, Arivalagan M, Pavithra KC, Roy TK, Gopal M, Shivashankara KS, Chowdappa P (2020) Nutritional profiling of coconut (Cocos nucifera L.) inflorescence sap collected using novel coco-sap chiller method and its value added products. J Food Meas Charact 14:2703–2712

Hebbar KB, Ramesh SV, Ghosh DK, Beegum PPS, Pandiselvam R, Manikantan MR, Mathew AC (2022) Coconut sugar-a potential storehouse of nutritive metabolites, novel bio-products and prospects. Sugar Tech 24(3):841–856

Hill C, Guarner F, Reid G, Gibson GR, Merenstein DJ, Pot B, Morelli L, Canani RB, Flint HJ, Salminen S (2014) Activity of cecropin P1 and FA-LL-37 against urogenital microflora. Nat Rev Gastroenterol Hepatol 11(8):506

Ho CW, Aida WMW, Maskat MY, Osman H (2007) Changes in volatile compounds of palm sap (Arenga pinnata) during the heating process for production of palm sugar. Food Chem 102(4):1156–1162

Ismail I, Singh R, Sirisinghe RG (2007) Rehydration with sodium-enriched coconut water after exercise-induced dehydration. Southeast Asian J Trop Med Public Health 38(4):769

Kantachote D, Ratanaburee A, Hayisama-ae W, Sukhoom A, Nunkaew T (2017) The use of potential probiotic Lactobacillus plantarum DW12 for producing a novel functional beverage from mature coconut water. J Funct Foods 32:401–408

Kumari V, Yadav BS, Yadav RB, Nema PK (2020) Effect of osmotic agents and ultasonication on osmo-convective drying of sweet lime (Citrus limetta) peel. J Food Process Eng 43(4):e13371

Lal G, Siddappa GS, Tandon GL (1960) Preservation of fruits and vegetables. Indian Council of Agricultural Research, New Delhi

Madhavan K, Arumuganathan T, Mathew AC (2010) Commercial production of coconut chips. CPCRI Tech Bull 62:14

Mahayothee B, Koomyart I, Khuwijitjaru P, Siriwongwilaichat P, Nagle M, Müller J (2016) Phenolic compounds, antioxidant activity, and medium chain fatty acids profiles of coconut water and meat at different maturity stages. Int J Food Prop 19(9):2041–2051

Manikantan MR, Pandiselvam R, Beegum S, Mathew AC (2018) Harvest and postharvest technology. In: The coconut palm (Cocos nucifera L.)—research and development perspectives. Springer, Singapore, pp 635–722

Manivannan A, Bhardwaj R, Padmanabhan S, Suneja P, Hebbar KB, Kanade SR (2018) Biochemical and nutritional characterization of coconut (Cocos nucifera L.) haustorium. Food Chem 238:153–159

Marina AM, Man YBC, Amin I (2009) Virgin coconut oil: emerging functional food oil. Trends Food Sci Technol 20(10):481–487

Nguyen VD, Harifara R, Shiro S (2016) Sap from various palms as a renewable energy source for bioethanol production. Chem Ind Chem Eng Q 22(4):355–373

Nimbkar S, Leena MM, Moses JA, Anandharamakrishnan C (2022) Medium chain triglycerides (MCT): state-of-the-art on chemistry, synthesis, health benefits and applications in food industry. Compr Rev Food Sci Food Saf 21(2):843–867

Pandiselvam R, Manikantan MR, Subhashree N, Mathew AC, Balasubramanian D, Shameena Beegum PP, Ramesh SV, Niral V, Ranjini TN, Hebbar KB (2019) Correlation and principal component analysis of physical properties of tender coconut (Cocos nucifera L.) in relation to the development of trimming machine. J Food Process Eng 42(6):e13217
Pandiselvam R, Mahanti NK, Manikantan MR, Kothakota A, Chakraborty SK, Ramesh SV, Beegum PPS (2022) Rapid detection of adulteration in desiccated coconut powder: Vis-NIR spectroscopy and chemometric approach. Food Control 133:108588
Pandiselvam R, Joseph LT, Manikantan MR, Khanashyam AC, Beegum PPS, Ramesh SV, Balasubramanian D, Neenu S, Gopal M, Mathew AC (2023) Physical, chemical and functional attributes of neera honey infused extrudates. Bioengineering 10(1):114
Plessas S, Nouska C, Karapetsas A, Kazakos S, Alexopoulos A, Mantzourani I, Chondrou P, Fournomiti M, Galanis A, Bezirtzoglou E (2017) Isolation, characterization and evaluation of the probiotic potential of a novel lactobacillus strain isolated from feta-type cheese. Food Chem 226:102–108
Prades A, Dornier M, Diop N, Pain J-P (2012a) Coconut water uses, composition and properties: a review. Fruits 67(2):87–107
Prades A, Dornier M, Diop N, Pain J-P (2012b) Coconut water preservation and processing: a review. Fruits 67(3):157–171
Prithviraj V, Pandiselvam R, Babu AC, Kothakota A, Manikantan MR, Ramesh SV, Beegum PPS, Mathew AC, Hebbar KB (2021) Emerging non-thermal processing techniques for preservation of tender coconut water. LWT 149:111850
Pummer S, Heil P, Maleck W, Petroianu G (2001) Influence of coconut water on hemostasis. Am J Emerg Med 19(4):287–289
Ray M, Ghosh K, Singh S, Mondal KC (2016) Folk to functional: an explorative overview of rice-based fermented foods and beverages in India. J Ethn Foods 3(1):5–18
Sangamithra A, John SG, Sorna Prema R, Chandrasekar V, Sasikala S, Hasker E (2013) Coconut: an extensive review on value added products. Indian Food Industry Mag 32:29–36
Sebastian KS (2017) Desiccated Coconut Powder export. Indian Coconut Journal 4
Seow CC, Gwee CN (1997) Coconut milk: chemistry and technology. Int J Food Sci Technol 32(3):189–201
Sethi S, Tyagi SK, Anurag RK (2016) Plant-based milk alternatives an emerging segment of functional beverages: a review. J Food Sci Technol 53:3408–3423
Shameena Beegum PP, Manikantan MR, Sharma M, Pandiselvam R, Gupta RK, Hebbar KB (2019) Optimization of processing variables for the development of virgin coconut oil cake based extruded snacks. J Food Process Eng 42(4):e13048
Silva PSA (2008) Manufacture of cabonated tender coconut water & development of a process for the utilization of coconut flesh. PhD diss., University of sri jayewardenepura, Nugegoda
Sindumathi G, Amutha S (2014) Processing and quality evaluation of coconut based jam. IOSR J Environ Sci Toxicol Food Technol 8(1):10–14
Trinidad TP, Mallillin AC, Sagum RS, Encabo RR (2010) Glycemic index of commonly consumed carbohydrate foods in the Philippines. J Funct Foods 2(4):271–274
Upadhyaya A, Sonawane SK (2023) Palmyrah palm and its products (Neera, Jaggery and Candy)—a review on chemistry and technology. Appl Food Res 3(1):100256
Uzodinma EO, Mbaeyi-Nwaoha IE, Onwurafor EU, Ochulor CE (2020) Influence of pasteurization on the quality of pineapple, watermelon and banana pulps-based smoothie flavoured with coconut milk. Am J Food Sci Technol 8(3):99–105
Vengaiah PC, Ravindrababu D, Murthy GN, Prasad KR (2013) Jaggery from Palmyrah palm (Borassus flabellifer L.)-Present status and scope
Walter EHM, Kuaye AY, Hoorfar J (2014) Case study on the safety and sustainability of fresh bottled coconut water. In: Global safety of fresh produce. Elsevier, Philadelphia, pp 367–382
Yong JWH, Ge L, Ng YF, Tan SN (2009) The chemical composition and biological properties of coconut (Cocos nucifera L.) water. Molecules 14(12):5144–5164

Chapter 11
Coconut: A Powerhouse of Nutraceuticals

Kiran Mishra, Muskan Beura, C. S. Keerthana, and Veda Krishnan

Abstract The coconut tree holds immense importance, serving as a vital resource for millions of individuals by providing sustenance, employment, and avenues for commerce. Recognized as the "miracle fruit," its fruit boasts a diverse array of macro and micro nutrients essential for human health and nutrition. From its water to meat, it is known for its nutraceutical abilities which are due to bioactives' presence. The state and type of nutrient being important, a few have only been extensively studied to date while other bio-actives have largely been ignored. This chapter aims to thoroughly analyze the present understanding of coconut nutraceuticals, distinguishing between promising areas for further research and unsupported assertions. Ultimately, the aim is to steer readers towards a well-informed comprehension of this captivating domain within the realms of health and nutrition. We comprehensively elaborate and conceptually explain the different bioactives and their clinical outcomes by defining the underlying phenomenon in this chapter.

Keywords Coconut bioactives · Nutraceuticals · Functional foods · MCFAs

K. Mishra
Department of Microbiology, SIES College of Arts, Science and Commerce, University of Mumbai, Mumbai, Maharashtra, India

M. Beura
Division of Biochemistry, ICAR-Indian Agricultural Research Institute (IARI), New Delhi, Delhi, India

Department of Plant Science, School of Biological Sciences, Central University of Kerala, Kasaragod, Kerala, India

C. S. Keerthana · V. Krishnan (✉)
Division of Biochemistry, ICAR-Indian Agricultural Research Institute (IARI), New Delhi, Delhi, India
e-mail: veda.krishnan@icar.gov.in

S. V. Ramesh, S. Praveen (eds.), *Coconut-Based Nutrition and Nutraceutical Perspectives*, https://doi.org/10.1007/978-981-97-3976-9_11

11.1 Introduction

Coconuts (*Cocos nucifera* L.) are versatile fruits that are not only a popular culinary ingredient but it is also recognized as the 'tree of abundance,' 'tree of heaven,' and 'tree of life' due to their diverse applications. It plays a vital role in providing sustenance, employment, and business prospects for millions of individuals. With its various parts offering a wealth of macro and micronutrients, the coconut is often selected as an alternative source of protein and fiber.

Coconut nutraceuticals have gained widespread recognition for their remarkable health-promoting properties, drawing from their rich nutritional profile. Different coconut products and by-products—such as coconut water, milk, copra, testa, flour, raw kernels, oil, and desiccated coconut have been reported to possess a range of bioactive components with potential health benefits. These dietary supplements can help to avoid nutrient deficiencies and provide health benefits and are rich in bioactives like medium chain triglycerides (MCTs), functional polysaccharides, polyphenols, vitamins, minerals, fiber, cytokinins, and phytosterols (Kannaian et al. 2020). According to proximate analysis, 100 g of coconut flour has 12.1% protein, 10.9% fat, 3.1% ash, 3.6% moisture, and 70.3% carbohydrates (Trinidad et al. 2006). Khan et al. (2015) reported that coconut meat contained 6.7% moisture, 1.55% ash, 14.3% protein, 54.0% fat, 20.50% fiber, and 23.40% carbohydrates. One of the key components contributing to the nutritional value of coconut nutraceuticals is the presence of MCTs. These unique fatty acids (FA) are easily absorbed by the body, provide a quick source of energy, and support various metabolic functions (Watanabe and Tsujino 2022). The lauric acid and other saturated fatty acids found in Virgin coconut oil (VCO) have been shown to have antibacterial properties (Mat et al. 2022). Such documented activities of various bioactive components of coconut make them promising candidates for combating oxidative stress and inflammation within the body.

In this comprehensive chapter, we delve into the bioactive components within a coconut (Table 11.1), exploring their mechanisms of action, therapeutic implications, and potential avenues for future research in the field of nutraceuticals. By unraveling the nutritional bounty of coconut, we aim to elucidate its role as a powerhouse of health-promoting compounds and pave the way for novel dietary interventions aimed at optimizing human health and well-being.

11.2 Bioactive Components in Coconut

Coconut is a versatile resource, with proteins, oil, water, and derived products like coconut palm sugar, inflorescence, haustorium, and nutraceuticals offering health benefits and addressing nutrient deficiencies. Coconut oil, particularly VCO, stands out for its medicinal values and antibacterial properties, owing to its components like lauric acid. VCO extraction precludes the refining process, thereby preserving

Table 11.1 Bioactive components of various parts of coconut, and their biochemical mechanism offer immense health benefits

S.No.	Coconut part/ component	Bioactive compound	Activity	References
1.	Tender	Medium-chain fatty acids	Increase blood HDL-cholesterol	Ngampeerapong and Chavasit (2019)
		Phenolic compounds and flavonoids	Anti-aging, anticancer, anti-inflammation, and reducing the risk of cardiovascular disease against damage from free radical	Ngampeerapong and Chavasit (2019)
		Lauric acid, capric acid, and myristic acid	Antimicrobial properties, immune support, cardiovascular benefits	Hewlings (2020)
2.	Water	Ascorbic acid, catechin and epicatechin, caffeic acid	Antioxidants and anti-aging agents	Halim et al. (2023)
		Potassium, sodium, calcium, magnesium ions	Hydration, cellular homeostasis, and rehydration during physical activity	Yong et al. (2009), Zhang et al. (2020)
		L-arginine and ascorbic acid	Reduces the generation of free radicals and has antioxidant activity. Decreases lipid peroxidation in rats	Lima et al. (2015)
		Phytoestrogen	Hormone replacement therapy, reducing the risk of dementia and in wound healing in postmenopausal women	Radenahmad et al. (2006)
3.	Oil	Lauric acid	Regulated consumption could reduce risk of type II diabetes (T2DM)	Ngampeerapong and Chavasit (2019)
		Monolaurin	Antiseptic effects and is used as an efficient, safe skin moisturizer effective against superficial skin infections	Agero and Verallo-Rowell (2004), Carpo et al. (2007)

(continued)

Table 11.1 (continued)

S.No.	Coconut part/ component	Bioactive compound	Activity	References
4.	Coconut flour	Lauric acid	Antimicrobial properties, oral infections such as mouth sores	Taheri et al. (2010)
		Dietary fiber (56 g insoluble and 4 g soluble per 100 g of flour)	Prebiotic, supports gut health, reduce LDL cholesterol levels, lower glycemic index	Trinidad et al. (2006)
5.	Copra	Potassium and phytochemicals	Anti-inflammatory, antioxidant, and reducing properties	Odenigbo and Otisi (2011)
6.	Testa	Phenolics and flavonoids	Antioxidant activity	Mat et al. (2022)
7.	Milk	Polyphenols	Associated with reduction in risk for cardiovascular diseases (CVD)	Ngampeerapong and Chavasit (2019)
		Phytosterols	Reduces cholesterol absorption in the small intestine	Ngampeerapong and Chavasit (2019)
		Amino acids and Vitamins E and C	Antioxidant activities	Ngampeerapong and Chavasit (2019)
8.	Fermented Coconut Milk	Organic acids (diacetyl, acetaldehyde, monolaurin)	Higher antibacterial activity compared to unfermented coconut milk	Qadi et al. (2023)
		Gamma-aminobutyric acid (GABA)	Antioxidant and antibacterial activity	Qadi et al. (2023)
		Amino acids (valine, arginine, methionine, aspartate, threonine, phenylalanine)	Nutrition sources	Qadi et al. (2023)
9.	*Neera* (non-alcoholic nectar)	Presence of ions such as Ca, Na, K, Mg, Fe, Zn, Cu, S, and Mn	Play vital role in normal physiological processes such as formation of strong bones, teeth, hemoglobin, etc.	Panonnummal et al. (2021)
		Vitamin C, phenolics, flavonoids, and tannins	Antioxidants	Panonnummal et al. (2021)

its natural qualities. The coconut industry benefits economically from VCO and expanded coconut flour production, contributing to the prevention of ailments such as diabetes, colon cancer, and cardiovascular disease (CVD). Additionally, the waste from the coconut, vegetable, and fruit industries, rich in nutrients, can be repurposed into value-added food products for significant economic gains. Among

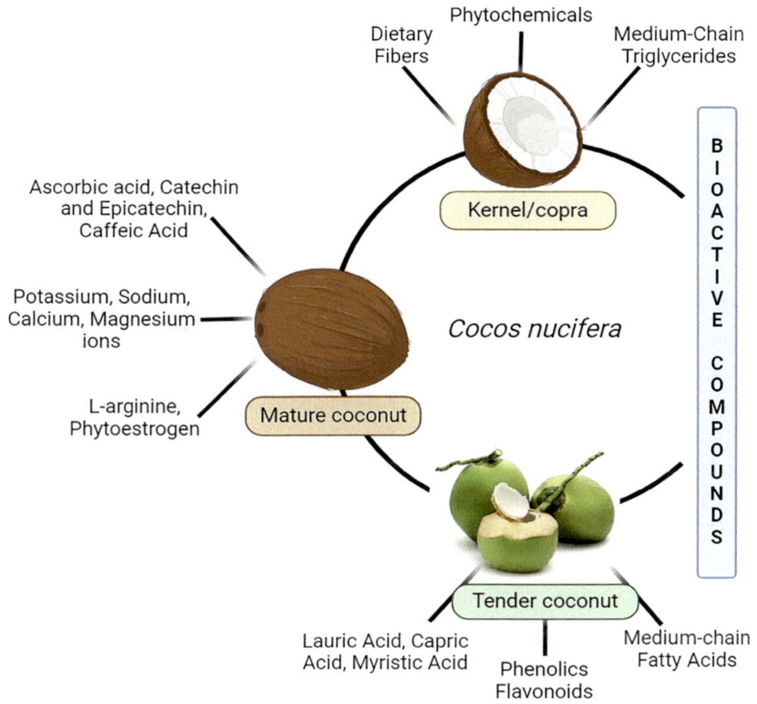

Fig. 11.1 Bioactive compounds found in coconut (*Cocos nucifera* L.). A plethora of bioactives are found in tender coconut, mature coconut, copra/kernel, and coconut water. The bioactivity depends on the dietary fibers, polysaccharides, phytochemicals, medium chain triglycerides (MCTs), medium chain fatty acids (MCFAs), phenolics, flavonoids, vitamins, and minerals

the nutraceuticals, MCTs, functional polysaccharides, polyphenols, phytosterols, and cytokinins are predominant (Fig. 11.1).

11.2.1 Medium Chain Triglycerides (MCTs)

Lipids are considered one of the crucial factors for normal body functioning and growth, predominantly existing as triglycerides offering essential FA. FA serves as a concentrated source of energy and is influenced by the source, and composition varying between plants and animals. MCT, a nutraceutical fat with health benefits, has medium-chain fatty acids (MCFAs) like caprylic, capric, and lauric acids. Natural sources of MCTs include coconut oil, palm kernel oil, and bovine milk. MCT, synthesized by esterification, provides fewer calories (8.4 kcal/g), a liquid state at room temperature, and unique physicochemical properties. The calorie intake is ideally healthy and has applications in clinical nutrition (Jadhav and

Annapure 2023). Lauric acid, an MCFA, is found abundantly in coconut. Coconut oil subjected to the refining process still has 46–54% of lauric acid, followed by 5–10% caprylic acid and 5–8% capric acid. The high concentration of lauric acid in coconut oil leads to the production of pharmacologically active compounds such as monolaurin through the hydrolysis of MCTs, which yields a significant amount of mono lauryl glycerol (Narayanankutty et al. 2018). The oil contains a triglyceride backbone with 55% MCFAs strategically positioned for rapid dietary absorption. This unique stereo-specific FA arrangement sets it apart from commonly available vegetable oils (Ramesh et al. 2021). In the 1950s, Babayan et al. pioneered industrial MCT production from low-melting-point FA in coconut oil, primarily C8:0 and C10:0. Commercial MCT production still focuses on these due to their superior nutrient absorption compared to alternatives. Initially developed as byproducts, MCTs have recently gained attention for their health benefits, becoming a potential nutraceutical solution. They stand out for minimal impact on postprandial blood triglycerides, stimulate acylated ghrelin for growth hormone secretion and appetite regulation, and influence incretin secretion for lowered postprandial blood glucose levels. MCTs show promise in various health issues like gastrointestinal malabsorption, epilepsy, and diabetes, and are being explored for addressing elderly health concerns. Clinical studies, particularly in animals, indicate immune modulation and antioxidative effects. In neurodegenerative disorders like Alzheimer's and in cancer treatment, MCTs combined with standard therapies offer encouraging results, underscoring their diverse health benefits (Jadhav and Annapure 2023).

11.2.2 Functional Polysaccharides and Fiber

Functional attributes, especially prebiotic and gut-friendly features, are majorly contributed by non-glycemic carbohydrates known as functional polysaccharides or dietary fibers. In coconut, the predominant ones are cellulose (13%), galactomannan (61%), and mannan (26%). Trinidad et al. (2006) state that coconut flour, recognized for its high dietary fiber content, produces short-chain fatty acids (SCFA) like butyrate, acetate, and propionate during fermentation. It comprises 56.8% insoluble and 3.8% soluble fibers, contributing to a total dietary fiber content of 60.9%. Research indicates that coconut flour exhibits variations in protein and fiber content depending on the processing method—dry processing yields high protein levels, while wet processing results in elevated fiber content. This versatile ingredient is employed in creating functional foods with diverse health benefits, given its potential to lower blood sugar and cholesterol levels, as well as increase fecal bulk volume.

Within the coconut, galactomannan is predominantly found in the kernel or meat. The chemical structure of galactomannans consists of a linear chain of mannose sugar units linked by β-1,4-glycosidic bonds, often with side branches containing galactose units. The specific ratio of mannose to galactose varies, influencing the functional properties of the galactomannan (Geronço et al. 2021). In practical applications, galactomannan extracted from coconut serves as a valuable thickening and gelling agent in the food industry. Its addition enhances the texture, stability, and viscosity of various food products (Seo 2022). Moreover, the dietary fiber content in coconut, including galactomannan, contributes to digestive health. Dietary fiber is known for its potential benefits, such as aiding in weight management, regulating blood sugar levels, and supporting heart health.

11.2.3 Polyphenols

Polyphenols are a group of diverse bioactives that include simple phenols, flavonoids, phenylethanoids, hydroxycinnamic acid, hydroxybenzoic acids, anthocyanins, and various others. Coconut oil has rich polyphenolics, especially VCO, which includes vanillic acid, caffeic acid, p-coumaric acid, ferulic acid, quercetin, catechins, and resveratrol. The method used for extracting coconut oil plays a crucial role in its phenolic content, highest in the VCO and least in refined-bleached-deodorized (RBD) oil. The results of the extraction method and retention of polyphenols have been well explained by Seneviratne and Sudarshana Dissanayake (2008), who found that the total phenol content in traditional coconut oil was approximately seven times higher compared to commercial coconut oil (Zeb 2021). On the other hand, Ramesh et al. (2020) demonstrated that VCO produced by a hot process, among the various variants of coconut oils, has high total phenolic and flavonoid content and strong antioxidant capacity.

The bioactive compound exhibits antioxidant activity such as 1,1-diphenyl-2-picrylhydrazyl (DPPH) radical scavenging, β-carotene-linoleate bleaching, and reducing power. In mouse model experiments, VCOs have been proven to enhance antioxidant enzymes such as catalase (CAT), glutathione peroxidase (GPx), glutathione reductase (GR), superoxide dismutase (SOD), glutathione content (GSH) and reduce the lipid peroxidation (Rohman et al. 2021). Apart from that, the polyphenols in the VCO account for the anti-inflammatory, cytoprotective, and lipid-lowering characteristics. The enrichment of polyphenols in coconut, and VCO can be a potential health-promoting factor for overall wellness (Zeng et al. 2024).

11.2.4 Phytosterols

Phytosterols are the phytonutrients and bioactive sterols from plants, resembling animal-derived cholesterol in their structure and activity. They have therapeutic implications widely in diet-related metabolic problems such as type II diabetes mellitus (T2DM) and cardiovascular disorders and have drawn global attention (Prasad et al. 2021). Phytosterols have been studied extensively in VCOs as they boast higher concentrations compared to coconut milk and commercially available coconut oil, attributed to their lipophilic nature. Apart from cholesterol-modulating behavior, they exhibit anti-inflammatory, anti-cancer, and immunomodulatory properties. β-sitosterol, a prominent sterol is known for inhibiting cancer cells and improving cognitive functions. β-sitosterols are highly capable of scavenging free radicals, modulating the activities of several antioxidant enzymes, and preventing the formation of superoxide radicals and peroxides. However, despite the promising effects of phytosterol, the total content of phytosterol and biological activity remains restricted to reducing blood cholesterol levels, thus opening further research opportunities (Zeng et al. 2022).

11.2.5 Cytokinins

The nutritional content of coconut water has been extensively documented by Ge et al. (2006), and the growth-promoting elements that tender coconut water as an effective nutrient medium for plant tissue culture have been recognized (Al-Khayri et al. 1992). Adoption of capillary electrophoresis-mass spectrometry (CE-MS/MS) as an analytical tool identified endogenous cytokinin nucleotides in purified extracts of coconut water. Kinetin-type cytokinins, which are signaling molecules present in coconut water, have demonstrated beneficial biomedical effects on mammalian cells (injected *in vitro*) with anti-cancer, anti-oxidative, anti-aging, cardioprotective, and DNA-repairing functions. Conversely, because of ethical reasons, there is no direct way of assessing the biomedical effects of coconut water when it is consumed orally by humans. Zeatin-type cytokinins, also present in coconut water, are the bio-active form of cytokinins in plants and are specifically driving growth and development in tissue cultures and biofertilizers. This is because they are signaling molecules that promote vital cellular processes (e.g., chloroplast formation) including appropriate cell cycle development and regulating key physiological functions (e.g., stomatal opening). Isopentenyladenine (iP), a cytokinin also present in coconut water, is a precursor to the biologically active form of cytokinin in plants and is also produced by bacteria. Kinetin-type and zeatin-type cytokinins, along with iP, all share the same biosynthesis and metabolic pathway.

11.2.6 Peptides

Bioactive peptides are short-chain amino acids found within the food proteins extending nutraceutical values and specific biological effects (Ulug et al. 2021). These peptides demonstrate multifunctional properties. Wang and Ng (2005) worked on the antifungal peptides from coconut and conducted experiments to prove the same on various fungal species. These pioneering studies prompted further exploration into the other properties of coconut peptides, including their potential antimicrobial, antioxidant, anti-inflammatory, and immunomodulatory effects. The nutritional profile of coconut, especially tender coconut and its water has led to several medicinal formulations and nutraceuticals. However, the peptides are the ones that are least explored. Continuing the antifungal peptide extraction from coconut fibers, Mandal et al. (2009) investigated the antimicrobial peptides (AMPs) from green coconut water. The team identified three novel peptides: Cn-AMP1, Cn-AMP2, and Cn-AMP3 showing antimicrobial properties against several human pathogenic bacteria. The Cn-AMPs reported are promising in the development of antibiotics. Further research focused on the angiotensin-I converting enzyme (ACE) inhibitory peptides for antihypertensive ability extracted from the coconut cake globulin hydrolysate (CCGH), a byproduct from the coconut oil (Li et al. 2016). Following this, coconuts have been thoroughly studied for the ACE-inhibitory peptides and their antioxidant activity. Zheng et al. (2019) found three novel ACE-inhibitory and antioxidant peptides from coconut cake albumin hydrolysate (CCAH) making coconut peptides a functional food component to control antioxidation and ACE activity.

11.2.7 Proanthocyanidins

Coconut husks, the fibrous outer layer of the coconut, are rich in proanthocyanidins, a type of antioxidant with potential health benefits. These antioxidants may help protect cells from damage, fight bacteria and fungi, reduce inflammation, and even promote wound healing. While research is ongoing, studies suggest these potential benefits. However, it's important to note that proanthocyanidins found in coconut huskis different from coconut oil which is extracted from the inner flesh of the coconut and doesn't contain these compounds. Other fruits like grapes, cranberries, and apples also contain proanthocyanidins (Padumadasa et al. 2016). It has also been shown that these proanthocyanidins can be used as corrosion inhibitors for carbon steel (Guedes et al. 2021).

11.2.8 Other Major Nutrients

Proteins: The coconut palm consists of various parts, including leaves, buds, flowers, fruit, and germinating nuts, some of which are rich in protein, offering health benefits. For instance, the edible white kernel of the coconut contains approximately 4.3% protein, primarily composed of globulin. The essential amino acids found in coconut globulin predominantly include arginine (31%) and lysine (4.8%) presented as a percentage of the total nitrogen. When incorporated into a well-rounded diet, coconut serves as a sufficient protein source, supporting growth even when it is the sole protein source. Lal et al. (2003) reported that proteins isolated from coconut kernels can reduce lipid content in experimental animals due to a low lysine-to-arginine ratio. Moreover, within the coconut endosperm, there exists a highly efficient natural coagulant protein that is water-soluble. Derived from coconuts, copra meat has proven to be a viable protein source for ruminants, pigs, and poultry. Conversely, the protein content in coconut sap (obtained from coconut flowers) is recorded at 0.26%, suggesting that coconut sap lacks the attributes necessary to be deemed a significant protein source (Mat et al. 2022). The properties shown above prove that some parts (e.g., coconut kernel and meal) of the coconut palm are rich in proteins while some (e.g. coconut milk, trunk, and leaves) contain little protein.

Vitamins and minerals: The richness of vitamins and minerals in coconut makes it a valuable addition to the diet. A significant amount of calcium, iron, zinc, potassium, sodium, vitamin C, and vitamin E is present which are highly crucial for health (Ishiaq 2012). Starting from coconut sap, green coconut, meat, and oil, all offer a diverse array of vitamins and minerals making it a nutrient powerhouse. The young/green/tender coconut is abundant in vital electrolytes like potassium and sodium. Additionally, it contains calcium, ascorbic acid (vitamin C), and vitamin B complex. Nursing mothers are often advised to consume tender coconut water to fulfill their infants' calcium needs. Moreover, the water of the green coconut is rich in various other minerals like iron, magnesium, potassium, copper, zinc, and phosphorus. Sodium is crucial for maintaining hydration levels in the body, while potassium plays a vital role in muscle function, and these two create balance in the electrolyte content of the body. Magnesium aids in muscle contraction and energy production; phosphorus supports bone health and nerve function; calcium facilitates muscle contraction and nerve transmission, and iron is essential for oxygen transport and cellular function. Copper acts as a cofactor for various enzymes and supports overall body function, while chloride helps maintain fluid balance and blood pH stability. Tender coconut houses several important vitamins such as nicotinic acid, pantothenic acid, biotin, riboflavin, folic acid, tocopherol (vitamin E), and thiamine along with B1, B2, B3, B5, B6, B7, and B9. Although the fruit is not very rich in vitamin E, the abundance of vitamin B and vitamin C fulfills the essential dietary requirements if consumed daily (Prades et al. 2012).

11.3 Mechanisms of Action of Coconut Bioactives

11.3.1 Physiological Implications and Metabolic Pathways of MCTs (Medium Chain Triglycerides)

MCTs are a distinctive class of fatty acids found in coconut oil. Their unique metabolic pathways and physiological implications have garnered significant attention in recent years (Jadhav and Annapure 2023). MCTs are absorbed directly into the bloodstream from the digestive tract, bypassing the lymphatic system and providing a rapid source of energy (Shah and Limketkai 2017). It differs from long-chain fatty acids (LCFAs) in their metabolism. While LCFAs are stored in adipose tissue, MCTs are hydrolyzed by human endogenous lipase enzymes, releasing MCFA from the glycerol backbone. Due to their hydrophilic nature and shorter carbon chain, these MCFA are promptly transported via the hepatic portal vein to the liver, where they undergo β-oxidation. This rapid metabolism of MCFA leads to the production of ketones in the body. These ketones serve as an alternative energy source, crossing the blood-brain barrier and supplying the brain with readily available and efficient fuel (Jadhav and Annapure 2023; Jensen et al. 2020). This metabolic process has notable implications for weight management, as MCTs have been shown to increase feelings of fullness, promote fat oxidation, and potentially reduce overall calorie intake, making them valuable in weight loss diets (Mumme and Stonehouse 2015; St-Onge et al. 2014; Jensen et al. 2020). Also, it was reported that hydrolyzed MCT does not go to the lymphatic system for re-synthesis of triglyceride molecules which can be stored in the form of fat in adipose tissue leading to obesity (Babayan 1968).

The conversion of MCTs into ketones has profound implications for neurological health. Ketones are known to have neuroprotective effects, and studies are exploring their potential in managing neurological conditions like epilepsy and Alzheimer's disease (AD) (Gough et al. 2021; Jensen et al. 2020). Research in this area is promising, offering hope for individuals seeking alternative approaches to neurodegenerative disease management. Additionally, the conversion of MCTs into ketones holds promise for neurological health, with research indicating neuroprotective effects and potential benefits in managing conditions like epilepsy and AD (Gough et al. 2021; Jensen et al. 2020). It can also be incorporated into various food products for critically ill patients unable to metabolize carbohydrates easily, while also being used in designer lipids for patients with cardiovascular issues, obesity, cancer, and inflammation; moreover, MCTs exhibit hydrophilic properties, making them effective solvents for food additives, and demonstrate antibacterial and antiviral activity. Consumption of MCT in the diet is also related to an increase in psychological health by boosting memory (Jadhav and Annapure 2023).

11.3.2 The Biochemical Functions of Coconut Bio-actives in Immune-Modulatory Responses

Lauric acid, the most abundant and potent MCFA in coconut, constitutes nearly 50% of coconut's fat content. Monolaurin is not formed in the body unless there is a source of lauric acid in the diet, and coconut is a rich source of monolaurin (DebMandal and Mandal 2011). Its significance lies in its effectiveness against a broad range of lipid-coated bacteria, due to its ability to disintegrate their lipid membranes. This property makes lauric acid and its derivatives, such as monoglycerides (MGs) found in coconut, valuable in combating various bacterial infections associated with stomach ulcers, sinusitis, dental cavities, oral infections, skin infections, food poisoning, and urinary tract infections (DebMandal and Mandal 2011; Taheri et al. 2010). A typical phenomenon involved in developing the disease atherosclerosis is an inflammatory process provoked by a pathogenic bacteria resulting in the oxidation of lipoproteins with induction of cytokines and production of proteolytic enzymes. As part of this process, certain pathogenic gram-negative bacteria can be effectively inactivated or killed by lauric acid, monolaurin, capric acid, and monocaprin when combined with an appropriate chelator (Enig 1999; Casillas-Vargas et al. 2021; Joshi et al. 2020). Sucrose monolaurate, a glycolipid compound found in coconut, exhibits anti-caries effects by inhibiting glycolysis and sucrose oxidation caused by *Streptococcus mutans* in a non-competitive manner, thereby preventing the formation of dental plaque *in vitro* (Barnabé et al. 2004).

Beyond antibacterial properties, lauric acid has demonstrated antiviral potential, especially against lipid-coated viruses such as visna virus, CMV, Epstein-Barr virus, influenza virus, etc. The MCFA in coconut oil primarily destroys these organisms by disrupting their membranes, interfering with virus assembly and maturation. Among the saturated fatty acids, lauric acid has greater antiviral activity than caprylic acid, capric acid, or myristic acid. Monolaurin acts by solubilizing the lipids and phospholipids in the envelope of the virus, causing the disintegration of the virus envelope (Arora et al. 2010). While more research is needed, this property suggests the possibility of using lauric acid in antiviral therapies (Angeles-Agdeppa et al. 2021; Ogedengbe et al. 2018). By enhancing the body's defenses against pathogens, lauric acid contributes to overall immune system health. Lauric acid is reported to improve digestion and metabolism, help stimulate immunity, and contribute to balancing a better serum lipid profile (Ramya et al. 2022). By enhancing the body's defenses against pathogens, bacteria, and fungus, lauric acid contributes to overall importance in promoting overall health and wellness, highlighting coconut's role as a natural source of beneficial compounds with therapeutic potential.

11.3.3 The Biochemical Functions of Coconut Bio-actives in Antioxidative Mechanisms

Coconut is not only a source of healthy fats but also a rich reservoir of phenolic compounds, which exhibit potent antioxidant properties (Karunasiri et al. 2020). Understanding the role of these compounds and their mechanisms is essential in appreciating the health benefits of coconut. Antioxidants play a crucial role in maintaining cellular health. They protect cells from oxidative damage, which is linked to various chronic diseases, including cancer, CVDs, and neurodegenerative disorders. Coconut's phenolic compounds contribute to this protection, potentially lowering the risk of such conditions (Narayanankutty et al. 2018). The antioxidant activity of coconut bioactives has been reported and phenolics play a major role. Phenolic compounds in coconut, including ferulic acid, p-coumaric acid, and gallic acid, possess strong antioxidant properties. They neutralize harmful free radicals in the body, reducing oxidative stress and inflammation. This antioxidative capacity is believed to underlie many of the health benefits associated with coconut consumption (Marina et al. 2009).

11.3.4 The Biochemical Functions of Coconut Bio-actives in Cellular Homeostasis

The clear liquid found inside young, green coconuts, known as coconut water, is frequently referred to as "nature's sports drink" because of its exceptional electrolyte profile. Since ancient times, this natural hydration source has been prized in tropical areas and is now known around the world for its advantages. Coconut water's electrolyte composition is similar to that of human plasma, making it an ideal hydrating solution. It contains essential electrolytes such as potassium, sodium, calcium, and magnesium. This balance of electrolytes not only aids in rehydration but also plays a vital role in maintaining cellular homeostasis (Yong et al. 2009; Zhang et al. 2020). Electrolytes are crucial for cellular function. They help regulate the flow of water in and out of cells, ensuring proper hydration. This is essential for maintaining cellular integrity, as dehydration can lead to cell shrinkage and dysfunction. Coconut water's electrolyte profile supports cellular hydration, benefiting various physiological processes (Campbell-Falck et al. 2000). During physical activity or in hot climates, the body loses electrolytes through sweat. Replenishing these electrolytes with coconut water helps restore fluid and electrolyte balance, preventing issues like muscle cramps and heat exhaustion.

11.3.5 The Biochemical Functions of Coconut Bio-actives and Digestive Health

Coconut contains dietary fiber, a component that has several notable effects on digestive health. Coconut fiber primarily consists of insoluble fiber that is rich in cellulose, hemicellulose, and lignin. Coconut meat provides about 9 g of fiber for every 100 g of consumption (FoodData Central—Coconut Meat n.d.). Dietary fiber, including that from coconut, adds bulk to the stool, which helps prevent constipation. It promotes regular bowel movements by softening the stool and encouraging its efficient passage through the digestive tract. This can relieve discomfort and reduce the risk of digestive issues (Khalid et al. 2022). Coconut fiber also plays a role in supporting a healthy gut microbiome. The fiber serves as a substrate for beneficial gut bacteria, allowing them to thrive and produce SCFAs, which have various health benefits. A balanced gut microbiome is associated with improved digestion and overall well-being (Fu et al. 2022). A diet rich in dietary fiber, such as that found in coconut, is linked to a reduced risk of digestive disorders like diverticulitis (Aune et al. 2011), irritable bowel syndrome (IBS) (Yan et al. 2020), and colorectal cancer (Masrul and Nindrea 2019). These health benefits highlight the importance of including fiber-rich foods like coconut in one's diet.

VCOs constitute an important part of the diet comprising triglycerides and lauric acid, get hydrolyzed by the lipase enzymes present in the gastrointestinal tract

(GIT), mainly in the stomach and intestine get effectively absorbed and transported in the body (Khalid et al. 2022).

11.4 Clinical and Therapeutic Applications

11.4.1 Cardiovascular System: Lipid Profiles, Atherogenic Index, and Endothelial Function

CVD is a primary concern worldwide, and coconut has garnered attention for its potential impact on various cardiovascular parameters. Studies have extensively investigated the effects of coconut consumption on lipid profiles. These include high-density lipoprotein cholesterol (HDL-C), low-density lipoprotein cholesterol (LDL-C), triglycerides, and total cholesterol. The hypercholesterolemic effect associated with coconut oil consumption is largely attributed to its elevated saturated fat content, which is believed to diminish LDL receptor activity and mRNA abundance. In comparison to butter, coconut oil presents a more favorable lipid profile by elevating HDL-C levels and lowering LDL-C levels. This distinction could be due to the differing chain lengths of fatty acids present in coconut oil and animal fats, despite both being saturated fat sources. While animal fats primarily contain LCFAs, coconut oil is abundant in MCFAs, particularly lauric acid. These MCFAs exhibit reduced potential for promoting insulin resistance, inflammation, and fat accumulation compared to LCFAs like stearic acid found in butter (Jayawardena et al. 2020). One significant discovery is coconut oil's capacity to elevate HDL-C, often referred to as "good" cholesterol. HDL-C plays a vital role in eliminating excess cholesterol from the bloodstream, thereby reducing the risk of atherosclerosis. The ability of coconut oil to boost HDL-C levels while maintaining LDL-C levels holds promise for cardiovascular health (Sekhar et al. 2022). However, the ongoing debate surrounding the potential benefits of coconut oil and its lipid components requires thorough examination for a definitive conclusion.

Another important feature includes the atherogenic index, which is considered as a valuable indicator of cardiovascular risk. It assesses the balance between beneficial HDL-C and harmful LDL-C (Dobiášová 2006). Coconut consumption, especially tender and mature coconut water, has shown hypocholesterolemic effects that favor the index by increasing the HDL-to-LDL cholesterol ratio. This shift towards a more favorable lipid profile suggests a potential protective effect against atherosclerosis and coronary artery disease (Sekhar et al. 2022).

Endothelial dysfunction is a hallmark of CVD. Impaired endothelial function contributes to the development of atherosclerosis and hypertension (Hadi et al. 2005). Nurul-Iman et al. (2013) treated rats with VCO confirming the supplementation was capable of preventing the elevation in the blood pressure. It, however, didn't influence the relaxation but significantly decreased vasoconstriction of the endothelial lines. These studies and emerging evidence suggest that certain components in coconut, particularly phenolic compounds (Mahayothee et al. 2016), may have a positive impact on endothelial function. These compounds can help improve the dilation and relaxation of blood vessels, promoting healthy blood flow and reducing the risk of hypertension (Di Pietro et al. 2020).

11.4.2 Neurological Insights: Potential Modulation of Amyloidogenic Pathways

Neurological disorder, AD is characterized by memory loss and cognitive decline, with the gradual death of the brain cells leading to the progressive development of mild dementia to severe impairments. The fundamental biochemical characteristics contributing to the pathogenesis of AD include the formation of extracellular amyloid β plaques and the accumulation of intracellular neurofibrillary tangles (Kocahan and Doğan 2017). CVD, marked by elevated LDL-C levels, hypertension, T2DM, obesity, and insulin resistance, represent significant risk factors associated with the rising incidence of AD, and evidence supports that MCTs present in coconut oil undergo metabolism and absorption processes that mitigate the severity of these physiological risk factors (Sandupama et al. 2022). Cholesterol acts as an antioxidant within the brain, for structural scaffolding of the neural network, as an electrical insulator to prevent ion leakage, and plays a pivotal role in the wrapping and synaptic delivery of neurotransmitters (Kappally et al. 2015). Hence cholesterol plays an important role in the formation and functioning of synapses in the brain. Recent research has explored the potential of coconut components to modulate amyloidogenic pathways, offering hope for AD management.

Ketones produced from the metabolism of coconut-derived MCTs (Jadhav and Annapure 2023) have demonstrated neuroprotective effects, providing an alternative fuel source for the brain. This shift in brain metabolism bypasses the energy deficits often seen in Alzheimer's patients, potentially slowing disease progression and improving cognitive function (Jensen et al. 2020). Additionally, a diet rich in saturated fats, such as those found in coconut oil, is essential for maintaining high HDL-C levels, particularly for individuals with deficiencies and neurological disorders (Rahilly et al. 2011). Coconut oil, rich in MCTs, offers a potential dietary intervention for AD by providing an alternative energy source in the form of ketones, which have been associated with improved cognitive function in patients (Reger et al. 2004).

AD, characterized by the accumulation of β-amyloid plaques in the brain, is a growing concern globally. Some studies suggest that phenolic compounds may inhibit the aggregation of amyloid β, a key player in Alzheimer's pathology (Hamaguchi et al. 2009). Phenolic compounds found in coconut, such as ferulic acid, p-coumaric acid, and gallic acid, have been shown to have strong antioxidant properties. These compounds may help neutralize free radicals in the brain, which are implicated in the formation of β-amyloid plaques. The antioxidative capacity of these phenolic compounds contributes to overall brain health (Sandupama et al. 2022). By preventing the formation of toxic amyloid plaques, coconut components may contribute to reducing the risk of AD or delaying its onset.

11.4.3 Immunological Responses: Anti-microbial, Anti-viral, and Inflammation Modulation

Coconut's bioactive components also exhibit remarkable immunological properties, impacting the body's ability to combat infections and manage inflammation.

Several studies have shown the potential antimicrobial effect of MCFAs especially lauric acid, a significant component of coconut and VCOs. The structural aspects and melting point of 40–45 °C interact effectively and disrupt the lipid membranes of bacteria, viruses, and fungi, rendering them susceptible to destruction. Incorporating coconut into the diet may support the body's defense against various pathogens (Casillas-Vargas et al. 2021). The monoglyceride from lauric acid, monolaurin, also exhibits potent antimicrobial activity against a wide range of pathogens. Coconut oil has shown effectiveness against a range of lipid-coated microorganisms, such as certain viruses and fungal species, expanding its antimicrobial spectrum. Studies have demonstrated coconut oil's ability to inhibit the growth of *Candida* species, and several bacteria and to reduce the growth rate of multi-antibiotic-resistant bacteria. From testing crude aqueous extracts of husk fibers against methicillin-resistant *Staphylococcus Aureus* (MRSA) and *S. aureus,* it has been found that the extracts are capable of limiting the growth of both organisms (Lima et al. 2015). These findings underscore the potential of coconut oil as a natural antimicrobial agent, prompting further exploration of its therapeutic applications (Deen et al. 2021). Recent studies have also shown that it helps in combating SARS-CoV-2 and reducing inflammatory markers like C-reactive protein (Nitbani et al. 2022).

Research indicates that lauric acid and monolaurin, along with other compounds in coconut, have antiviral properties, particularly against enveloped viruses. The MCFAs from coconut oil destroy and break the membranes and interfere with viral maturation (Lima et al. 2015). The promising results in clinical trials for its antiviral effects include reducing HIV viral load and increasing CD4+ T lymphocyte counts in HIV-infected patients have been confirmed due to the presence of lauric acid. Not only that, these studies provided a base for the treatment of novel viruses including SARS-CoV-2 (Deen et al. 2021). These findings open doors to potential antiviral therapies or preventive measures, particularly in the context of emerging viral infections (Angeles-Agdeppa et al. 2021).

Coconut's phenolic compounds contribute to its anti-inflammatory properties. Studies involving VCOs have demonstrated their anti-inflammatory properties by reducing the expression of inflammatory genes such as cyclooxygenase-2 (COX-2), inducible nitric oxide synthase (iNOS), and interleukin-6 (IL-6) (Deen et al. 2021).

Aqueous crude extracts of husk fiber consisting of multiple polyphenols are used to treat arthritis and other inflammatory illnesses in Northeastern Brazil's traditional medicine (Esquenazi et al. 2002). The inflammatory affection, both acute and chronic, reduces oxidative stress and inflammatory responses in the body. Chronic inflammation is implicated in various chronic diseases, and coconut's potential to modulate inflammation is a promising avenue for health promotion (Mahayothee et al. 2016).

11.4.4 Metabolic Modulation: Insights into Glycemic Control and Thermogenesis

Metabolic health is a critical aspect of overall well-being, and coconut components may play a role in modulating key metabolic processes. Emerging research suggests that MCTs found in coconut oil may aid in glycemic control. Consuming MCTs can lead to improved insulin sensitivity and better blood sugar regulation, making coconut a potential dietary choice for individuals with diabetes or those at risk of developing the condition (Thomas et al. 2019). Lauric acid and its effect on glucose uptake, mitochondrial function, and mitochondrial biogenesis in insulin-resistant macrophages have been reported. Lauric acid has been reported with the potential to improve insulin sensitivity and mitochondrial dysregulation in insulin-resistant macrophages (Tham et al. 2020). Coconut oil supplementation has been found to have a favorable effect on glycemic control, possibly through phenolic compounds mediating anti-inflammatory effects. A systematic meta-analysis study by Dhanasekara et al. (2022), revealed the effect of acute and long-term (i.e., >10 days) effects of coconut fat on glycemic control. Coconut fat in meals seems to be associated with a diminished postprandial insulin response, resulting in a subtle increase in the postprandial glycemic response. However long-term intake of coconut fat was observed with increased insulin resistance, yet does not seem to be beneficial for long-term glycemic control. The effect of lauric acid and the amino acid, tryptophan ('Trp') and its additive effect to reduce blood glucose are also reported. The duodenal infusion study by McVeay et al. (2019) moderately reduced plasma glucose compared with the control ($p < 0.05$). C12 + Trp, but not C12 or Trp, stimulated insulin and increased the insulin-to-glucose ratio ($p < 0.05$).

MCTs have been linked to increased thermogenesis, the process by which the body generates heat and burns calories, primarily occurring in brown adipose tissue (BAT). These tissues have high concentrations of mitochondria that are rich in iron coupled with the action of uncoupling protein 1 (UCP1) also known as thermogenin. The activation of BAT thermogenesis and the subsequent metabolic effect is linked to weight management and fat loss offering a potential mechanism for obesity prevention. Literature analysis has shown the ability of fatty acids to activate the UCP1 and the MCFAs found in coconut oil bring benefits in mitigating diabetes-related complications by reducing adiposity and preserving insulin sensitivity in muscle and adipose tissue. However, studies on coconut oil's effects on cholesterol levels yield conflicting results. Despite this, research on traditional coconut-consuming populations indicates favorable lipid profiles and lower heart disease rates, hinting at potential cardioprotective effects (Fabien et al. 2014). These metabolic effects may contribute to weight management and fat loss. Incorporating coconut oil or MCTs into the diet can potentially support individuals aiming to achieve and maintain a healthy body weight (LaBarrie and St-Onge 2017).

The safety of long-term consumption of coconut and its derivatives has been a subject of interest. Studies suggest that coconut can be a part of a healthy diet when consumed in moderation (Hewlings 2020). However, individuals with specific health conditions, such as CVDs, diabetes, or liver disorders, may need to monitor their coconut intake (Eyres et al. 2016). It is crucial to consider variations in individual responses, and consulting healthcare professionals for personalized advice is recommended.

11.5 Conclusion

Coconut is a fruit that has bioactive components with promising health-promoting properties starting from choir, meat, water, and the oils extracted from various parts within. The rich array of bioactive especially has led to the extraction of oil from coconut, VCO, that stands out for its medicinal and antibacterial properties, particularly attributed by MCFAs such as lauric acid. The MCFAs contribute to other health benefits due to the presence of dietary fibers among the functional polysaccharides, proteins, polyphenols, vitamins, and phytosterols. Studies based on MCTs in the oil have shown unique metabolic pathways that provide rapid energy, help in weight management, and may have therapeutic implications for neurological conditions like epilepsy and AD. VCOs are popular for their antioxidant and anti-inflammatory effects while phytosterols modulate the cholesterol in the body. Cytokinins present in coconut water have shown biomedical effects on mammalian cells and are essential for plant growth and development. Not only that, the impact of coconut on the lipid profiles, atherogenic index, and endothelial function suggests a potential role in cardiovascular health, though ongoing research is needed for definitive conclusions. Coconut has the potential to be a 'one-stop food' option in the near future as the essential nutrients exert antioxidant, anti-inflammatory, lipid-lowering, and immune-modulating effects supporting overall wellness. Several coconut-based products like coconut milk, coconut flour, and VCOs have been ruling the market due to their therapeutic importance. Moreover, coconut wastes can be reused for the production of diverse value-added food products, opening the potency of economic prosperity and environmental sustainability.

References

Agero ALC, Verallo-Rowell VM (2004) A randomized double-blind controlled trial comparing extra virgin coconut oil with mineral oil as a moisturizer for mild to moderate xerosis. DERM, 15(3), pp.109–116

Al-Khayri JM, Huang FH, Morelock TE, Busharar TA (1992) Spinach tissue culture improved with coconut water. HortScience 27(4):357–358

Angeles-Agdeppa I, Nacis JS, Capanzana MV, Dayrit FM, Tanda KV (2021) Virgin coconut oil is effective in lowering C-reactive protein levels among suspect and probable cases of COVID-19. J Funct Foods 83:104557

Arora R, Chawla R, Marwah R, Arora P, Sharma RK, Kaushik V, Goel R, Kaur A, Silambarasan M, Tripathi RP, Bhardwaj JR (2010) Potential of complementary and alternative medicine in preventive management of novel H1N1 flu (Swine flu) pandemic: thwarting potential disasters in the bud. Evid Based Complement Altern Med 2011:586506

Aune D, Chan DS, Lau R, Vieira R, Greenwood DC, Kampman E, Norat T (2011) Dietary fibre, whole grains, and risk of colorectal cancer: Systematic review and dose-response meta-analysis of prospective studies. BMJ 343:d6617

Babayan VK (1968) Medium-chain triglycerides-their composition, preparation, and application. J Am Oil Chem Soc 45:23–25

Barnabé W, de Mendonça NT, Pimenta FC, Pegoraro LF, Scolaro JM (2004) Efficacy of sodium hypochlorite and coconut soap used as disinfecting agents in the reduction of denture stomatitis, streptococcus mutans and Candida albicans. J Oral Rehabil 31(5):453–459

Campbell-Falck D, Thomas T, Falck TM, Tutuo N, Clem K (2000) The intravenous use of coconut water. Am J Emerg Med 18(1):108–111

Carpo BG, Verallo-Rowell VM, Kabara JJ (2007) Novel antibacterial activity of monolaurin compared with conventional antibiotics against organisms from skin infections: an in vitro study. J Drugs Dermatol 10:991–998

Casillas-Vargas G, Ocasio-Malavé C, Medina S, Morales-Guzmán C, Del Valle RG, Carballeira NM, Sanabria-Ríos DJ (2021) Antibacterial fatty acids: an update of possible mechanisms of action and implications in the development of the next-generation of antibacterial agents. Prog Lipid Res 82:101093

DebMandal M, Mandal S (2011) Coconut (Cocos nucifera L.: Arecaceae): in health promotion and disease prevention. Asian Pac J Trop Med 4(3):241–247

Deen A, Visvanathan R, Wickramarachchi D, Marikkar N, Nammi S, Jayawardana BC, Liyanage R (2021) Chemical composition and health benefits of coconut oil: an overview. J Sci Food Agric 101(6):2182–2193

Dhanasekara CS, Nelson A, Spradley M, Wynn A, Robohm-Leavitt C, Shen CL, Kahathuduwa CN (2022) Effects of consumption of coconut oil or coconut on glycemic control and insulin sensitivity: a systematic review and meta-analysis of interventional trials. Nutr Metab Cardiovasc Dis 32(1):53–68

Di Pietro N, Baldassarre MPA, Cichelli A, Pandolfi A, Formoso G, Pipino C (2020) Role of polyphenols and carotenoids in endothelial dysfunction: an overview from classic to innovative biomarkers. Oxidative Med Cell Longev 2020:1–19

Dobiášová M (2006) AIP—atherogenic index of plasma as a significant predictor of cardiovascular risk: from research to practice. Vnitr Lek 52(1):64–71

Enig MG (1999) Coconut: in support of good health in the 21st century. In 36th meeting of APCC

Esquenazi D, Wigg MD, Miranda MM, Rodrigues HM, Tostes JB, Rozental S, da Silva AJ, Alviano CS (2002) Antimicrobial and antiviral activities of polyphenolics from Cocos nucifera Linn. (Palmae) husk fiber extract. Res Microbiol 153(10):647–652

Eyres L, Eyres MF, Chisholm A, Brown RC (2016) Coconut oil consumption and cardiovascular risk factors in humans. Nutr Rev 74(4):267–280

Fabien DDF, Annie NN, Adélaide DM, Florian S, Inocent G (2014) Effect of heating and of short exposure to sunlight on carotenoids content of crude palm oil. J Food Process Technol 5(4):1

FoodData Central—Coconut Meat (n.d.) [National Website]. https://fdc.nal.usda.gov/fdc-app.html#/food-details/170169/nutrients. Accessed 10 July 2023
Fu J, Zheng Y, Gao Y, Xu W (2022) Dietary fiber intake and gut microbiota in human health. Microorganisms 10(12):2507
Ge L, Yong JWH, Tan SN, Yang XH, Ong ES (2006) Analysis of cytokinin nucleotides in coconut (Cocos nucifera L.) water using capillary zone electrophoresis-tandem mass spectrometry after solid-phase extraction. J Chromatogr 1133(1–2):322–331
Geronço MS, da Silveira Ramos IF, da Silva Filho EC, dos Santos Rizzo M, Ribeiro AB, da Costa MP (2021) Are structurally modified galactomannan derivatives biologically active? Polysaccharides 2(1):1–15
Gough SM, Casella A, Ortega KJ, Hackam AS (2021) Neuroprotection by the ketogenic diet: evidence and controversies. Front Nutr 8:782657
Guedes D, Martins GR, Jaramillo LYA, Simas Bernardes Dias D, da Silva AJR, Lutterbach MTS, Reznik LY, Sérvulo EFC, Alviano CS, Alviano DS (2021) Proanthocyanidins with corrosion inhibition activity for AISI 1020 carbon steel under neutral pH conditions of coconut (Cocos nucifera L.) husk fibers. ACS Omega 6(10):6893–6901
Hadi HAR, Carr CS, Al Suwaidi J (2005) Endothelial dysfunction: cardiovascular risk factors, therapy, and outcome. Vasc Health Risk Manag 1(3):183–198
Halim HH, Pak Dek MS, Hamid AA, Saari N, Mohd Lazim MI, Abas F, Ngalim A, Ismail A, Jaafar AH (2023) Novel sources of bioactive compounds in coconut (Cocos nucifera L.) water from different maturity levels and varieties as potent skin anti-aging strategies and anti-fatigue agents. Food Biosci 51:102326
Hamaguchi T, Ono K, Murase A, Yamada M (2009) Phenolic compounds prevent Alzheimer's pathology through different effects on the amyloid-β aggregation pathway. Am J Pathol 175(6):2557–2565
Hewlings S (2020) Coconuts and health: different chain lengths of saturated fats require different consideration. J Cardiovasc Dev Dis 7(4):59
Ishiaq O (2012) Bio-nutritional constituents of coconut fruit and its possible medicinal applications. African J Plant Sci 6:309–313
Jadhav HB, Annapure US (2023) Triglycerides of medium-chain fatty acids: a concise review. J Food Sci Technol 60(8):2143–2152
Jayawardena R, Swarnamali H, Lanerolle P, Ranasinghe P (2020) Effect of coconut oil on cardio-metabolic risk: a systematic review and meta-analysis of interventional studies. Diabetes Metab Syndr 14(6):2007–2020
Jensen NJ, Wodschow HZ, Nilsson M, Rungby J (2020) Effects of ketone bodies on brain metabolism and function in neurodegenerative diseases. Int J Mol Sci 21(22):8767
Joshi S, Kaushik V, Gode V, Mhaskar S (2020) Coconut oil and immunity: what do we really know about it so far? J Assoc Physicians India 68(7):67–72
Kannaian UPN, Edwin JB, Rajagopal V, Shankar SN, Srinivasan B (2020) Phytochemical composition and antioxidant activity of coconut cotyledon. Heliyon 6(2):e03411
Kappally S, Shirwaikar A, Shirwaikar A (2015) Coconut oil—a review of potential applications. Hygeia J D Med 7(2):34–41
Karunasiri AN, Gunawardane M, Senanayake CM, Jayathilaka N, Seneviratne KN (2020) Antioxidant and nutritional properties of domestic and commercial coconut milk preparations. Int J Food Sci 2020:1–9
Khalid W, Arshad MS, Jabeen A, Muhammad Anjum F, Qaisrani TB, Suleria HAR (2022) Fiber-enriched botanicals: a therapeutic tool against certain metabolic ailments. Food Sci Nutr 10(10):3203–3218
Khan M, Mahesh C, Semwal A, Sharma G (2015) Effect of virgin coconut meal (VCM) on the development of rice-based extruded snacks. Int J Adv Res 3:717–725
Kocahan S, Doğan Z (2017) Mechanisms of Alzheimer's disease pathogenesis and prevention: the brain, neural pathology, N-methyl-D-aspartate receptors, tau protein and other risk factors. Clin Psychopharmacol Neurosci 15(1):1

LaBarrie J, St-Onge M-P (2017) A coconut oil-rich meal does not enhance thermogenesis compared to corn oil in a randomized trial in obese adolescents. Insights Nutr Metab 1(1):30–36
Lal J, Kumar CS, Indira M (2003) Coconut palm. In: Caballero B (ed) Encyclopedia of food sciences and nutrition, 2nd edn. Academic Press, London, pp 1464–1475
Li Y, Zheng Y, Zhang Y, Liu L, Zhao S (2016) Purification, characterization, synthesis, in vivo and in vitro antihypertensive activity of bioactive peptides derived from coconut (Cocos nucifera L.) cake globulin hydrolysates. RSC Adv 6(95):92688–92698
Lima E, Sousa C, Meneses L, Ximenes N, Santos Júnior M, Vasconcelos G, Lima N, Patrocínio M, Macedo D, Vasconcelos S (2015) Cocos nucifera (L.) (Arecaceae): a phytochemical and pharmacological review. Braz J Med Biol Res 48(11):953–964
Mahayothee B, Koomyart I, Khuwijitjaru P, Siriwongwilaichat P, Nagle M, Müller J (2016) Phenolic compounds, antioxidant activity, and medium chain fatty acids profiles of coconut water and meat at different maturity stages. Int J Food Prop 19(9):2041–2051
Mandal SM, Dey S, Mandal M, Sarkar S, Maria-Neto S, Franco OL (2009) Identification and structural insights of three novel antimicrobial peptides isolated from green coconut water. Peptides 30(4):633–637
Marina AM, Che Man YB, Nazimah SAH, Amin I (2009) Antioxidant capacity and phenolic acids of virgin coconut oil. Int J Food Sci Nutr 60(Suppl 2):114–123
Masrul M, Nindrea RD (2019) Dietary fibre protective against colorectal cancer patients in Asia: a meta-analysis. Open Access Maced J Med Sci 7(10):1723–1727
Mat K, Abdul Kari Z, Rusli ND, Che Harun H, Wei LS, Rahman MM, Mohd Khalid HN, Mohd Ali Hanafiah MH, Mohamad Sukri SA, Raja Khalif RIA, Mohd Zin Z, Mohd Zainol MK, Panadi M, Mohd Nor MF, Goh KW (2022) Coconut palm: food, feed, and nutraceutical properties. Animals 12(16):2107
McVeay C, Fitzgerald PCE, Horowitz M, Feinle-Bisset C (2019) Effects of duodenal infusion of lauric acid and l-tryptophan, alone and combined, on fasting glucose, insulin and glucagon in healthy men. Nutrients 11(11):2697
Mumme K, Stonehouse W (2015) Effects of medium-chain triglycerides on weight loss and body composition: a meta-analysis of randomized controlled trials. J Acad Nutr Diet 115(2):249–263
Narayanankutty A, Illam SP, Raghavamenon AC (2018) Health impacts of different edible oils prepared from coconut (Cocos nucifera): a comprehensive review. Trends Food Sci Technol 80:1–7
Ngampeerapong C, Chavasit V (2019) Nutritional and bioactive compounds in coconut meat of different sources: Thailand, Indonesia and Vietnam. Chiang Mai Univ J Nat Sci 18(4):562–573
Nitbani FO, Tjitda PJP, Nitti F, Jumina J, Detha AIR (2022) Antimicrobial properties of lauric acid and monolaurin in virgin coconut oil: a review. ChemBioEng Rev 9(5):442–461
Nurul-Iman BS, Kamisah Y, Jaarin K, Qodriyah HMS (2013) Virgin coconut oil prevents blood pressure elevation and improves endothelial functions in rats fed with repeatedly heated palm oil. Evid Based Complement Alternat Med 2013:629329
Odenigbo UM, Otisi CAO (2011) Fatty acids and phytochemical contents of different coconut seed flesh in Nigeria. Int J Plant Physiol Biochem 3(11):176–182
Ogedengbe OO, Naidu ECS, Akang EN, Offor U, Onanuga IO, Peter AI, Jegede AI, Azu OO (2018) Virgin coconut oil extract mitigates testicular-induced toxicity of alcohol use in antiretroviral therapy. Andrology 6(4):616–626
Padumadasa C, Dharmadana D, Abeysekera A, Thammitiyagodage M (2016) In vitro antioxidant, anti-inflammatory and anticancer activities of ethyl acetate soluble proanthocyanidins of the inflorescence of Cocos nucifera L. BMC Complement Altern Med 16(1):345
Panonnummal R, Gopinath D, Thankappan Presanna A, Viswanad V, Mangalathillam S (2021) Non alcoholic palm nectar from Cocos nucifera as a promising nutraceutical preparation. J Food Biochem 46(4):e13900
Prades A, Dornier M, Diop N, Pain JP (2012) Coconut water uses, composition and properties: a review. Fruits 67(2):87–107
Prasad M, Jayaraman S, Eladl MA, Abdelrahman MA, Veeraraghavan VP, Vengadassalapathy S, Umapathy VR, Jaffer Hussain SF, Krishnamoorthy K, Sekar D, Palanisamy CP, Mohan SK,

Rajagopal P (2021) A comprehensive review on therapeutic perspectives of phytosterols in insulin resistance: a mechanistic approach. Molecules 27(5):1595

Qadi W, Mediani A, Benchoula K, Wong E, Misnan N, Sani N (2023) Characterization of physicochemical, biological, and chemical changes associated with coconut milk fermentation and correlation revealed by 1H NMR-based metabolomics. Foods 12(10):1971

Radenahmad N, Vongvatcharanon U, Withyachumnarnkul B, Connor RJ (2006) Serum levels of 17β-estradiol in ovariectomized rats fed young-coconut-juice and its effect on wound healing. Songklanakarin J Sci Technol 28(5):897–910

Rahilly TCR, Spiro A, Vokonas P, Gaziano JM (2011) Relation between high-density lipoprotein cholesterol and survival to age 85 years in men. Am J Cardiol 107(8):1173–1177

Ramesh S, Krishnan V, Praveen S, Hebbar K (2021) Dietary prospects of coconut oil for the prevention and treatment of Alzheimer's disease (AD): a review of recent evidences. Trends Food Sci Technol 112:201–211

Ramesh SV, Pandiselvam R, Thushara R et al (2020) Engineering intervention for production of virgin coconut oil by hot process and multivariate analysis of quality attributes of virgin coconut oil extracted by various methods. J Food Process Eng 43:e13395. https://doi.org/10.1111/jfpe.13395

Ramya V, Shyam KP, Kowsalya E, Balavigneswaran CK, Kadalmani B (2022) Dual roles of coconut oil and its major component lauric acid on redox nexus: focus on cytoprotection and cancer cell death. Front Neurosci 16:833630

Reger MA, Henderson ST, Hale C, Cholerton B, Baker LD, Watson GS, Hyde K, Chapman D, Craft S (2004) Effects of betahydroxybutyrate on cognition in memory-impaired adults. Neurobiol Aging 25(3):311–314

Rohman A, Irnawati, Erwanto Y, Lukitaningsih E, Rafi M, Fadzilah NA, Windarsih A, Sulaiman A, Zakaria Z (2021) Virgin coconut oil: extraction, physicochemical properties, biological activities and its authentication analysis. Food Rev Int 37(1):46–66

Sandupama P, Munasinghe D, Jayasinghe M (2022) Coconut oil as a therapeutic treatment for Alzheimer's disease: a review. J Future Foods 2(1):41–52

Sekhar S, Makaram Ravinarayan S, Kashmer D, Yu A, Kilic F, Dhawan R, Sidhu R, Elazrag SE, Bijoora M, Mohammed L (2022) Are we nuts over coconuts? Studying the effects of coconut oil on low-density lipoprotein and cardiovascular diseases: a systematic review. Cureus 14(4):e24212

Seneviratne KN, Sudarshana Dissanayake DM (2008) Variation of phenolic content in coconut oil extracted by two conventional methods. Int J Food Sci Technol 43:597–602

Seo CW (2022) Effect of galactomannan addition on rheological, physicochemical, and microbial properties of cultured sour cream. Food Sci Biotechnol 31(5):571–577

Shah ND, Limketkai BN (2017) The use of medium-chain triglycerides in gastrointestinal disorders. Pract Gastroenterol 160:20–25

St-Onge M-P, Mayrsohn B, O'Keeffe M, Kissileff HR, Choudhury AR, Laferrère B (2014) Impact of medium and long chain triglycerides consumption on appetite and food intake in overweight men. Eur J Clin Nutr 68(10):1134–1140

Taheri JB, Espineli FW, Lu H, Asayesh M, Bakhshi M, Nakhostin MR, Hooshmand B (2010) Antimicrobial effect of coconut flour on oral microflora: an in vitro study. Res J Biol Sci 5(6):456–459

Tham YY, Choo QC, Muhammad TST, Chew CH (2020) Lauric acid alleviates insulin resistance by improving mitochondrial biogenesis in THP-1 macrophages. Mol Biol Rep 47:9595–9607

Thomas DD, Stockman M-C, Yu L, Meshulam T, McCarthy AC, Ionson A, Burritt N, Deeney J, Cabral H, Corkey B, Istfan N, Apovian CM (2019) Effects of medium chain triglycerides supplementation on insulin sensitivity and beta cell function: a feasibility study. PLoS One 14(12):e0226200

Trinidad TP, Mallillin AC, Valdez DH, Loyola AS, Askali-Mercado FC, Castillo JC, Encabo RR, Masa DB, Maglaya AS, Chua MT (2006) Dietary fiber from coconut flour: a functional food. Innov Food Sci Emerg Technol 7:309–317

Ulug SK, Jahandideh F, Wu J (2021) Novel technologies for the production of bioactive peptides. Trends Food Sci Technol 108:27–39
Wang HX, Ng TB (2005) An antifungal peptide from the coconut. Peptides, 26(12), pp.2392–2396
Watanabe S, Tsujino S (2022) Applications of medium-chain triglycerides in foods. Front Nutr 9:802805
Yan R, Murphy M, Genoni A, Marlow E, Dunican IC, Lo J, Andrew L, Devine A, Christophersen CT (2020) Does Fibre-fix provided to people with irritable bowel syndrome who are consuming a low FODMAP diet improve their gut health, gut microbiome, sleep and mental health? A double-blinded, randomised controlled trial. BMJ Open Gastroenterol 7(1):e000448
Yong JW, Ge L, Ng YF, Tan SN (2009) The chemical composition and biological properties of coconut (Cocos nucifera L.) water. Molecules 14(12):5144–5164
Zeb A (2021) A comprehensive review on different classes of polyphenolic compounds present in edible oils. Food Res Int 143:110312
Zeng J, Xiao T, Ni X, Wei T, Liu X, Deng ZY, Li J (2022) The comparative analysis of different oil extraction methods based on the quality of flaxseed oil. J Food Compos Anal 107:104373
Zeng Y-Q, He J-T, Hu B-Y, Li W, Deng J, Lin Q-L, Fang Y (2024) Virgin coconut oil: a comprehensive review of antioxidant activity and mechanisms contributed by phenolic compounds. Crit Rev Food Sci Nutr 64(4):1052–1075
Zhang X, Peng L, Dai Y, Sheng X, Chen S, Xie Q (2020) Effects of coconut water on retina in diabetic rats. Evid Based Complement Alternat Med 2020:1–7
Zheng Y, Li Y, Li G (2019) ACE-inhibitory and antioxidant peptides from coconut cake albumin hydrolysates: purification, identification and synthesis. RSC Adv 9(11):5925–5593

Chapter 12
Policy Issues and Trade Potential of Coconut: A Global Outlook

S. Jayasekhar and Vimala Thomas

Abstract Policymakers and planners from the world's coconut-growing nations face formidable challenges from the liberalization of the coconut sector's marketing and trade regimes. At a time when the global coconut industry is confronting numerous difficult problems such as low productivity, pest and disease outbreaks, price swings, unstable domestic marketing systems, a recession in the trade sector, and so on, this is especially true. Topics covered in this chapter include the current state of affairs in coconut sector on a global scale, the difficulties encountered by the world's leading coconut-producing nations, the state of international trade, the level of global competitiveness, the analysis of prices, and the outlook for the future of the global coconut economy. The analysis utilized various data sources, including the UN Comtrade database, Statistical Year Book of International Coconut Community, and regional data sets. The high level of concentration in the production, exports, and imports of the coconut sector indicates that the sector is highly vulnerable to even minor disruptions in supply and market conditions.

Keywords Coconut productivity · Product diversification · Economic analysis · Trade dynamics

12.1 Introduction

Given the importance of coconuts as a source of income and employment in rural areas, they play a significant role in the national economies of countries that grow them. This vital sector, not only supports the livelihoods of millions, but also contributes significantly to global trade and commerce. According to recent statistics, the global area of coconut spans over 12 million hectares, with Asia-Pacific nations like Indonesia, the Philippines, and India leading in cultivation, accounting for over

S. Jayasekhar (✉) · V. Thomas
ICAR-Central Plantation Crops Research Institute, Kasaragod, Kerala, India
e-mail: jayasekhar.s@icar.gov.in

S. V. Ramesh, S. Praveen (eds.), *Coconut-Based Nutrition and Nutraceutical Perspectives*, https://doi.org/10.1007/978-981-97-3976-9_12

90% of the world's coconut production. Annually, the coconut sector yields a staggering output of over 66 billion nuts, catering to a burgeoning demand for coconut-based products both domestically and internationally. In the past decade, coconut production, productivity, and trade have remained stagnant, despite the economic significance of the coconut palm (Jayasekhar and Chandran 2021; Sairam and Jayasekhar 2018). Global plantation economies were integrated after the World Trade Agreement (WTA) and the ASEAN Treaty regime, leading to intense competition among producing nations. Currently, coconut farmers face greater vulnerability to economic risks and uncertainties due to the significant volatility in prices. In order to improve the future of the coconut industry, it is crucial to reduce its reliance on coconut oil, and increase the production of a variety of higher-value products (Sportel and Véron 2016; Muralidharan et al. 2019). The recent trend has shown a significant increase in the production of various value-added products derived from coconut processing. The processing sectors across the coconut growing regions in the world, and the international trade in particular have been experiencing the new dynamics. Researching the global competitiveness, performance, and trade patterns of coconuts and coconut products is essential for every country that grows coconuts if they want to capitalize on these new opportunities in the global market. Against this backdrop, there arises a compelling need for a comprehensive study to delve into the complexities of the global coconut sector. The chapter attempts to illustrate the global scenario of the coconut sector by narrating the production, trade, competitiveness, and price aspects of the sector. Multiple data sources such as UN Comtrade database, statistical year book of international coconut community, and regional data sets were used for the data gathering (UN Comtrade 2024).

12.2 Area, Production, and Productivity of Coconut

Coconut cultivation is geographically widespread, with countries such as the Philippines, Indonesia, India, Sri Lanka, and Papua New Guinea playing a significant role. Analysis of the spatial data provides interesting revelations about changing cultivation areas and trends in productivity, which have a significant impact on global supply dynamics. The Philippines has the highest share of coconut cultivation worldwide, representing 29.75% of the total area, with Indonesia closely following at 27.53%. India has a cultivation area that accounts for 17.94% of the total, making it the third largest coconut growing region in the world. Sri Lanka follows with 3.62% and Papua New Guinea with 1.81% (Fig. 12.1). The Philippines and Indonesia have exhibited comparable trend in areas, with a slight decrease observed for the latter in recent times (Fig. 12.2).

Coconut production (in whole nuts), exhibits variation among different countries. India takes the lead with 31% of the global production, followed by the Philippines (22%), and Indonesia (21%). Sri Lanka and Papua New Guinea account for 4.6% and 2.2% of the global production, respectively. India has consistently outperformed other countries in terms of production, while Indonesia and the

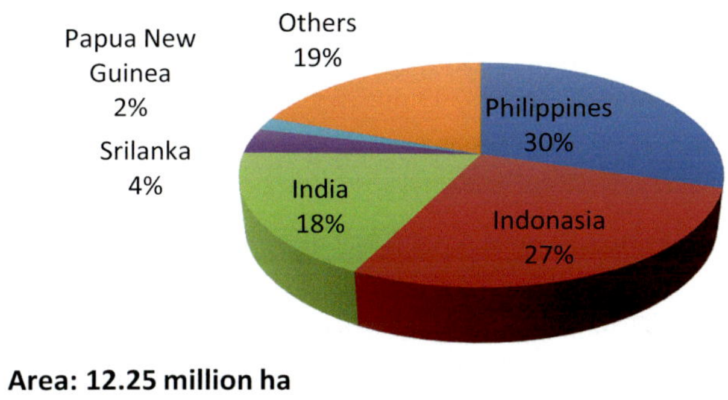

Fig. 12.1 Global distribution of area under coconut cultivation

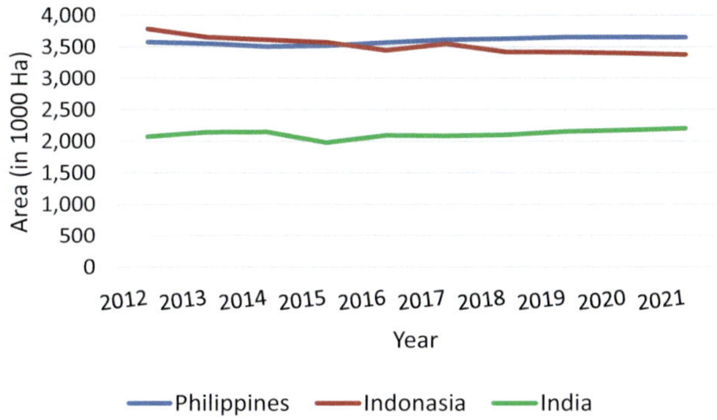

Fig. 12.2 Trend in area among major coconut producing countries

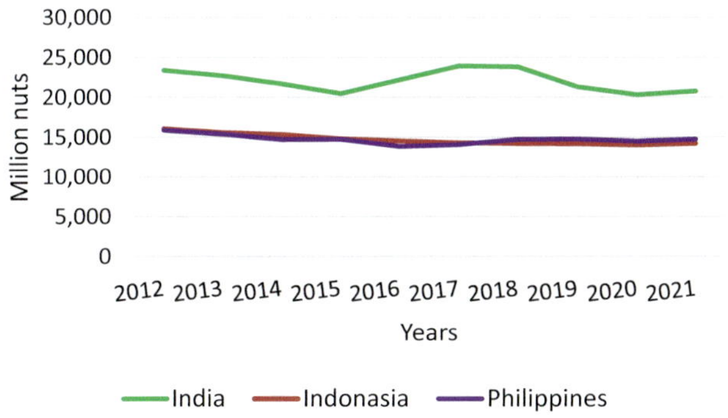

Fig. 12.3 Trend in production among major coconut producing countries

Philippines have exhibited a comparable pattern (Fig. 12.3). Regarding productivity, Jamaica has the highest yield with 10,438 nuts/ha, followed by India with 9430 nuts/ha, and Vietnam with 8393 nuts/ha.

12.3 Trade Dynamics of Coconut and Coconut Products

12.3.1 Production and Consumption

The coconut sector includes several value added products, mainly, coconut oil, copra, desiccated coconut, coconut milk, and coconut shell charcoal, in addition to raw coconuts. Comprehending the patterns of production for these products offers significant understanding of the dynamics of value chains and the respective economic contributions of various countries. Over the years, there has been a consistent increase in the global production of copra and coconut oil, suggesting a rising demand for these coconut products. On the other hand, the production of desiccated coconut has remained relatively stable, consistently staying below one million tonnes per year (Fig. 12.4). The variation in production patterns implies different levels of demand and utilization, for various coconut products in the global market.

After carefully examining the data sources, it turns out that the Philippines is the leading producer of coconut oil, with a production of 1297 thousand tonnes. Followed by Indonesia with 777 thousand tonnes and India with 567 thousand tonnes. The Philippines is the top producer of desiccated coconut, with a production of 234,000 tonnes. Indonesia follows closely with 187,000 tonnes, and India comes in third with 138,000 tonnes. Furthermore, it is noteworthy that the European Union is the largest estimated domestic consumer of coconut oil, while the Philippines holds the highest estimated domestic consumption of desiccated coconut.

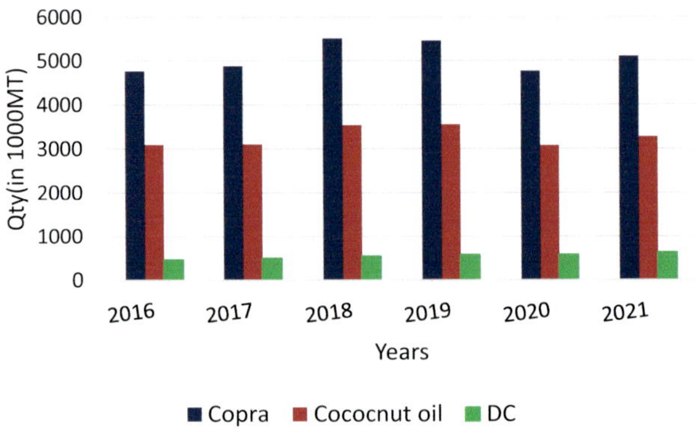

Fig. 12.4 Temporal pattern of production in major coconut products

12.3.2 Global Scenario of Exports and Imports

Trade patterns within the coconut sector further exemplify its global significance, with countries engaging in both export and import activities to meet domestic demands and capitalize on international markets. Analysis of trade data uncovers the leading exporters and importers of various coconut products, highlighting competitive advantages, market dynamics, and emerging trends.

According to the data source, the top three countries for coconut oil exports globally are the Philippines (42%), Indonesia (30%), and Malaysia (9%). Despite minor fluctuations in export volumes over the years, these countries consistently maintain their positions (Fig. 12.5). Conversely, in the case of desiccated coconut, the trend reveals the dominance of the Philippines (30%), followed by Indonesia (25%), and Sri Lanka (7%). Although the Philippines experienced a decline in exports in 2015, it has since rebounded and emerged as a potential competitor to Indonesia on the global stage, as depicted in Fig. 12.6. Vietnam and Indonesia emerge as potential export competitors in the coconut shell charcoal industry. Thailand leads in coconut milk exports (37%), followed by Indonesia (24%), and Sri Lanka (17%). Thailand is the leading country worldwide in terms of coconut sugar exports, with a dominant market share of 78%.

The global import scenario for the coconut sector is characterized by intricate supply chains and diverse consumer preferences. Various countries engage in importing coconut products to meet domestic demands, supplement local production, and capitalize on specific market niches. According to recent observations, Europe stands out as the primary importer of coconut oil, accounting for 39% of global imports, followed by the United States of America at 26%, with Asia constituting 15% of the total imports. Notably, both the US and Asia have experienced decline in coconut oil imports over time (Fig. 12.7). In the case of desiccated coconut, the United States holds the largest share of imports at 29%, followed by Europe at 25% and Asia at 17%. While the trend in desiccated coconut imports has shown continuous growth for the United States and Asia, there has been a slight decrease for Europe (Fig. 12.8).

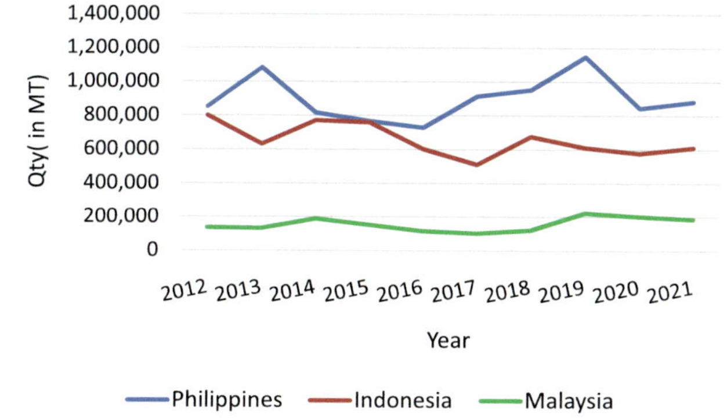

Fig. 12.5 Trend in coconut oil exports among major exporters (2012–2021)

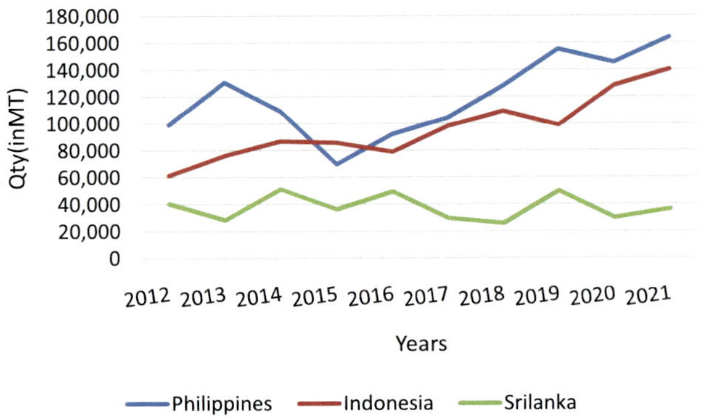

Fig. 12.6 Trend in desiccated coconut exports among major exporters (2012–2021)

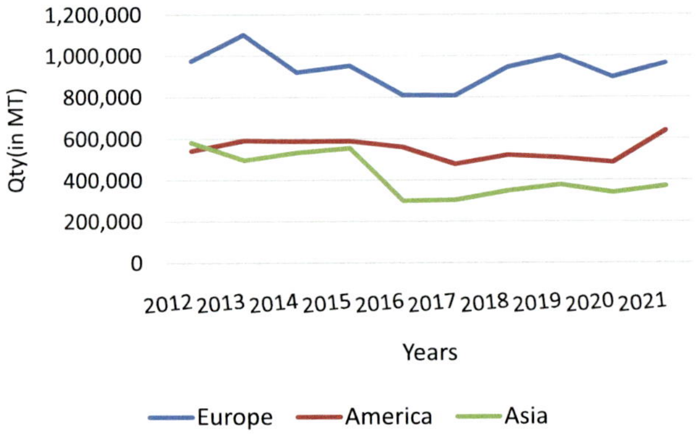

Fig. 12.7 Trend in coconut oil imports among major importers (2012–2021)

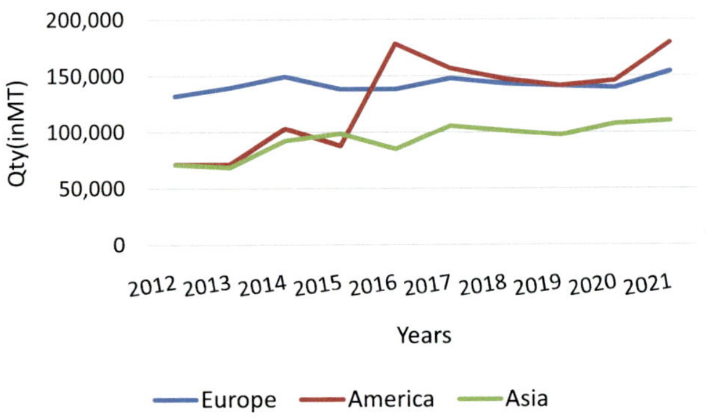

Fig. 12.8 Trend in desiccated coconut imports among major importers (2012–2021)

12.4 Price Analysis of Coconut Products

An analysis of the average annual price of coconut and its products can provide valuable insights into the trends and fluctuations in pricing dynamics. Analyzing the compound annual growth rate (CAGR) of coconut prices over 2012–2021 reveals the comparative price pattern of major coconut products (Table 12.1). Copra prices, with a CAGR of 0.089, show a moderate growth trend, indicating a low but consistent demand of copra over the specified time period. Coconut oil prices have shown a CAGR of 0.282, suggesting a slightly better growth rate compared to copra. However, both copra and coconut oil prices have demonstrated a positive growth trend, albeit at a slower pace. The CAGR of copra meal is −0.084, indicating a negative growth rate. The prices of desiccated coconut show a CAGR of 0.0551, implying the highest growth trend in prices among all other coconut products. Coconut milk has a negative CAGR of −0.814, which may be indicative of challenges or shifts in consumer preferences affecting the coconut milk market.

Products with positive growth rates in prices, such as copra, coconut oil, and desiccated coconut, indicate potential opportunities for expansion and increasing market demand. On the other hand, the observed negative growth rate for coconut milk and copra meal underscores the necessity for additional analysis to comprehend the factors causing the decline and investigate strategies for improved price realization.

Along with the growth rates, the stability analysis of the prices of coconut products is also pertinent. The price fluctuations (instability) in major coconut products were analyzed using the Coppock Instability Index (CII), which is calculated as the antilog of the square root of the logarithmic variance of the prices over a period of time (Coppock 1962; Radhakrishnan et al. 2016; Rajani et al. 2023). The Coppock instability index is a close approximation of the average year-to-year percentage variation adjusted for trend. A higher numerical value for the index represents greater instability, and vice versa. The instabilty indices of the prices of coconut products over the period 2012–2021 are depicted in Table 12.1.

The volatility of coconut oil prices has been significantly higher than that of other major coconut products during the period being analyzed. It is worth mentioning that the prices of all other coconut products, with the exception of coconut oil, have undergone similar fluctuations between 2012 and 2021.

Table 12.1 Compound annual growth rates and price instability of major coconut products (2012–2021)

S.No.	Coconut product	CAGR	Coppock's instability index
1	Copra	0.089	40.58
2	Coconut oil	0.282	46.90
3	Copra meal	−0.084	38.40
4	Desiccated coconut	0.551	39.21
5	Coconut milk	−0.814	38.67

Over recent decades, there has been a significant surge in both the supply and demand of coconuts and coconut-derived products globally, making the industry a key contributor to the economies of producer nations. However, like other agricultural sectors, the coconut industry has grappled with price fluctuations, highlighting the importance of reliable price modeling and forecasting techniques to alleviate pressure on stakeholders along the value chain.

Current coconut price forecasting primarily relies on time series models, predominantly univariate ones, which limit the analysis to a single variable despite the complex interactions inherent in coconut pricing systems. A major drawback of existing price modeling studies is the oversight of interconnected factors such as prices, production, climatic variables, and their interactions within the system. Therefore, there's a pressing need to enhance current approaches to coconut price modeling and forecasting by adopting a systems approach, integrating other influential variables. This holistic approach aims to produce more realistic forecast values, enabling the industry to adapt effectively to its evolving circumstances (Abeysekara and Waidyarathne 2020).

12.5 Coconut Sector of Major Countries

An in-depth examination of the coconut sectors in the Philippines, Indonesia, and India offers a comprehensive understanding of the global coconut industry. These countries, distinguished by their extensive coconut cultivation areas, substantial production volumes, and significant economic contributions, provide adequate economic insights into the dynamics of coconut sector.

12.5.1 Philippines

With its sprawling coconut plantations, lush landscapes, and millions of smallholder farmers, the Philippines boasts a rich and vibrant coconut sector that has been integral to the country's economy and cultural heritage for centuries. The Philippines stands as the global leader in coconut cultivation, with a vast area of 3.647 million hectares of coconuts, comprising nearly 29.75% of the world's total coconut acreage. With a production capacity of 14,717 million nuts, the nation balances its domestic demand, which consumes 4305 million coconut nuts annually with productivity of 4035 nuts/ha. Emerging as a formidable force in the international market, the Philippines contributes significantly to its economy, with coconut products constituting 3.4% of the country's total export earnings. Notably, coconut oil spearheads the export volume at 50%, closely trailed by copra meal at 18%, and desiccated coconut at 9% (Table 12.2). While the export of coconut oil exhibits a fluctuating trend with a recent downturn, desiccated coconut and shell charcoal maintain relatively stable export volumes, each hovering around 0.2 million metric

Table 12.2 Export volume (share) of coconut products from Philippines

S.No.	Coconut product	Export volume (MT)	Export share (%)
1	Coconut oil	881,085	50
2	Copra meal	323,806	18
3	Desiccated coconut	163,811	9
4	Coconut shell charcoal	113,618	7
5	Coconut milk(liquid)	22,623	1
6	Coco fiber products	111,681	6
7	Coconut water	13,364	1
9	Others	137,497	8
	Total	1,775,165	100

Source: UNCOMTRADE (https://comtradeplus.un.org/)

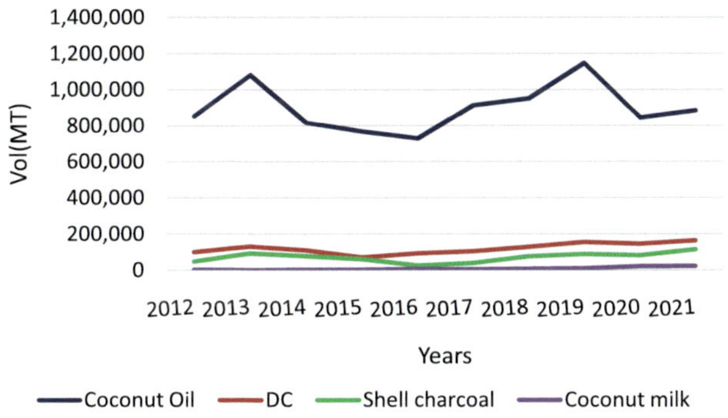

Fig. 12.9 Trend in exports of coconut products from the Philippines (2012–2021)

tonnes. In contrast, coconut milk demonstrates consistent and stable production over the span of a decade (Fig. 12.9). European nations, followed by America, emerge as the primary destinations for most coconut products in the Philippines' export market.

The current capacity utilization rates for coconut oil mills in the Philippines stand at 56%, while desiccated coconut mills operate at 41% capacity. A comparative analysis of average annual domestic prices against global annual prices facilitates a fair understanding of potential income enhancement avenues across various coconut products. Domestic coconut oil prices demonstrate close integration with global annual prices, with recent upticks observed in the international market (Fig. 12.10). Conversely, world desiccated coconut prices consistently surpass domestic prices over an extended duration, showcasing a pattern of integration with occasional divergences (Fig. 12.11). This juxtaposition highlights opportunities for strategic pricing adjustments to maximize revenue streams in the desiccated coconut sector.

It is pertinent to note that, in addition to traditional coconut products, the Philippines has diversified its export portfolio to include innovative offerings such as coconut acid oil, Makapuno, and coconut water, each commanding a significant

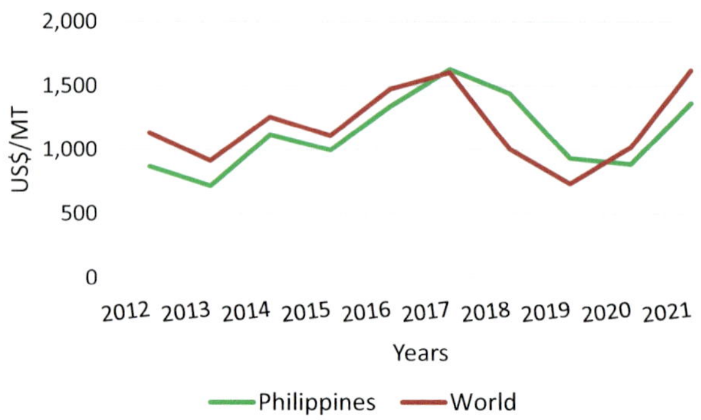

Fig. 12.10 Price movement of coconut oil (Philippines & World)

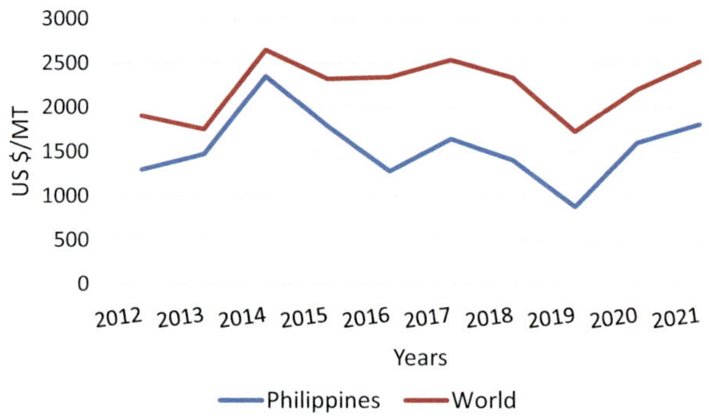

Fig. 12.11 Price movement of desiccated coconut (Philippines & World)

market share. Despite being one of the world's largest coconut producers, the Philippines struggles with outdated farming practices, pest infestations, and the need for replanting initiatives to rejuvenate aging coconut plantations.

12.5.2 Indonesia

Indonesia, with its vast archipelago spanning thousands of islands, stands as a significant player in the global coconut industry. The coconut sector in Indonesia is not only a vital component of the country's agricultural landscape but also plays a crucial role in rural livelihoods, economic development, and global trade. Indonesia has 3.374 million ha of area for coconut cultivation, which is almost 27.53% globally. They produce around 14,200 million nuts, with an estimated consumption of 8112 million nuts and 4209 nuts/ha as productivity. They are a potential competitor to the Philippines in the coconut industry. Exports of coconut products contribute almost 0.7% to the national export earnings. Coconut oil shows a major share in coconut exports at about 34%, followed by copra meal (13%), and coconut shell charcoal (9%) (Table 12.3).

While observing the export trend of coconut products from Indonesia, coconut oil has shown an increasing trend in recent years. However, over the past 10 years, the exports of coconut oil have exhibited more or less a cyclical pattern, with frequent ups and downs. Coconut shell charcoal has shown a recent decline in exports. Desiccated coconut and coconut milk have shown an increasing trend in exports, especially in the recent period (Fig. 12.12). Europe and America are the major export markets for most of Indonesia's coconut products.

Coconuts and coconut products have become crucial export commodities for tropical nations like Indonesia. However, the export dynamics are heavily influenced by external factors such as foreign income, with coconut prices playing a negligible role. Economic crises tend to have a significantly negative impact. Interestingly, an uptick in the average Gross National Income of coconut-importing countries correlates with increased value in Indonesia's coconut exports, particularly post the 1997 economic downturn (Mulyadi et al. 2019).

12.5.3 India

In India, coconut contributed about rupees 10,707 crores in crop output in 2020–2021, and the coconut industry directly or indirectly employs about 12 million people. Coconut is a major plantation crop of coastal regions of Kerala, Tamil Nadu, Karnataka, and Andhra Pradesh. These top-four producers accounted for 90% of total production and about 89.5% of total production acreage in the country in the year 2020–2021 (Table 12.4). Other important coconut producing States in the country includes West Bengal, Odisha, Gujarat, Maharashtra, Assam and Bihar, which account for nearly 8% of production. Among the four major coconuts growing States, Andhra Pradesh had the highest productivity (13,969 nuts/ha), followed by Tamil Nadu with 12,280 nuts/ha. While Kerala, which accounts for the largest

Table 12.3 Export volume (share) of coconut products from Indonesia

S.No.	Coconut products	Export volume (MT)	Export share (%)
1	Coconut oil	611,452	34
2	Copra meal	229,644	13
3	Desiccated coconut	139,932	8
4	Coconut shell charcoal	154,524	9
5	Coconut milk(liquid)	111,279	6
6	Coco fiber products	37,084	2
9	Others	494,818	28
10	Total	1,778,733	100

Source: ICC (2023)

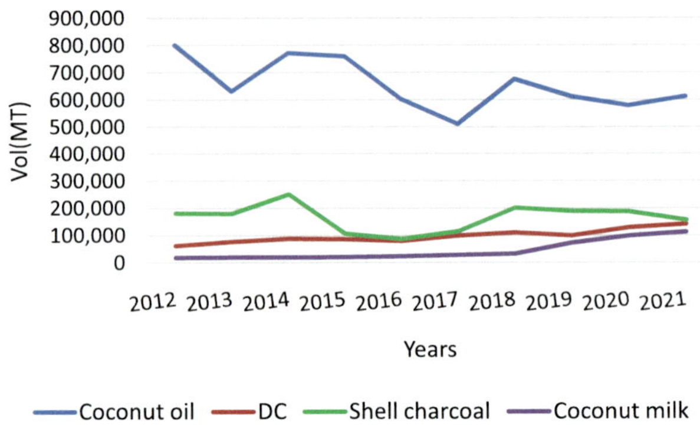

Fig. 12.12 Trend in exports of coconut products from Indonesia (2012–2021)

Table 12.4 State-wise statistics of coconuts in India

State/UT'S	Area ('000 Ha)	% share	Production (million nuts)	% share	Productivity (nuts/ha)
Tamil Nadu	437.57	20.1	5373.21	26.5	12,280
Karnataka	624.03	28.7	4300.69	21.2	6892
Kerala	760.78	35.0	6980.30	34.4	9175
Andhra Pradesh	111.38	5.2	1555.82	7.7	13,969
Others	221.40	11.0	1718.96	10.3	–
All India	**2173.28**	**100.00**	**20308.70**	**100.00**	**9345**

Source: Horticulture Division, Dept. of Agriculture & Cooperation, Govt. of India (Govt. of India 2023)

share in production in the country, had average productivity of 9175 per hectare in 2020–2021, marginally lower than the all-India yield of 9345 nuts/ha. The productivity level in Karnataka (6892 nuts/ha) was significantly lower than the all India average and other major producers (Coconut Development Board 2024).

Coconut is predominantly cultivated in small and marginal holdings. These tiny fragmented holdings suffer from socio-economic and bio-physical resource limitations. They are unable to effectively utilize the potential of available technologies for generating sufficient income to meet the family requirement. Presently coconut growers are more exposed to economic risks and uncertainties owing to the high degree of price fluctuations.

The exports of coconut and its products from India have significantly increased during the last few years. As per the DGCI's data, exports of coconut products (excluding coir and coir products) increased by over 41% in 2021–2022 and by 9.8% in 2022–2023 (Table 12.5). It is notable that the uninterrupted growth in exports of coconut products in 2022–2023 was due to increase in exports earnings from coconut (fresh), other coconut excluding (fresh/dried), coconut oil (crude), dried endocarp, other endocarp, activated carbon and copra.

Table 12.5 Exports of coconut and its products from India

Year	Value (Rs Crore)	% Variation over previous year
2014–2015	1312.38	13.52
2015–2016	1450.24	10.5
2016–2017	2061.7	42.16
2017–2018	1764.31	−14.42
2018–2019	2045.36	15.93
2019–2020	1762.17	−13.85
2020–2021	2294.81	30.23
2021–2022	3236.83	41.05
2022–2023	3554.23	9.81

Source: CDB (https://coconutboard.gov.in/export.htm)

12.6 Conclusions and Way Forward

The growing awareness of coconuts as a healthy food source suggests a potential rise in foreign demand for coconut products. However, domestic supply shortages could hinder exports, necessitating a long-term strategy from the government to revitalize existing coconut plantations and incentivize farmers to establish new ones. Moreover, government support for research and development is crucial to harness the increasing importance of coconuts in the global market.

Suggestions for future research include comprehensive studies on the determinants of export demand for coconut and its products using cross-country and micro-level data. Additionally, coconut-producing nations are encouraged to diversify coconut-based products and promote the consumption of healthy coconut products through intensified campaigns.

To ensure the profitability of the coconut industry, it is necessary to significantly increase the scale of processing and value addition in the coconut sector in all countries where coconuts are grown, as part of the ongoing trade liberalization efforts. The decreasing worldwide production and productivity of coconuts is a worrisome issue that requires individual attention from each coconut producing country. It is important to prioritize participatory research that involves farmer groups in order to refine and fine-tune technologies for higher efficiency in the coconut sector. This is because coconuts are a smallholder crop, unlike other plantations around the world. The countries that grow coconuts should take stock of their SWOT (strengths, weaknesses, opportunities, and threats) and use that information to create a time-bound, action-oriented strategy for the development of their coconut industries. An effective strategic framework must take into account the current trade complexities, food safety regulations, and market preferences of the primary trade destinations for coconut products. It is important to carefully consider the coconut value chain in each coconut-growing country and make sure that the farmers, who are the main players at the initial stage of the chain, receive a fair portion of the revenue generated throughout the entire chain. Amidst the current competitive landscape, it is recommended to operate as agricultural collectives in order to achieve the most efficient economies of scale and minimize marketing expenses. In addition, research organizations should emphasize coconut-based farming systems that are economically feasible and potentially connected to processing units. Coconut cultivation should be given high priority in the agricultural policies and developmental agendas of countries where coconuts are grown. It is critical to replicate the successful models across the coconut growing tracts in the world to proliferate the benefits to the marginalized coconut farming community in the endeavor to empower them through women initiatives. The recent focus on product diversification, value addition, and the utilization of by-products has led to the creation of numerous high-value coconut products. These efforts not only enhance competitiveness but also contribute significantly to addressing food security, providing nutrition, promoting health, and ensuring social well-being. One notable area of opportunity lies in leveraging the positive health effects of monolaurin derived from coconuts. Monolaurin, a compound found in coconut, has been associated with various health benefits. By fully capitalizing on these positive effects, the coconut industry can further enhance the value proposition of its products and contribute to improving public health outcomes. Overall, continued investment in innovation, research, and development within the coconut sector, along with a focus on product quality and market competitiveness, will play a crucial role in realizing the full potential of coconut as a versatile and valuable resource for both economic and societal advancement. Hence, it is of paramount importance to streamline plausible and workable policy frame under the overarching ambit of ICC to realize the long term goal of economic enhancement and social empowerment of vulnerable coconut farmers (as well as entrepreneurs) across the world.

References

Abeysekara MGD, Waidyarathne K (2020) The coconut industry: a review of price forecasting modelling in major coconut producing countries. CORD 36:17–26. https://doi.org/10.37833/cord.v36i.422

Coconut Development Board (2024) Statistics/prices. Ministry of Agriculture & Farmers Welfare, Govt. of India. https://coconutboard.nic.in/

Coppock JD (1962) International economic instability: the experience after World War II, Economics handbook series. McGraw-Hill, New York

Govt. of India (2023) Horticultural statistics at a glance 2021. Government of India Ministry of Agriculture & Farmers' Welfare, Horticulture Statistics Division, New Delhi

ICC (2023) Coconut statistical year book-2021. International Coconut Community, Jakarta

Jayasekhar S, Chandran KP (2021) World economic importance. In: The coconut genome. Springer, Cham, pp 1–12. https://doi.org/10.1007/978-3-030-76649-8_1

Mulyadi H, Nazamuddini BS, Seftarita C (2019) What determines exports of coconut products? The case of Indonesia. Int J Acad Res Econ Manage Sci 8(2):12–24

Muralidharan K, Subramanian P, Mathew AC, Thamban C, Jayasekhar S, Krishnakumar V, Madhavan K (2019) Upgrading a coconut value chain: empirical evidence from North Kerala. Int J Innov Hortic 8(1):72–80

Radhakrishnan K, Tesfom MA, Infantina AJ, Krishnan M, Velmurugan R (2016) Marine fisheries growth, performance and institutional arrangements in Tamil Nadu. Int J Fish Aquat Stud 4(5):342–346

Rajani M, Balasubramanian A, Sudhakar O (2023) Estimation of growth and instability in shrimp production of Andhra Pradesh and India. Pharma Innov J 12(12):1582–1589

Sairam CV, Jayasekhar S (2018) World coconut economy: sectoral issues, markets and trade. In: The coconut palm (Cocos nucifera L.)—research and development perspectives. Springer, Singapore, pp 801–820

Sportel T, Véron R (2016) Coconut crisis in Kerala? Mainstream narrative and alternative perspectives. Dev Chang 47(5):1051–1077

UN Comtrade (2024) UN Comtrade database, United Nations. https://comtrade.un.org/

Chapter 13
Coconut Biomolecules-Future Perspectives

S. V. Ramesh and Shelly Praveen

Abstract Coconut, being a versatile crop, offers numerous opportunities for value-added products utilizing various parts of the plant. Although coconut products have been used as food since time immemorial, they have achieved greater significance in the realm of nutraceuticals or nutrition-driven value addition only in recent decades. Biochemical characterization of coconut and its products has mainly concentrated on macromolecules like fatty acids, proteins, and fiber fractions. However, considering its nutraceutical potential, various bioactives of coconut have been unearthed, and clinical trials are underway. In this context, this chapter presents the future perspectives of coconut-derived biomolecules with special emphasis on human nutrition.

Keywords Coconut nutrition · Nutritional biomolecules · Bio peptides · Functional foods

Coconut and its derivatives have gained significant attention in both traditional media and the digital sphere, with medical professionals endorsing their health benefits and describing coconut oil as a highly valuable and healthy option. The distinctive nutritional profile of coconut oil has been associated with positive effects on reducing cardiovascular disease, as well as exhibiting anti-inflammatory and anti-oxidative properties. However, discussions surrounding the potential health benefits of coconut oil, particularly in mitigating cardiovascular diseases, managing hyperglycemic conditions, and exhibiting neuroprotective properties, tend to focus solely on its fatty acid composition (i.e. medium chain fatty acids), disregarding other crucial phytonutrients like phenolic acids or phytosterols, known for their established health-promoting effects. Therefore, it's vital to investigate the nutraceutical

S. V. Ramesh (✉)
ICAR-Central Plantation Crops Research Institute, Kasaragod, Kerala, India

S. Praveen (✉)
ICAR-Indian Agricultural Research Institute (ICAR-IARI), New Delhi, Delhi, India
e-mail: ramesh.sv@icar.gov.in

S. V. Ramesh, S. Praveen (eds.), *Coconut-Based Nutrition and Nutraceutical Perspectives*, https://doi.org/10.1007/978-981-97-3976-9_13

effects of phenolic acids or phytosterols derived from coconut oil in this context. Hence further investigation is needed to identify coconut polyphenols and unique bioactive fractions, to establish a safe and effective intake levels, and define underlying mechanisms of action. In addition, adoption of scientific rigor in clinical trials and assessment of gut microbiome profiles would provide meaningful information with respect to human health. While animal experiments have demonstrated the medicinal potential of coconut and its products, further validation is required through solid evidence regarding their therapeutic properties and mechanisms of action in treating specific diseases.

Given the increasing demand for virgin coconut oil (VCO), it is vital to conduct studies aimed at enhancing the quality characteristics of the oil. In recent years, there has been a growing focus on exploring the synergy between coconut oil and nanoparticles. This research has revealed that combining coconut oil with nanoparticles enhances its properties, such as stability, lubrication, and antimicrobial activity (Yin et al. 2024).

Given the positive role of coconut oil derived MCTs in alleviating the symptoms of Alzheimers Disease (AD), it is vital to design MCTs-based nutraceutical drug formulations and to assess the cognition stability of AD subjects in large scale clinical trials (Ramesh et al. 2021a). The development of coconut oil-based products personalized for various applications is crucial. However, concerns about the relatively high cost of coconut oil have raised issues regarding potential adulteration, leading to significant interest in methods for detecting its purity. To efficiently detect adulterated VCO in both commercial and consumer settings, utilizing specialized sensors and adopting appropriate software for data collection and analysis is recommended to enhance efficacy and speed. Development of coconut oil derived diacyl glycerol (CO-DAG) based non-dairy or vegan creamer, without trans fat, and low fat coconut milk devoid of saturated fatty acids have opened up avenues for incorporation of coconut derived biomolecules in non-conventional food products and novel applications (Liu et al. 2023; Cheirsilp et al. 2023). Thus, the prevailing areas of research interest and the evolving trends in the application of coconut oil is aptly presented in keywords overlay clustering map of coconut oil (Yin et al. 2024) (Fig. 13.1). For the coconut industry, transitioning away from solely focusing on the oil sector could prove beneficial, exploiting its health and nutritional attributes, particularly amidst intense competition from other vegetable oils.

Also, the dearth of knowledge concerning the functional and biological attributes of individual coconut proteins or protein groups has constrained their practical applications. Peptides with ACE-inhibitory and/or antioxidant properties have been isolated and characterized from proteins found in food sources. In light of these circumstances, identification and characterization of coconut kernel or storage proteins utilizing a high-throughput proteomic approach is imperative to elucidate their functional and biological activities. Moreover, bioinformatics analyses are required to unveil the bioactive peptides of globulins and antioxidant proteins and disclose their potential functions. Antimicrobial peptides were discovered in green coconut water, while various ACE-inhibitory (Angiotensin Converting Enzyme-inhibiting) and antioxidant peptides were found in coconut cake globulin and albumin hydrolysates. Despite their many health benefits, incorporating these peptides into food products presents challenges due to their instability and bitter taste. Effective processing methods are necessary to enhance food formulations with these bioactive peptides and create functional products (Görgüç et al. 2020; Sarabandi et al. 2024).

Coconut water based probiotic foods and defatted coconut residue (DCR) derived polysaccharides as prebiotics are suggested as a beneficial dietary approach for enhancing host health by regulating the composition and functions of the gut microbiota community. Research efforts towards the development of coconut-based psychobiotics, referring to live microorganisms that confer health benefits to individuals experiencing psychological distress through the 'microbiota-gut-brain axis,' are also an important way forward (Casertano et al. 2022).

Nanoformulations of active compounds, utilizing biodegradable or semisynthetic nanocarriers like polymeric matrices, micelles, liposomes, nanoemulsions, solid lipid nanoparticles, nanostructured lipid carriers, or appropriate inorganic matrices, offer an advantageous solution. These nanoformulations not only enhance stability but also often facilitate controlled release of nutrients. In this context application of coconut oil based nano-oil emulsion as a suitable carrier of bioactive components have opened up avenues to utilize coconut oil or VCO based

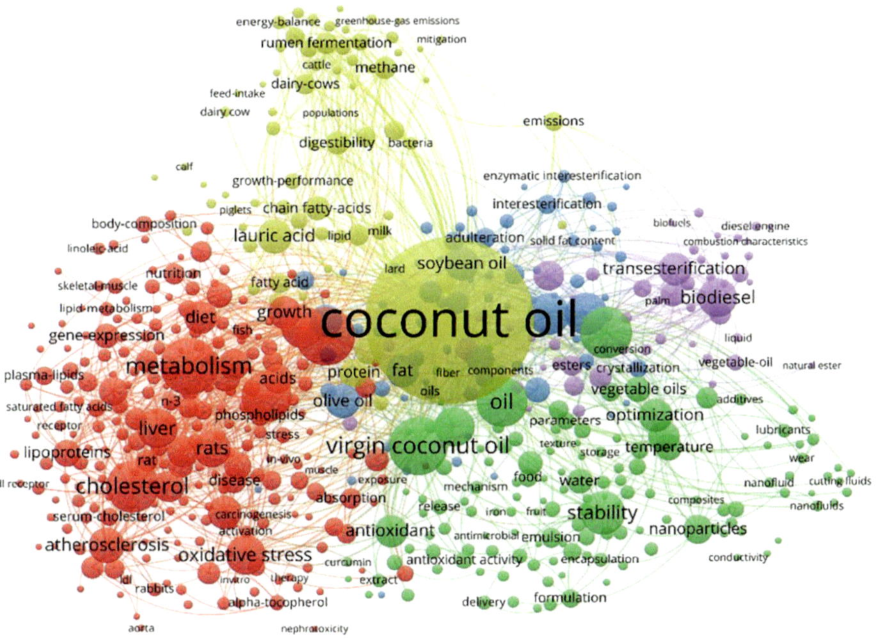

Fig. 13.1 Cluster map depicting the research priorities in coconut. Clustering analysis using 'coconut oil' as a keyword revealed that research areas such as nutritional evaluation of coconut oil, its applications as an emulsifier and lubricant, and adulteration detection predominate. (Source: https://doi.org/10.53388/FH2024005, under CC-BY license. https://creativecommons.org/licenses/by/4.0/)

nanoemulsion in food, beverages, and health care industries (Widianingrum et al. 2023). Also, the prospect of using the coconut testa-derived phytonutrients in developing a nutraceutical product utilizing the principles of nanoencapsulation is an exciting area of research (Ramesh et al. 2021a) (Fig. 13.2).

The growing public awareness of the adverse effects of chemical-based farming has implications for consumers who prefer eco-friendly organic products. Given the volatile and flavor profile of VCO and coconut sugar, products obtained from

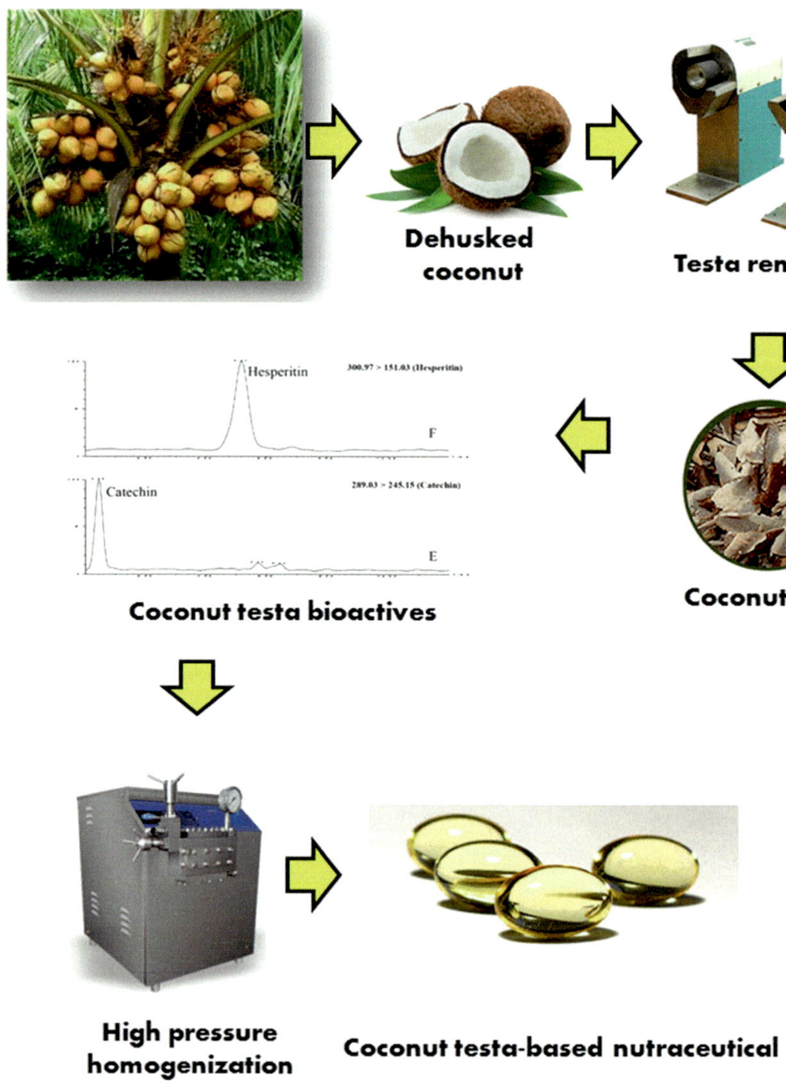

Fig. 13.2 Development of coconut testa based nutraceutical product using the principles of nanoencapsulation (Source: Ramesh et al. 2021b; https://doi.org/10.1007/s13197-021-05310-2)

organically cultivated coconuts would likely command a premium in the international market (Restianto et al. 2021). The biochemical profile of coconut products, especially VCO, sugar, coconut milk, and coconut flour obtained from organically cultivated orchards, and development of quality attributes matrix would greatly contribute to in the popularity of some of the specialty varieties of coconut. Certainly, the emergence of certified organic and/or fair-trade coconut products presents a promising opportunity for the coconut industry in the future. By meeting the growing demand for sustainably sourced and ethically produced goods, producers can attract environmentally conscious consumers and tap into premium markets. This shift not only aligns with the global trend towards responsible consumption but also has the potential to improve livelihoods for coconut farmers and promote environmentally friendly practices throughout the supply chain (Parisi et al. 2024).

The elite coconuts, including 'makapuno' and aromatic varieties, are in high demand due to their rarity, as well as their delicious taste and nutritional benefits for consumers. Makapuno endosperm is utilized in various culinary creations, or incorporated as a flavor enhancer in ice cream and baked goods. Advancements in pertinent food processing methods will enhance the potential for these distinct coconut varieties to access markets beyond tropical regions, opening up new opportunities for distribution and consumption (Nguyen et al. 2016).

Adoption of nutrigenomics and nutrigenetics including epigenetics techniques in the context of coconut derived biomolecules and human nutrition is a major future research strategy. Such an approach is warranted in the realms of coconut nutrition and cognitive enhancement, coconut and anti-obesity effects, coconut and anti-aging phenomenon among others. Recent research results depicting the pleiotropic effects of coconut derived lauric acid in modulating Liver Receptor Homolog1 (LRH 1) signaling is encouraging (Caudill and Moore 2021).

13.1 Concluding Remarks

Coconut is naturally packed with a wide range of nutrients and renowned for its versatility, as every part of the fruit offers nutritional benefits. It becomes a crucial dietary component by supplying essential nutrients such as calories, protein, fat, vitamins, and minerals. Coconut is a valuable crop not only for its oil production but also for its various by-products, making it beneficial for coconut growers in generating income. Currently, research on coconut should focus on the identification of novel bioactive compounds of health and nutritional importance. Adoption of novel bioactive extraction techniques and formulation of food products with nutraceutical potential, nutrigenomics of dietary lipids and biopeptides are the need of the hour.

References

Casertano M, Fogliano V, Ercolini D (2022) Psychobiotics, gut microbiota and fermented foods can help preserving mental health. Food Res Int 152:110892. https://doi.org/10.1016/j.foodres.2021.110892

Caudill MSR, Moore DD (2021) Coconut oil goes nuclear: the nutrigenomics of LRH-1. https://www.texaschildrens.org/sites/default/files/uploads/documents/symposia/2021/posters/137.pdf

Cheirsilp B, Wannathip K, Rakmai J, Jongpanyareat B (2023) Production of low-fat coconut milk using β-cyclodextrin column for selective removal of saturated fatty acids. Naresuan Univ J Sci Technol 31(4):93–102

Görgüç A, Gençdağ E, Yılmaz FM (2020) Bioactive peptides derived from plant origin by-products: biological activities and techno-functional utilizations in food developments—a review. Food Res Int 136:109504

Liu X, Xu W, Wang W, Luo R, Yang B, Lan D, Wang Y (2023) Physicochemical properties and feasibility of coconut oil-based diacylglycerol as an alternative fat for healthy non-dairy creamer. Food Chem X 19:100749

Nguyen QT, Bandupriya HD, Foale M, Adkins SW (2016) Biology, propagation and utilization of elite coconut varieties (makapuno and aromatics). Plant Physiol Biochem 109:579–589

Parisi S, Parisi C, Varghese SM (2024) Value addition and coconut-based beverages: current perspectives. Beverages 10(1):14

Ramesh SV, Krishnan V, Praveen S, Hebbar KB (2021a) Dietary prospects of coconut oil for the prevention and treatment of Alzheimer's disease (AD): a review of recent evidences. Trends Food Sci Technol 112:201–211

Ramesh SV, Pandiselvam R, Shameena Beegum PP et al (2021b) Review of *Cocos nucifera* L. testa-derived phytonutrients with special reference to phenolics and its potential for encapsulation. J Food Sci Technol 60:1–10. https://doi.org/10.1007/s13197-021-05310-2

Restianto YE, Dinanti A, Naufalin LR (2021) Enhancing organic continuance intentions of organic coconut sugar technology. CAL 22(184):138–147

Sarabandi K, Dashipour A, Akbarbaglu Z, Peighambardoust SH, Ayaseh A, Kafil HS, Jafari SM, Mousavi Khaneghah A (2024) Incorporation of spray-dried encapsulated bioactive peptides from coconut (*Cocos nucifera* L.) meal by-product in bread formulation. Food Sci Nutr. https://doi.org/10.1002/fsn3.4120

Widianingrum DC, Khasanah H, Purnamasari L, Krismaputri ME, Hwang SG (2023) Antimicrobial activities of nano-emulsion of virgin coconut oil. Vet Med 68(1):27

Yin JJ, Huang H, Jiang XM et al (2024) Coconut oil research: past, present, and future directions. Food Health 6(1):5. https://doi.org/10.53388/FH2024005

Printed by Printforce, the Netherlan